Education in Anesthesia

MW00636191

Education in Anesthesia

How to Deliver the Best Learning Experience

Edited by

Edwin A. Bowe
University of Kentucky College of Medicine

Randall M. Schell
University of Kentucky College of Medicine

Amy N. DiLorenzo
University of Kentucky College of Medicine

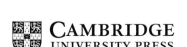
CAMBRIDGE
UNIVERSITY PRESS

CAMBRIDGE
UNIVERSITY PRESS

University Printing House, Cambridge CB2 8BS, United Kingdom

One Liberty Plaza, 20th Floor, New York, NY 10006, USA

477 Williamstown Road, Port Melbourne, VIC 3207, Australia

314–321, 3rd Floor, Plot 3, Splendor Forum, Jasola District Centre, New Delhi – 110025, India

79 Anson Road, #06-04/06, Singapore 079906

Cambridge University Press is part of the University of Cambridge.

It furthers the University's mission by disseminating knowledge in the pursuit of
education, learning, and research at the highest international levels of excellence.

www.cambridge.org
Information on this title: www.cambridge.org/9781316630389
DOI: 10.1017/9781316822548

© Cambridge University Press 2018

This publication is in copyright. Subject to statutory exception
and to the provisions of relevant collective licensing agreements,
no reproduction of any part may take place without the written
permission of Cambridge University Press.

First published 2018

Printed in the United Kingdom by TJ International Ltd. Padstow Cornwall

A catalogue record for this publication is available from the British Library.

Library of Congress Cataloging-in-Publication Data
Names: Bowe, Edwin A., 1949– editor. | Schell, Randall M., 1960– editor. |
DiLorenzo, Amy N., 1972– editor.
Title: Education in anesthesia : how to deliver the best learning experience /
edited by Edwin A. Bowe, Randall M. Schell, Amy N. DiLorenzo.
Description: Cambridge, United Kingdom; New York, NY:
Cambridge University Press, 2018. | Includes bibliographical references and index.
Identifiers: LCCN 2017044980 | ISBN 9781316630389 (pbk.)
Subjects: | MESH: Anesthesiology – education | Anesthesia – methods | Teaching
Classification: LCC RD81 | NLM WO 18 | DDC 617.9/6–dc23
LC record available at https://lccn.loc.gov/2017044980

ISBN 978-1-316-63038-9 Paperback

Cambridge University Press has no responsibility for the persistence or accuracy of URLs
for external or third-party internet websites referred to in this publication and does not
guarantee that any content on such websites is, or will remain, accurate or appropriate.

Contents

Contents

A supplementary chapter, Training Physician-Scientists in Anesthesiology and Perioperative Medicine: Challenges, Opportunites and Strategies for Success by Brian J. Gelfand, Frederic T. Billings IV, Pratik Pandharipande, Edward Sherwood, and Matthew D. McEvoy, can be found at www.cambridge.org/9781316630389

Contributors

Frederic T. Billings IV, MD
Co-Director B. H. Robbins Scholars Program, Department of Anesthesiology, Vanderbilt University Medical Center and Assistant Professor of Anesthesiology, Vanderbilt University School of Medicine, Nashville, TN

Jeanna D. Blitz, MD
Assistant Professor and Director, Preoperative Evaluation Clinic, Department of Anesthesiology, Perioperative Care and Pain Medicine, New York University School of Medicine, New York, NY

Edwin A. Bowe, MD
Professor, Department of Anesthesiology, University of Kentucky College of Medicine, Lexington, KY

Amanda R. Burden, MD
Associate Professor of Anesthesiology, Vice Chair of Faculty Affairs, Director of Clinical Skills and Simulation, Cooper Medical School of Rowan University, Cooper University Hospital, Camden, NJ

Stephen F. Dierdorf, MD
Professor of Clinical Anesthesia, Department of Anesthesiology and Perioperative Medicine, Medical University of South Carolina, Charleston, SC

Amy N. DiLorenzo, MA
Assistant Dean for Graduate Medical Education and Senior Lecturer, Department of Anesthesiology, University of Kentucky College of Medicine, Lexington, KY

Brian S. Donahue, MD, PhD
Professor of Anesthesiology and Pediatrics, Department of Anesthesiology, Monroe Carell Jr Children's Hospital at Vanderbilt, Vanderbilt University Medical Center, Nashville, TN

John H. Eichhorn, MD
Professor, Department of Anesthesiology, University of Kentucky College of Medicine and Provost's Distinguished Service Professor, University of Kentucky, Lexington, KY

Robert Gaiser, MD
Professor and Chair, Department of Anesthesiology, University of Kentucky, Lexington, KY

Jason Gatling, MD
Associate Professor, Department of Anesthesiology, Loma Linda University Medical Center, Loma Linda, CA

Brian J. Gelfand, MD
Associate Vice-Chair for Educational Affairs and Program Director, Department of Anesthesiology, Vanderbilt University Medical Center and Associate Professor of Anesthesiology and Surgery, Vanderbilt University School of Medicine, Nashville, TN

Rebecca M. Gerlach, MD, FRCPC
Assistant Professor and Director, Anesthesia Perioperative Medicine Clinic, Department of Anesthesia and Critical Care, University of Chicago, Chicago, IL

Marc Hassid, MD
Assistant Professor of Anesthesia, Department of Anesthesiology and Perioperative Medicine, Medical University of South Carolina, Charleston, SC

Stephanie B. Jones, MD
Associate Professor of Anaesthesia, Harvard Medical School and Vice Chair for Education and Faculty Development, Department of Anesthesia, Critical Care, and Pain Medicine, Beth Israel Deaconess Medical Center, Boston, MA

Ryan Ivie, MD
Assistant Professor and Assistant Program Director Regional Anesthesia and Acute Pain Medicine Fellowship, Oregon Health and Science University, Portland, OR

Robert Maniker, MD
Assistant Professor, Columbia University School of Medicine, New York, NY

Susan M. Martinelli, MD
Associate Professor, Department of Anesthesiology, University of North Carolina, Chapel Hill, NC

Robina Matyal, MD
Associate Professor of Anaesthesia, Harvard Medical School and Staff Anesthesiologist, Department of Anesthesia, Critical Care, and Pain Medicine, Beth Israel Deaconess Medical Center, Boston, MA

Richard E. Mayer, PhD
Distinguished Professor, Department of Psychological and Brain Sciences, University of California, Santa Barbara, CA

Matthew D. McEvoy, MD
Vice-Chair for Educational Affairs, Department of Anesthesiology, Vanderbilt University Medical Center and Professor of Anesthesiology, Vanderbilt University School of Medicine, Nashville, TN

John D. Mitchell, MD
Associate Professor of Anaesthesia, Harvard Medical School and Residency Program Director, Department of Anesthesia, Critical Care, and Pain Medicine, Beth Israel Deaconess Medical Center, Boston, MA

Jordan Newmark, MD
Chairman, Department of Anesthesiology and Director (Interim), Pain & Functional Restoration Clinic, Alameda Health System, Adjunct Clinical Assistant Professor, Department of Anesthesiology, Perioperative and Pain Medicine, Division of Addiction Medicine, (by courtesy), Stanford University School of Medicine, Stanford, CA

Pratik Pandharipande, MD
Chief, Division of Anesthesiology Critical Care Medicine, Department of Anesthesiology, Vanderbilt University Medical Center and Professor of Anesthesiology, Vanderbilt University School of Medicine, Nashville, TN

Manuel Pardo Jr., MD
Professor and Vice Chair for Education and Residency Program Director, University of California, San Francisco, Department of Anesthesia and Perioperative Care, San Francisco, CA

Davinder Ramsingh, MD
Associate Professor, Department of Anesthesiology, Loma Linda University Medical Center, Loma Linda, CA

Matthew Reed, MD, MSPH
Assistant Professor, University of California Davis, Department of Psychiatry and Behavioral Sciences, Behavioral Health Clinic, Sacramento, CA

John J. Schaefer III, MD
Professor of Anesthesia and Associate Dean for Statewide Clinical Effectiveness Education, Department of Anesthesiology and Perioperative Medicine, Medical University of South Carolina, Charleston, SC

Randall M. Schell, MD, MACM
Professor and Vice Chair for Education and Program Director, Department of Anesthesiology, University of Kentucky College of Medicine, Lexington, KY

Edward Sherwood, MD, PhD
Vice-Chair for Research, Department of Anesthesiology, Vanderbilt University Medical Center and Cornelius Vanderbilt Chair in Anesthesiology and Professor of Anesthesiology, Pathology, Microbiology and Immunology, Vanderbilt University School of Medicine, Nashville, TN

Naileshni Singh, MD
Assistant Professor, Division of Pain Medicine, University of California Davis, Department of Anesthesiology and Pain Medicine, Sacramento, CA

Gary R. Stier, MD, MBA
Professor of Anesthesiology, Internal Medicine, and Critical Care, Department of Anesthesiology, Loma Linda University Medical Center, Loma Linda, CA

BobbieJean Sweitzer, MD, FACP
Professor of Anesthesiology and Director, Perioperative Medicine, Department of Anesthesiology, Northwestern University, Chicago, IL

John E. Tetzlaff, MD
Professor of Anesthesiology, Cleveland Clinic
Lerner College of Medicine of Case Western Reserve
University and Staff Anesthesiologist, Department of
General Anesthesia, Cleveland Clinic, Cleveland, OH

J. Scott Walton, MD
Associate Professor of Anesthesia, Department of
Anesthesiology and Perioperative Medicine, Medical
University of South Carolina, Charleston, SC

Glenn Woodworth, MD
Editor of Anesthesia Education Toolbox, Associate
Professor, and Director, Regional Anesthesia and
Acute Pain Medicine Fellowship, Oregon Health and
Science University, Portland, OR

Chapter

1

Creating (and Choosing) an Optimal Learning Environment

Randall M. Schell and Amy N. DiLorenzo

I never teach my pupils. I only attempt to provide the conditions in which they can learn.

– Albert Einstein

Introduction

Anesthesiology educators and accreditation organizations devote considerable effort to establish and periodically reassess what knowledge and skills an anesthesiology resident must demonstrate to become a competent practitioner. Evidence in education (e.g., active learning [Chapter 15], test-enhanced learning [Chapter 18]) is being used more to inform and guide how teachers deliver educational content. Excellent educators, however, recognize that many things influence anesthesiology learners beyond "what" they teach and "how" they teach. "Where" they teach is the learning environment – the context or setting – in which the anesthesiology curriculum exists.

Anesthesiology residents beginning training bring their individual skills, foundations of knowledge, work ethic, and attitudes into the larger context of the healthcare delivery system, program, and institution. This larger context of the everyday world surrounding residents during training has a strong influence on a resident becoming a competent practitioner, including their future performance. Accrediting organizations (Association of American Medical Colleges, AAMC; Accreditation Council for Graduate Medical Education, ACGME) have recognized this.[1]

Learning cannot be separated from its physical, social, and psychological context (the atmosphere or culture pervading the setting where faculty teach and residents learn). Teaching is as much about creating the optimal learning environment as it is about conveying knowledge or sharing expertise.

What Is a "Learning Environment"?

The characterization of a learning environment extends beyond physical structures, equipment, classrooms, and available technology.[2,3] The learning environment includes the conditions (social, emotional, intellectual) and surroundings (physical) in which learning takes place. It is *where* educators teach as opposed to *what* they teach. Other learners, their faculty, the residency program, the curriculum, the department, and the healthcare system among others influence the learning environment of individual anesthesiology residents. The learning environment is also influenced by the individual anesthesiology resident and may include many interwoven elements that are dynamic and difficult to quantify. The elements of quality of supervision, instructors, and spatial conditions, and working and learning environments have been aggregated under the term *learning climate*.

The learning environment may be experienced differently by different learners. For example, assume two residents are sitting side by side in a lecture. The physical environment is identical. They are hearing the same lecture from the same individual. One resident has a good relationship with the faculty member and perceives a very positive learning environment. The other resident had a negative interaction with the faculty member the prior day and therefore perceives the learning environment to be negative. Thus, the optimal learning environment or climate might be defined as the "best conditions in which an individual learner can learn."

Components of the Learning Environment

The resident learner is one of many microlearning "environments" embedded in a macrolearning environment that they influence. The macrolearning environment includes many physical and sociocultural elements that have an influence on the learner (Figure 1.1).

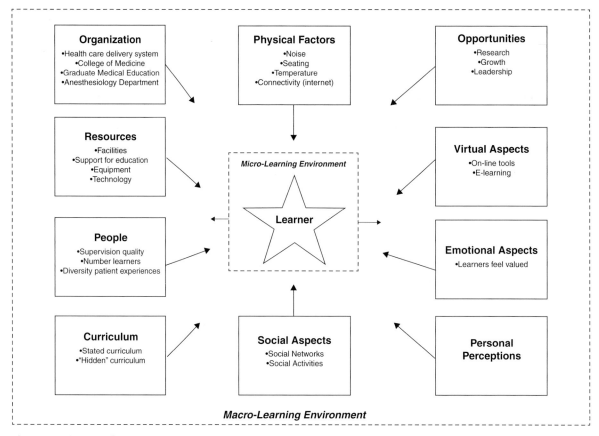

Figure 1.1 Elements of the learning environment.

The elements of a learning environment include but are not limited to the:

1. Organization (e.g., healthcare delivery system, college of medicine, graduate medical education, anesthesiology department);
2. Resources (e.g., facilities, financial support for education, simulators, equipment, technology);
3. People (e.g., quality of supervision, number of students, mix of patients available for learning);
4. Teaching or learning activities (e.g., stated or written curriculum);
5. Social aspects (e.g., teacher role modeling, social networks, activities);
6. Personal perceptions (e.g., perceptions of workload, faculty members, classmates);
7. Emotional aspects (e.g., perception of being valued);
8. Web-based aspects (e.g., online tools, podcasts, e-learning, see Chapter 16);
9. Opportunities (e.g., research, growth, leadership);
10. Physical factors, (e.g., noise, temperature, seating); and
11. The hidden curriculum (e.g., implicit, unwritten, tacit dimensions of medical learning, see Chapter 19).

Within this complex educational environment, the teacher (including actions, attitudes, enthusiasm, and interest) is one of the most powerful variables.

The learning environment has also been divided into three broad domains:

1. **Personal development or goal direction dimensions**: clarity about learning objectives, relevant learning content, and constructive criticism;

2. **Relationship dimensions:** open communication, friendliness, social and interpersonal support, cohesion and feelings of spirit; and

3. **System maintenance and system change dimensions:** orderly, clear expectations, thoughtful response to change, organizational structure, role clarity, teacher control, student influence and innovation, work pressure, and physical comfort.

In the future, we are likely to develop a better understanding of what elements comprise a learning environment, understand what is most conducive to teaching and learning, and better define what roles the teacher and learner have. A better comprehension of learning environments may improve outcomes including not only knowledge, skills, and attitudes of the learner but also patient care outcomes of safety and quality.

Importance of the Learning Environment

It has been said there are two principal influences on physician behavior: (1) how they are paid and (2) how they are trained. A positive training environment helps anesthesiology residents succeed, influences physician behavior, models a humanistic approach to medicine, may improve wellness and reduce burnout, and imprints a model of safety and quality.

The learning environment surrounding residents during training is purported to have a strong influence on patient care outcomes as well as training outcomes. A recent study demonstrated that completing graduate medical education training in hospitals with lower rates of complications is associated with achieving better patient outcomes throughout a physician's career.[1] This finding of imprinting of the learning environment on individual physician career performance and an understanding that the learning environment for medical education shapes the patient care environment has been recognized by the AAMC and ACGME and resulted in current initiatives to improve the clinical learning environment.

The AAMC Statement on the Learning Environment reads in part: "We believe that the learning environment for medical education shapes the patient care environment. The highest quality of safe and effective care for patients and the highest quality of effective and appropriate education are rooted in human dignity … We affirm our commitment to shaping a culture of teaching and learning that is rooted in respect for all. Fostering resilience, excellence, compassion, and integrity allows us to create patient care, research, and learning environments that are built upon constructive collaboration, mutual respect, and human dignity."[1] The AAMC (AAMC Optimizing Graduate Medical Education 2014), in a five-year road map for America's medical schools, teaching hospitals, and health systems, stated as a priority goal to define the critical elements of the optimal learning environment and to define the critical components of an optimal environment for faculty at academic institutions. Priority #4 is "Define and foster optimal learning environments in AAMC member institutions," and #5 is "Improve the environment for teaching faculty."

The ACGME recognizes that the clinical setting in which residents and fellows learn directly impacts the quality of their training (CLER 2016 Executive Summary).[4] The Clinical Learning Environment Review (CLER) initiative was established by the ACGME in 2012[2] and is designed to assess and provide formative feedback to hospitals, medical centers, and ambulatory care sites that serve as clinical learning environments for ACGME-accredited residency and fellowship programs. The CLER provides formative feedback to inform graduate medical education (GME) and executive leadership (institutional) of the clinical learning environments in six main areas:

1. Patient safety;
2. Healthcare quality, including healthcare disparities;
3. Care transitions;
4. Supervision;
5. Fatigue management, fatigue mitigation, and duty hours; and
6. Professionalism.

There are many factors in the learning environment that impact learner outcomes. The tone of the environment (i.e., respectful, welcoming, sarcasm, ridicule) impacts learning and performance through motivation and emotions. Emotions can disrupt

---

1 https://www.aamc.org/download/408212/data/learning environmentstatementdownload.pdf (accessed November 18, 2017).
2 www.acgme.org/What-We-Do/Initiatives/Clinical-Learning-Environment-Review-CLER (accessed November 18, 2017).

cognitive processes (e.g., anger, anxiety) or support them (e.g., positive feedback, empathy). Emphasizing the importance of good role modeling, attitudes are learned through observation of those in relative power (see Chapter 19). A supportive, learner-oriented culture is of great importance in developing competent physicians. For GME to be truly excellent it must be embedded within an optimal clinical learning environment.

Optimal Learning Environment: Didactic and Clinical

At the foundation of the ideal learning environment are safety for patients and support for learners and educators in a culture of caring compassion. Select characteristics of an optimal learning environment are listed in Table 1.1.

Creating a Climate for Learning in Didactic Education

Setting the context or climate for didactic learning is as important as imparting knowledge. Learner comfort and safety, enthusiasm of the teacher, and a mutual respect between teacher and learner are critical for a positive learning environment.

The process and scientific-based methods to optimize knowledge acquisition in a learning environment are graphically represented in Figure 1.2.

For learning to maximally occur, there must be a convergence of learner, teacher, environment, and assessment, and anesthesia educators must develop a comprehensive approach to teaching. The point is to get learners to remember (retention) and transfer knowledge into practice resulting in improvement in skills development and clinical practice.

Table 1.1 Select characteristics of optimal learning environments

Institutions and Anesthesiology Departments

Expressly state the importance of the educational mission

Allocate resources to adequately support the educational mission

Provide structured learning, assessment, and feedback as part of the educational mission

Provide diversity of patient experiences, optimize work hours, and provide appropriate levels of supervision and autonomy for the learners

Deal effectively with concerns

Understand the importance of the physical and mental health of teachers and learners and support wellness initiatives within their programs that cultivate a sense of meaning and purpose, mutual appreciation, and teamwork

Establish a positive, nurturing, social environment

Continuously reevaluate their educational mission, evaluate their educational outcomes, and make changes as necessary

Teachers

Have a positive attitude toward teaching and create a positive environment for learning

Model safe, effective, and systems-based approach to patient care

Model professionalism, humanism, and wellness

Provide supervision with appropriate levels of autonomy

Provide individualized and specific feedback to learners

Are committed to the educational mission of the organization

Learners

Are committed to excellence in patient care and learning

Feel welcomed, cared about, and emotionally supported

Respect their teachers and others in the interdisciplinary patient care team

Feel safe and comfortable expressing themselves

Provide critical appraisal of their learning environment and use feedback to make change as needed

Are motivated to diagnose their own needs, develop their own learning objectives, execute their learning plans, and self-reflect on their learning performance/outcomes

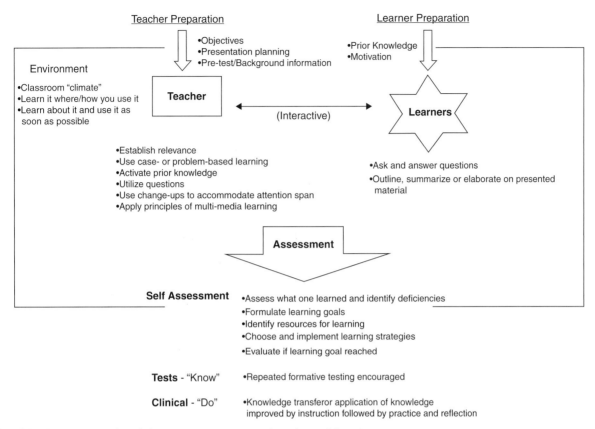

Figure 1.2 Optimizing knowledge acquisition, retention, and transfer in a didactic learning environment.

Teacher and learner must be prepared for learning. Effective teachers understand that learning and the learner, and not teaching and the teacher, are at the center of the educational process. Learning objectives should be determined in advance and the teacher should avoid attempts to provide exhaustive content on a topic. Background information (e.g., short podcast, video lecture, significant paper) may be used in preparation for an interactive learning session emphasizing direct applicability of the knowledge to practice.

Each learner brings preexisting knowledge to the learning environment. Learners should take advantage of educational content provided by the teacher in advance of an interactive educational session. This educational content may provide pertinent knowledge or activate prior knowledge.

Motivation drives learning. Motivation will be increased if (1) the learner perceives that the planned topic and information are relevant to what they currently need to know for practice; (2) the learner understands how the knowledge they are expected to learn will later be assessed and believes that their specific actions (e.g., attending an educational session, studying) will bring about a desired outcome (e.g., passing a test, gaining clinical competency); and (3) the teacher is enthusiastic about his or her topic.

The learning environment, context, and timing of learning are also important. Success in learning is more likely if:

1. There are no other competing responsibilities for the learner or teacher;
2. Knowledge acquisition and application occur as close together in time as possible (e.g., learn it and immediately use it);
3. Classroom "climate" is one where a learner is not afraid of being "wrong" and where learners trust the teacher (e.g., resist single answers, supportive);

4. Planned educational session is not of long duration; and

5. Learning environment and application environment are similar ("context-specific learning"). If the goal is for learners to retrieve and use information in actual real-life situations, it is important that the context in which learning the information occurs approximates the real clinical situation as closely as possible (e.g., learning about malignant hyperthermia in an immersive simulation session versus hearing a class on the same subject).

Following teacher and learner preparation, and in the appropriate learning environment, the teacher and learner are optimally ready to instruct and learn, respectively. The teacher may motivate and guide the learner by initially stating what the learner should learn from the lesson (e.g., learning objectives) and by providing examples of test items. Assessing and activating prior knowledge of the learner can be accomplished by sample audience response system (ARS) questions (see Chapter 15) and providing a short review of familiar material before new material is introduced. Instructional techniques to guide cognitive processing during learning include:

1. **Establish relevance:** Show how what is being learned is relevant to their future performance as anesthesiologists.

2. **Manipulate knowledge:** Focus on case-based and problem-based learning because acquiring knowledge through a professional problem or situation leads to more accessible knowledge.

3. **Activate prior knowledge and assist encoding:** Use analogies, compare and contrast, and present examples that connect to students' existing knowledge to ensure that new information can be meaningfully situated in the context of what learners already understand and will more likely be encoded into long-term memory.

4. **Utilize questions:** Insert questions (e.g., ARS, Socratic) before a section of a lesson to focus learners on parts of the lesson that help answer the questions, and insert questions after each section of a lesson to help learners focus on the most important information presented in the lesson.

5. **Use periodic activities (change-ups) to accommodate audience attention span:** Adult learners can stay attentive for approximately 15–20 minutes at a time and that is only at the beginning of a presentation. Reviewing what has been learned at natural breaks in presentation material and asking questions (e.g., ARS) at key points throughout the lecture are examples of effective change-ups.

6. **Apply principles of multimedia learning** (see Chapter 14): Use conversational style, combine words and pictures in presentation, use spatial layout such as outlines or headings to help learners organize information and increase retention, emphasize words or concepts in the lesson by use of highlighting (e.g., color, font, bold), accompany a visual with spoken description rather than on-screen captions, and keep corresponding printed words and pictures near rather than far from each other on screen or page.

The learners will facilitate and remain engaged in their own learning and improve retention by asking and answering questions during the presentation and outlining, summarizing, or elaborating on presented material.

Retention of knowledge is better if:

1. Demonstrations are used during the educational session rather than exclusively a formal lecture format;

2. The session includes interactive learning with a multimodal approach (e.g., images, figures, pictures, cases, problems, questioning);

3. Practical application of knowledge is emphasized; and

4. Repeated formative testing is used.

Evidence suggests that information retained through repeated practice or formative testing surpasses that of repeated studying, especially if testing is spaced over time (see Chapter 18). The practical application of this is for a learner to utilize sample practice questions or tests on multiple occasions rather than simply restudying a topic to retain knowledge better. Instruction, practice, and reflection are required for improved application or transfer of knowledge into clinical practice.

Creating a Climate for Learning in the Operating Room

A large component of clinical teaching in anesthesiology occurs in the perioperative environment including the operating room.[5] However, many aspects of this learning environment act as a barrier to effective learning.

Teaching in the operating room (see Chapters 5 and 7) is demanding and requires balancing teaching activities with the primary responsibility for patient safety. The operating room learning environment is frequently stressful and noisy, there is a lack of learner privacy, and time allotments for teaching are unpredictable. High levels of learner anxiety associated with patient care are an impediment to learning, divert attention, and decrease learning. Residents may be reluctant to challenge negative hierarchy. A negative hierarchical system, that is, one laden with fear and intimidation, can not only adversely affect resident learning but also unfavorably impact patient safety as well as team functioning and should not be tolerated.

Excellent clinical teachers demonstrate clinical competence and a passion for teaching. They are clear and organized, utilize multiple teaching methods, are self-reflective, target their teaching to the learner's level of knowledge, are kind, and demonstrate integrity and respect for others.

Some suggestions for the teacher in the operating room setting are listed in Box 1.1.

A starting point for creating an optimal learning environment in the operating room is an enthusiasm expressed by the teacher for what is being taught and an eagerness to transmit this enthusiasm to the learner. Adequate supervision and accessibility of the teacher is expected and this can reduce workplace stress that might distract from structured learning activities.

Teaching in the operating room is likely to be more effective when the residents choose topics that are of interest to them, when learning topics directly apply to the clinical situation, and when the teacher considers all aspects of the operating room clinical learning environment.

Assessing the Anesthesiology Learning Environment

Residents' perception of program quality is related to the relevancy of training (exposure to patients, education), quality of the faculty, collegiality of the group, and the social environment. Learners' perceptions of the quality of the educational environment influence their involvement, satisfaction, success, and motivation. However, residents differ widely in the importance they place on different aspects of residency training programs and they are often less satisfied with conditions in the working environment that should be more easily addressed (computer systems, clerical support) than those in the educational environment. One can see how difficult it may be to quantitatively or qualitatively measure a learning environment that is unlikely to be static, nor experienced in the same way by every learner.

Residents' assessment of their learning environment is an important element of residency accreditation and a strong predictor of resident satisfaction. The annual ACGME Resident/Fellow Survey (Box 1.2) is a useful tool for evaluating the learning environment of residency programs. The annual ACGME Faculty Survey focuses on faculty perceptions of the learning environment and determining alignment of the Resident versus Faculty Survey results may be of benefit. The results of the ACGME Resident Survey and ACGME Faculty Survey may be particularly useful to assess the departmental learning environment.

The ACGME established the CLER[3] in 2012 as part of the Next Accreditation System (NAS) to provide feedback to inform GME and institutional executive leadership of the clinical learning environments in six main areas (see Box 1.3).

The data from this review might be particularly useful as one measure of the clinical learning environment of the institution.

Box 1.1 The teacher in the perioperative environment should

- Set clear goals.
- Ask the learner what they would like to learn that day.
- Provide adequate supervision.
- Be accessible and responsive to the learner.
- Provide meaningful, specific, and prompt feedback.
- Create a low-stress learning environment where uncertainty and mistakes are used as teaching moments.
- Demonstrate genuine concern for the learner's progress toward independent practice.

---

[3] www.acgme.org/What-We-Do/Initiatives/Clinical-Learning-Environment-Review-CLER (accessed September 14, 2017).

Box 1.2 Aspects of the learning environment assessed in the ACGME Resident/Fellow Survey

- Clinical experience and education;
- Faculty;
- Evaluation;
- Educational content;
- Resources;
- Patient safety;
- Teamwork.

Box 1.3 CLER categories

1. Patient safety;
2. Healthcare quality, including healthcare discrepancies;
3. Care transitions;
4. Supervision;
5. Fatigue management, fatigue mitigation, and duty hours; and
6. Professionalism.

Instruments used to measure clinical learning environments have recently been reviewed.[6,7] Several of these instruments measure learners' perceptions about teachers, teaching, atmosphere, academic self-perceptions, and social self-perceptions. Instruments include the Postgraduate Hospital Educational Environment Measure (PHEEM), Anaesthetic Theatre Educational Environment Measure (ATEEM), Surgical Theatre Educational Environment Measure (STEEM), Dutch Residency Educational Climate Test (D-RECT), and the Dundee Ready Educational Environment Measure (DREEM). The DREEM is a 50-item questionnaire with five domains ([1] students' perception of teaching, [2] students' perceptions of teachers, [3] students' academic self-perceptions, [4] students' perceptions of atmosphere, and [5] students' self-perceptions) used to measure the educational environment in health professional education programs. It was recently used to measure anesthesiology residents' perceptions of their educational environment and to evaluate the association between year of residency training and perception of the learning environment.[8] The learning program studied was measured to be positive overall and interestingly, there was no association between the year of training

and the overall DREEM score or subscores for the five DREEM domains.

Surveys or instruments, as well as focused interviews with teachers and learners, can help provide a snapshot in time of the learning environment. They also can be used to assess the alignment of the formal and informal curricula and to assess strengths and weaknesses of individual departments. Factor analysis often suggests that teaching quality, instructor mentoring, and social support are very important.

Choosing a Learning Environment: Teachers and Learners

Many discussions about learning environment or culture start with the teacher (faculty member) already in an academic position or a learner (resident) already in a graduate residency training program. Creating the learning environment may not be a temporal or positional option and choosing from various learning environments you desire to join may be important. How might one who values excellence in the learning environment seek to determine if education and training are a valued part of the organizational structure?

Select elements from the educational environment can be used to help an anesthesiologist being recruited to an academic position evaluate the learning environment and are listed in Table 1.2.

A medical student desiring to choose a residency training program in anesthesiology with an optimal learning environment should interview multiple residents and faculty within the program and inquire about similar areas as did the potential faculty member discussed previously. The student's questions might focus on those things listed in Table 1.3.

Wellness and the Learning Environment

The intensive clinical workload, difficulties of communicating within multiprofessional teams, inadequacy of support and mentoring, and psychological stress associated with the practice of medicine not only threaten learning environments and learning effectiveness, but also the physical and mental health of resident trainees.

Burnout and satisfaction with work-life balance have worsened in US physicians over the last several

Table 1.2 Select elements from the educational environment that a potential faculty member might use to assess the learning environment

Health Care Institution mission statement
College of Medicine and Graduate Medical Education (GME) mission statements
Department of Anesthesiology mission statement
Results of institutional and departmental physician surveys
Results of GME learning environment surveys
Pattern of commitment of department to education (time, finances, technology, equipment)
Previous action(s) of the department when clinical service and education were in conflict
Pattern of supervision of learners
Availability of mentoring and record of faculty development
Wellness focus and emphasis (welcomed, valued, emotionally supported, care about all aspects of person/learners)
Specific examples where administrative leaders put education first
Record of retention of academic faculty
Pattern of using feedback to guide change when change is needed
Frequency of social activities
Examples of response to failures by individual faculty or programs
Examples where concerns were raised (standard of care, education) without fear of adverse consequences and where those concerns were addressed in a timely and effective way
Examples of how administrative leadership request feedback and how the results of feedback have been used to effect positive change

Table 1.3 Select elements from the educational environment that a potential resident might use to assess the learning environment

Program accreditation status
Availability of mentors
Examples of the department commitment to wellness of the residents
Examples of the way the department supported learners having difficulties
Evidence of departmental commitment to education
Examples of the way the program seeks feedback and utilizes the feedback to make change(s) as needed
A review of the results of surveys of learners and faculty (ACGME Annual Resident Survey, ACGME Annual Faculty Survey; www.acgme.org/Data-Collection-Systems/Resident-Fellow-and-Faculty-Surveys; accessed November 19, 2017)

years with more than one-half of US physicians now experiencing burnout.[9]

The percent of anesthesiologists reporting burnout is just slightly above the mean of physicians as a whole. Anesthesiology residents are not immune. In one study, 22 percent of anesthesiology residents screened positive for major depressive disorder and 5 percent reported suicidal ideation in the past two weeks, which is more than twice the rate of their age-matched peers in the general US population. Moreover, those survey respondents with high burnout and depression risk reported more multiple medication errors in the last year compared with low-risk respondents, suggesting an association between burnout and decreased patient safety.[10]

The ACGME's CLER Program outlines an expectation that institutions both educate residents about burnout and measure burnout annually. Efforts to improve the residency learning environment as it relates to wellness could begin with a focus on Maslach's six areas of work stress that can contribute to burnout (Box 1.4).

Leaders in anesthesiology programs should consider wellness initiatives (Figure 1.3) that cultivate a sense of meaning and purpose, mutual appreciation, and teamwork.

Box 1.4 Maslach's six areas of work life related to burnout

1. **Workload**: The extent to which work demands spill into personal life, the social pressures, as well as the physical and intellectual burden of job demands.
2. **Control**: The opportunity to make choices and decisions, to solve problems, and to contribute to the fulfillment of responsibilities.
3. **Balance between effort and reward**: Recognition, financial and social, you receive for your contribution on the job.
4. **Community**: The quality of the social context in which you work, encompassing your relationships with managers, colleagues, subordinates, and service recipients.
5. **Fairness**: The extent to which the organization has consistent and equitable rules for everyone, or the quality of justice and respect at work.
6. **Values**: The consistency between the values of the person that they bring to the profession and the values inherent in the organization where they work.

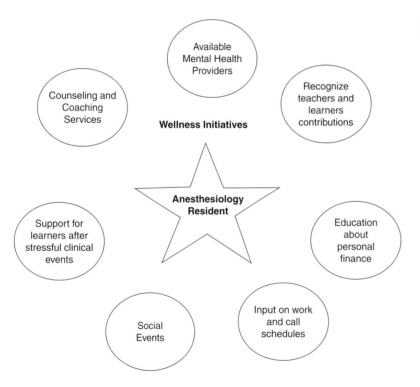

Figure 1.3 Wellness initiatives to support residents during training.

Select practical suggestions include (1) having mental health providers (psychiatrists, counseling services) who are unaffiliated with the institution available by appointment; (2) making counseling or coaching services available for those with life stressors; (3) developing an organized department response to support learners after stressful clinical events such as a death in the operating room; (4) providing opportunities for social bonding outside of work; (5) giving residents some sense of control and input on work and call schedules when possible; (6) providing education about personal finance (financial stress is associated with burnout and decreased quality of life); and (7) frequently providing mutual recognition of teachers' and learners' hard work and contributions.

Summary Points

- The learning environment consists of the conditions (social, emotional, intellectual) and surroundings (physical) in which learning takes place.
- Elements of the learning environment include the organization, resources, people, curriculum (stated and hidden), social aspects, emotional aspects, and physical factors.
- Because learning cannot be separated from its physical, social, and psychological context, teaching is as much about creating the optimal learning environment as it is about conveying knowledge or sharing expertise.
- A positive training environment helps anesthesiology residents succeed, influences physician behavior, models a humanistic approach to medicine, may improve wellness and reduce burnout, and imprints a model of safety and quality on the learner that is associated with similar practice patterns of safety and quality after graduation from training.
- The optimal learning environment or climate might be described as the "best conditions in which a learner can learn."
- A supportive, learning-oriented culture is an environment where learners are welcomed, valued, involved in the design and implementation of their own learning, emotionally supported, and where respect, collegiality, kindness, and cooperation among healthcare team members are embraced.
- Successful learning outcomes in the didactic learning environment are more likely if (1) there are no other competing responsibilities for the learner or teacher; (2) knowledge acquisition and application occur as close together in time as possible; (3) classroom "climate" is one where the learners are encouraged to inquire and trust the teacher; (4) planned educational sessions are not of long duration; and (5) evidence-based methods of teaching and learning are utilized.
- The clinical (operating room) learning environment is improved when there is enthusiasm for what is being taught and an eagerness to transmit this enthusiasm to others; a mutual goal of both teacher and learner for excellence in patient care and resident learning; professionalism and mutual respect; adequate supervision; attempts to decrease noise in the work environment; a reduction in learner anxiety; and structured learning that uses the patient situation/conditions to guide brief learning opportunities.
- Tools to measure or assess the learning environment include the annual ACGME Resident/Fellow Survey (resident assessment), the annual ACGME Faculty Survey (faculty assessment), the ACGME CLER (institutional assessment), and survey instruments determining self-perceptions of the learning environment (e.g., DREEM).
- An anesthesiologist evaluating an academic position or medical student choosing a residency training program can use select elements from the educational environment (e.g., mission statements, survey results) and interviews to determine whether education and training is a valued part of the organizational culture and to assess the learning environment.
- The percent of anesthesiologists reporting burnout is slightly higher than the mean of other physicians, and burnout has been associated with decreased patient safety. Wellness initiatives within departments might focus on Maslach's six areas of work stress: workload, control, balance between effort and reward, community, fairness, and values.

Conclusion

Great teachers take deliberate actions to foster a positive learning environment. Accreditation organizations also recognize the importance of the learning environment where graduate medical education is occurring. In 2016 the ACGME launched a new shared learning collaborative as part of its larger CLER initiative. The collaboration, called Pursuing Excellence in Clinical Learning Environments, aims to improve teaching practices and patient care in the hospitals, medical centers, and ambulatory care sites where residents and fellows pursue their formal clinical training. The goal is to stimulate changes that will broadly improve patient care and clinical learning environments across the nation.[10]

> The process through which residents become competent practitioners has as much to do with the everyday world surrounding their training as it has to do with their own brainpower and hard work.
>
> – T. Hoff (Academic Medicine 2004)

It is, I think, not easy to exaggerate the importance of the informal social element in the promotion of science and learning.

– Abraham Flexner 1930

References

1. D. A. Asch, S. Nicholson, S. Srinivas et al. Evaluating obstetrical residency programs using patient outcomes. *JAMA* 2009; 302: 1277–83.

2. R. Isba. Creating the Learning Environment. In K. Walsh, ed. *Oxford Textbook of Medical Education*. Oxford: Oxford University Press, 2013; 100–10.

3. J. P. Hafler, A. R. Ownby, B. M. Thompson et al. Decoding the learning environment of medical education: A hidden curriculum perspective for faculty development. *Acad Med* 2011; 86: 440–4.

4. ACGME. Clinical Learning Environment Review (CLER). National Report of Findings 2016 Issue Brief No.1: Executive Summary.

5. L. Viola, D. A. Young. How to teach anesthesia in the operating room. *Int Anesth Clin* 2016; 54: 18–34.

6. D. Soemantri, C. Herrera, A. Riquelme. Measuring the educational environment in health professions studies: A systematic review. *Med Teach* 2010; 32: 947–52.

7. N. A. Smith, D. J. Castanelli. Measuring the clinical learning environment in anaesthesia. *Anaesth Intensive Care* 2015; 43: 199–203.

8. E. Riveros-Perez, R. Riveros, M. Zimmerman, A. Turan. Anesthesiology residents' perception of educational environment: Comparison between different years of training. *J Clin Anesth* 2016; 35: 376–83.

9. T. D. Shanafelt, O. Hasan, L. N. Dyrbye et al. Changes in burnout and satisfaction with work-life balance in physicians and the general US working population between 2011 and 2014. *Mayo Clin Proc* 2015 Dec; 90: 1600–13.

10. G. S. De Oliveira, R. Change, P. C. Fitzgerald et al. The prevalence of burnout and depression and their association with adherence to safety and practice standards: A survey of United States anesthesiology trainees. *Anesth Analg* 2013; 117: 182–93.

11. R. Wagner, K. M. Weiss, M. L. Passiment, T. J Nasca. Pursuing excellence in clinical learning environments. *J Grad Med Educ* 2016; 8: 124–7.

Further Reading

1. K. D. Holt, R. S. Miller, I. Philibert et al. Resident's perspectives on the learning environment: Data from the Accreditation Council for Graduate Medical Education resident survey. *Acad Med* 2010; 85: 512–18.

2. Association of American Medical Colleges. AAMC Statement on the Learning Environment. 2017. www.aamc.org/initiatives/learningenvironment/ (accessed November 18, 2017).

3. M. C. Holt, S. Roff. Development and validation of the anesthetic theatre educational environment measure (ATEEM). *Med Teach* 2004; 26: 553–8.

4. M. Mitchell, M. Srinivasan, D. C. West et al. Factors affecting resident performance: Development of a theoretical model and a focused literature review. *Acad Med* 2005; 80: 376–89.

5. J. Schonrock-Adema, T. Bouwkamp-Timmer, E. A. van Hell, J. Cohen-Schotanus. Key elements in assessing the educational environment: Where is the theory? *Adv Health Sci Educ Theory Pract* 2012; 17: 727–42.

6. M. L. Jennings, S. J. Slavin. Resident wellness matters: Optimizing resident education and wellness through the learning environment. *Acad Med* 2015; 90: 1246–50.

7. T. J. Hoff, H. Pohl, J. Bartfield. Creating a learning environment to produce competent residents: The role of culture and context. *Acad Med* 2004; 79: 532–40.

8. M. D. Bould, S. Sutherland, D. T. Sydor et al. Residents' reluctance to challenge negative hierarchy in the operating room: A qualitative study. *Can J Anaesth* 2015; 62: 576–86.

9. T. D. Shanfelt, O. Hasan, L. N. Byrbye et al. Changes in burnout and satisfaction with work-life balance in physicians and general US working population between 2011 and 2014. *Mayo Clinic Proceedings* 2015; 90: 1600–13.

10. T. J. Daskivich, D. A Jardine, J. Tseng et al. Promotion of wellness and mental health awareness among physicians in training: Perspective of a national, multispecialty panel of residents and fellows. *J Grad Med Educ* 2015; 7: 143–7.

Learning Styles in Anesthesiology Education

Randall M. Schell and Amy N. DiLorenzo

Introduction

The learning-styles approach attempts to classify learners into theoretically distinct types or groups. The origins of learning-styles theories can be traced back to the development of the Myers-Briggs Type Indicator (MBTI) Test from the ideas of the psychiatrist and psychoanalyst C. G. Jung. The MBTI, which categorizes people into several groups (e.g., introvert vs. extrovert), became very popular beginning in the 1940s and remains so today (Box 2.1).

Despite the lack of objective studies supporting the assumption that people cluster into distinct groups, the appeal of finding out what type of person you are and the group into which you fit became popular and promoted the development of type-based learning-style assessments.

This chapter will discuss background concepts related to learning styles, emphasize the current lack of evidence for the learning-style hypothesis that claims instruction should be provided in the mode that matches the learner's style, and suggest that educational efforts in anesthesiology would do well to focus on evidence-based methods of teaching and learning (i.e., active learning [Chapter 15], test-enhanced learning, and spaced learning [Chapter 18]) that benefit learners independent of their learning-style preferences.

Box 2.1 **MBTI personality types**

Based on the following four characteristics, 16 different personality types (identified by four letters, one from each characteristic) are described.

Four characteristics:

Focus: Extroversion/Introversion;

Information: Sensing/Intuition;

Decisions: Thinking/Feeling;

Structure: Judging/Perceiving.

Learning Styles

The idea that individuals have distinct learning styles refers to the view that different people learn information in different ways (Table 2.1). The claim at the core of learning-styles theories is that not only can students be divided into types or groups by the way they prefer to learn, but that matching instruction with the preferred learning mode (e.g., visual learners taught visually) will improve overall learning.

Well more than 70 different learning schemes have been identified that attempt to group individuals into widely diverse domains.[1] One of the most popular current concepts of learning styles equates each different style with the preferred bodily sense through which one accumulates information (visual, auditory, kinesthetic).

There is a large amount of published research and many Internet sites, frequently linked with a commercially available learning-style test, dedicated to the topic of learning styles. Two influential articles on learning styles include a commissioned assessment of the scientific evidence underlying learning styles authored by several prominent cognitive psychologists and a systematic and critical review of the literature on learning styles.[1,2] Within graduate medical education (e.g., surgery, pediatrics), several studies about learning-style preferences in residents have been performed. The associated publications attempt to link learning-style preferences to various aspects of performance. A search of PubMed (accessed November 7, 2017) using the search term "anesthesiology education and learning styles" revealed a paucity of published research and a review article.[3]

Assessment of Learning Styles

If asked, students will volunteer preferences about how they prefer information to be presented to them and how they prefer to study. There are a large number and variety of learning-style models based on

Table 2.1 Example learning styles and preferences for presented information

Modality	Example Preferences for Presented Information
Visual Learners	• Pictures and graphics • Computer-assisted learning • Written instructions
Auditory Learners	• Oral reading • Listening to podcasts, tapes, CDs • Discussion, dialog, debate
Tactile Learners	• Hands-on learning (labs, skill learning) • Learn while doing (walking around, exercising) • Like to touch or manipulate what is being learned
Active Learners	• Doing, discussing, or explaining rather than listening and watching • Team competitions
Reflective Learners	• Reflective observation • Time to think about concepts quietly before any action

extremely wide and discrepant dimensions. In 2004, a nonexhaustive list of 71 assessment instruments were identified.[1] Some of the most popular include:

- VARK; visual, aural/auditory, read/write, kinesthetic (http://vark-learn.com/introduction-to-vark/the-vark-modalities/; accessed November 15, 2017)
- Kolb's Learning Styles Inventory; diverging, assimilating, converging, accommodating (http://store.kornferry.com/store/lominger/en_US/pd/productID.5124936000; accessed November 15, 2017)
- Dunn and Dunn Learning Styles Model (www.learningstyles.net; accessed November 15, 2017)
- Honey and Mumford's Learning Styles Questionnaire; activist, theorist, pragmatist, reflector (www.talentlens.co.uk/assets/lsq/downloads/learning-styles-helpers-guide-quick-peek.pdf; accessed November 15, 2017)

The existence of learning preferences does not by itself imply educational value or that optimal instruction for an individual student would need to take this preference into account.

Popularity and Intuitive Appeal of Learning Styles

The learning-styles approach is pervasive, with wide acceptance among the general public and some educators. This approach is also actively promoted by commercial vendors of learning-styles tests.

The popularity and prevalence of the learning-styles approach could be due to demonstrated effectiveness or possibly other factors. People like to identify themselves and others by type and want to be different. A goal of understanding self and others better, attempting to identify important differences between individual learners, and treating learners as unique individuals is laudable. It is also appealing to think that all have the potential to learn effectively and easily if teachers would just match their instruction to the learners' individual learning style. Although there is strong intuitive appeal in the idea that teachers and those designing educational curriculum should pay closer attention to individual students' learning styles and design teaching and learning interventions around them, the evidence that this approach is more effective and fosters better learning is not available.[2]

Instruction Tailored to Individual Learning Styles

If one were to incorporate the learning-styles hypothesis into individualized instruction, they would administer one or more assessment instruments (e.g., VARK, Kolb's Learning Styles Inventory) to a learner (Figure 2.1), determine the preferred mode of learning of the individual, and then individualize instruction in the mode that matches that learner's style (Table 2.1).

The premise of the learning-styles hypothesis is that learning will be less efficient or even ineffective if learners receive instruction that does not consider their learning style. The meshing hypothesis is

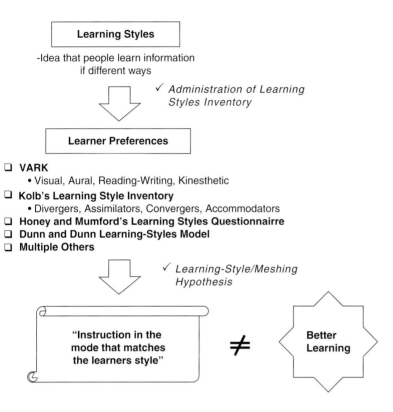

Figure 2.1 "Learning styles" refers to the concept that individuals differ regarding what mode of instruction or study is most effective for them. Students do have preferences about how they learn (e.g., visual, auditory), and these can be determined by one of a multitude and widely diverse commercially available instruments. The learning-styles hypothesis that learning can be improved by matching the mode of instruction to the preferred learning style of the student is not evidence based. Learning is equivalent whether or not students learn in their preferred mode.

a specific version of the learning-styles hypothesis and is the idea that instruction should be provided in the mode that matches the learner's style. In other words, the idea that individualizing instruction to the learner's preferred style can allow people to achieve better learning outcomes. The implications of this would be that a learner who prefers auditory learning should be provided information in an auditory format (podcasts) while a learner who prefers visual learning should be provided information in a visual format (figures, pictures).

In 2008, a group of prominent cognitive psychologists was commissioned by Psychological Science in the Public Interest to assess the scientific evidence underlying practical application of learning-styles assessment.[2] They concluded that individuals "will, if asked, express preferences in how they prefer information to be presented" but there is "no adequate evidence base to justify incorporating learning-styles assessment into general educational practice." Based on their review, they stated that "the belief that learning-style assessments are useful in educational contexts appears to be just that – a belief" and that "widespread use of learning-style measures in

educational settings is unwise and a wasteful use of limited resources."

Potential Consequences of Trying to Teach to Learning Styles

Some have suggested that learning-styles assessments might be a way to start discussions about learning strategies and for acknowledging diversity. However, one might also imagine the economic consequences of attempting to instigate the premise of the meshing hypothesis.

To individualize teaching based on learning styles, an anesthesiology department would need to provide assessments for all learners and faculty development for all instructors. Learners would need to be grouped by learning style and then provided some form of customized instruction. This would require additional instructor training and the validation of whatever instructional activities are being used for each learning style. There would have to be very strong evidence in support of the learning-styles hypothesis to warrant the economic costs alone of instituting teaching to learning styles. This evidence is not available. An indirect cost of attempting to teach to learning styles might be less time spent and less focus on what is evidence based and most important for learning outcomes.

Practical Application of Current Evidence

It is more important that the instructional style match the nature of the subject being taught than that the instructional style match the learning style. Some have used the example of teaching geometry with visual instruction and poetry with verbal instruction. An example from medicine might be an emphasis on visual instruction for regional anesthesia and auditory for learning to differentiate heart sounds.

Learners do have different interests, backgrounds, and abilities. One of the single most important individual difference measures for learning is prior knowledge. As an extreme example, if you are teaching cardiac pharmacology to an advanced resident who has previously spent months of training in the cardiac operating room, spent months in the cardiac intensive care unit, and has had instructional didactic sessions on the topic, you would appropriately teach differently and expect different learning outcomes than if the learner were a third-year medical student without previous exposure to clinical medicine.

In the absence of evidence that validates learning-styles theory, it makes more sense to emphasize teaching and learning strategies that are evidence based (e.g., spaced learning, active learning [Chapter 15], test-enhanced learning [Chapter 18], interleaving) and that benefit learners regardless of their style preferences.

Summary Points

- The idea that individuals have distinct **learning styles** refers to the view that different people learn information in different ways.
- If asked, students will volunteer **preferences** about **how** they **prefer information** to be **presented** to them and how they prefer to study.
- The existence of learning preferences does not by itself imply educational value or that optimal instruction for an individual student would need to take this preference into account.

- There are a large number and variety of **learning-styles models** based on extremely wide and discrepant dimensions. One of the most popular (**VARK**) equates style with the **preferred bodily sense** through which one **receives information: visual, auditory, read/write,** or **kinesthetic.**
- Belief in the learning-styles doctrine is pervasive among the general public and some educators and is actively promoted by vendors of learning-styles tests/inventories.
- **Learning-styles hypothesis:** The claim that individualizing instruction to the learner's preferred style can allow people to achieve better learning outcomes.
- **Meshing hypothesis:** The idea that instruction should be provided in the mode that matches the learner's style. For example, auditory instruction for an auditory learner and visual instruction for a visual learner.
- **The literature on learning styles is extensive and evidence is NOT available to validate learning-styles theory.** Learning is equivalent whether students learn in their preferred mode.
- Current evidence does not justify the major investment of time and money that would be required to assess anesthesiology learners and attempt to individualize instruction around learning styles.
- Educational efforts in anesthesiology should focus on evidence-based methods of teaching and learning (i.e., active learning, test-enhanced learning, and spaced learning) that benefit learners independent of their learning-style preferences.

References

1. F. Cofield, D. Moseley, E. Hall, K. Ecclestone. Learning styles and pedagogy in post-16 learning. In *A Systematic and Critical Review*. London: Learning and Skills Research Centre, 2004.

2. H. Pashler, M. McDaniel, D. Rohrer, R. Bjork. Learning styles: Concepts and evidence. *Psychol Sci Public Interest* 2008; 9(3):105–19.

3. J. M. Vollers. Teaching and learning styles. *Int Anesth Clin* 2008; 46(4):27–40.

Clinical Reasoning

Edwin A. Bowe

Background

Consider the circumstance in which a patient develops profound hypotension and markedly reduced end-tidal carbon dioxide (ETCO$_2$) concentrations due to a pulmonary embolism immediately after induction of general anesthesia (Box 3.1). The method necessary to achieve the correct diagnosis is the process of clinical reasoning. It is an essential part of clinical care, especially in the situation of an unanticipated adverse consequence. If the wrong diagnosis is made, there is a low probability that the treatment instituted will be beneficial.

Clinical reasoning has been described as "naming and framing" the patient's problems (i.e., establishing the diagnosis) that forms the basis for initiating treatment. Some studies report that as many as 20 percent of autopsies reveal a cause of death that was not suspected by the treating physician and that, if recognized and treated appropriately, could have prevented the patient's demise at that time.[1] Combining all the available information (history, physical examination, monitoring data, complications associated with the surgical procedure,

drug effects and possible interactions, laboratory results) and recognizing that not all results can be achieved in a timely manner, presents a serious intellectual challenge. It is imperative that residents learn the process of clinical reasoning and the operating room (OR) is the location where that process is most commonly taught.

Clinical medicine is being driven by progressively more guidelines, protocols, and algorithms. More and more the practice of medicine is proceeding to the point where it is little more than a function of establishing a diagnosis and adhering to algorithms or guidelines for patient management. Because the tendency is to rigidly adhere to those algorithms, it becomes even more important to make certain that the diagnosis is correct. (Example: Although the algorithm for the treatment of malignant hyperthermia is one of the most widely agreed upon treatment protocols, it is unlikely to be beneficial if the cause of the patient's hyperthermia, hypercarbia, tachycardia, and acidosis is thyroid storm instead of malignant hyperthermia.) The extensive use of treatment

---

Box 3.1 Clinical scenario

A patient with a history of colon cancer, type II diabetes, and peripheral vascular disease develops hypotension accompanied by a decrease in ETCO$_2$ immediately after induction of anesthesia for skin grafting necessary due to infiltration of chemotherapy drugs at an intravenous site. Because the most common etiology of hypotension immediately after induction of general anesthesia relates to drug administration, initial attempts at treatment will focus on reversing the hemodynamic effects of the drugs. When initial interventions do not produce the desired response, alternative diagnoses must be considered. Treatment of the patient is guided by the diagnoses under consideration and the probability of each. (Example: Drug dosages are reviewed by examining the syringes to make certain the correct volume was administered. Syringes may be checked to make certain that the label on the syringe is consistent with the intended drug administration.) Some diagnoses are moved down on the list of probable etiologies or dropped from the list completely. (Example: Tension pneumothorax is rejected when auscultation of the chest reveals breath sounds that are equal bilaterally and there is no increase in peak inspiratory pressure. Anaphylaxis is deemed less likely when there is no evidence of bronchospasm, the peak inspiratory pressure has not increased, and there are no cutaneous manifestations.) The experienced clinician is constantly reevaluating the patient and revising the items in the differential diagnosis based on the patient's condition and response to interventions. Tests (e.g., arterial blood gas, transesophageal echocardiogram) are ordered based on the likely diagnoses and the probability that the results of the test will help establish the diagnosis.

Table 3.1 Forms of reasoning used in clinical practice

Type of Reasoning	Characteristics
Hypothetico-Deductive	Begins with hypothesis, generates arguments, reaches conclusion; unless there is a pathognomic feature of a disease, this is useful only in ruling out a disease
Inductive	Uses specific observations to reach a general conclusion; conclusions are probable, not guaranteed.
Abductive	Uses signs, symptoms, laboratory results to try to select hypothesis that best explains available aggregated evidence
Rule-based/Categorical/Deterministic	Individualized established routines used on a regular basis
Probabilistic	Uses estimated base rates and conditional probabilities to modify hypotheses; unfortunately, data on base rates and conditional probabilities are imprecise
Causal	Uses medical knowledge to confirm or refute hypotheses

Source: From *ABC of Clinical Reasoning.*

protocols, in whatever guise, has the potential to result in the clinician simply complying with those recommendations without constantly questioning the accuracy of the diagnosis.

Incoming residents are generally ill-prepared to practice clinical reasoning. All medical students have courses on physiology and pharmacology and rotations on medicine and surgery. Few, if any, medical schools devote any time to teaching clinical reasoning. Because testing clinical-reasoning skills is difficult, even if exposed to this subject, students are more likely to spend time studying content with a higher probability of appearing on standardized tests. Even the American Board of Anesthesiology/Accreditation Council on Graduate Medical Education (ABA/ACGME) Milestones document[1] addresses clinical reasoning only by inference in the crisis management and critically ill patient sections. Although the OR can be used to teach fact-based information (e.g., the induction dose of propofol), the OR experience is an ideal setting of a "real-world" scenario in which to teach clinical reasoning.

Types of Clinical Reasoning

Most authors see physicians using several different types of reasoning (Table 3.1).

Consider as an example a patient who develops a high fever, tachycardia, and increased carbon dioxide production during a general anesthetic for a total hip replacement. Propofol was used for induction of anesthesia, succinylcholine was used to achieve tracheal

intubation, and sevoflurane is being used for maintenance of anesthesia.

Deductive Reasoning

As demonstrated in the following example, the validity of conclusions drawn from deductive reasoning depends on the underlying premises.

Example

Premise: Patients with an abnormality of the ryanodine receptor type 1 (RYR1) gene have malignant hyperthermia.

Fact: This patient has a documented abnormality of the RYR1 receptor.

Conclusion: This patient has malignant hyperthermia.

The problem with this process is that there are more than 400 documented RYR1 variations but fewer than 10 percent of those are known to be associated with malignant hyperthermia.

Hypothetico-Deductive Reasoning

With hypothetico-deductive reasoning the physician generates a list of possible diagnoses and compares each with the patient's presentation.

Sample Differential Diagnosis

Thyroid storm: Fever, tachycardia, and increased carbon dioxide production are consistent with thyroid storm but the diagnosis is not likely because the patient had no history of thyroid disease and the preoperative evaluation did not reveal any evidence of hyperthyroidism;

---

[1] www.acgme.org/Portals/0/PDFs/Milestones/Anesthe siologyMilestones.pdf?ver=2015-11-06-120534-217 (accessed November 18, 2017).

baseline vital signs prior to induction of anesthesia provided no evidence of tachycardia or temperature elevation.

Sepsis: Fever, tachycardia, and increased carbon dioxide production are consistent with sepsis but the diagnosis is not likely because the patient is undergoing a total hip replacement and there is no evidence of infection at the surgical site.

Malignant hyperthermia: Presentation is consistent and a triggering agent was administered.

Note that as described in the preceding text, this type of reasoning is useful for eliminating possibilities from a differential diagnosis, but does not provide a definitive diagnosis.

Abductive Reasoning

The following example demonstrates beginning with the manifestations and working to a diagnosis.

High fever, tachycardia, and increased carbon dioxide production are consistent with a diagnosis of malignant hyperthermia. In the absence of a history of thyroid disease or evidence of sepsis, malignant hyperthermia is the most likely diagnosis.

Rule-Based/Categorical/Deterministic Reasoning

This form of reasoning is applicable to familiar problems. Accordingly, the example of the patient who develops a fever during a "triggering" anesthetic is not particularly useful. A better example would be

something like, "When the patient without a history of lung disease develops an increase in peak inspiratory pressure and a decrease in oxygenation during a general anesthetic, one of the first things I do is to auscultate the lungs to make certain that the tracheal tube has not migrated to a position below the carina."

Probabilistic Reasoning

As noted in Table 3.1, the data necessary to determine the conditional probabilities of thyroid storm versus sepsis versus malignant hyperthermia are not known. This limits the validity of this type of reasoning.

Although the cognitive theories that form the basis for clinical reasoning are beyond the scope of this chapter, there is general agreement that there are two different processes used in clinical reasoning. The "fast" (nonanalytical) process is subconscious, generally effortless, and relies on pattern recognition. The "slow" (analytical) process is a conscious process that requires effort. Over time, physicians organize information into large aggregations termed "illness scripts." Reliance on these illness scripts allows fast thinking; development of these scripts should be one of the objectives of residency. It is widely believed that experienced physicians predominantly use nonanalytic thinking dealing with problems commonly seen in their practices. Providing a focus on the common presentations of common problems (e.g., inadvertent endobronchial intubation, Box 3.2) facilitates the development of illness scripts by the resident. The more illness scripts a physician has, the more likely the correct diagnosis will be achieved.

Box 3.2 "Illness script" for assessing the possibility of an inadvertent endobronchial intubation

How deep is the tracheal tube?

What is the peak inspiratory pressure?

Is an elevated peak inspiratory pressure caused by an increase in airway resistance or a decrease in lung compliance?

Is chest excursion equal on both sides?

Does auscultation reveal bilaterally equal breath sounds?

Is the capnography waveform normal?

Is the oxygen saturation what would be expected?

Is the partial pressure of oxygen in arterial blood what would be expected?

These questions may be translated into "The tracheal tube is placed at 22 cm in a normal-sized male. The pressure-time curve shows a peak inspiratory pressure of 22 cmH_2O and a plateau pressure of 21 cmH_2O. Simple observation suggests that the chest excursion is equal bilaterally. Auscultation reveals good breath sounds that are equal bilaterally. The capnometry waveform is normal and the patient's oxygen saturation is 99 percent with $FiO_2 = .30$." Based on these findings, the probability of an inadvertent endobronchial intubation is low and there is no need to obtain an arterial blood gas or a chest radiograph to confirm that the tracheal tube is above the carina.

This occurs either because the presentation is consistent with one of the physician's scripts or because variance from that script rules out a potential diagnosis.

It should be evident from the preceding discussion that a sound understanding of the disease processes involved is essential to effective clinical reasoning. There is no substitute for clinical experience; the events occurring while administering an anesthetic add to the foundational knowledge necessary to develop new or to expand preexisting illness scripts. Residents need to see many different situations; by definition, the decreased number of hours spent in patient care since the implementation of the ACGME duty hours rules results in decreased clinical experience that, in most circumstances, compromises the acquisition of the experience that is the foundation for clinical reasoning. With this constraint, it is incumbent upon residency training programs to try to maximize the value of the time residents spend in the OR. But knowledge alone is not sufficient; to be effective, residents require instruction in clinical reasoning.

Teaching Clinical Reasoning

In undergraduate and graduate medical education, it has been customary for learners (medical students or residents) to have no specific instruction in clinical reasoning other than that obtained by working with a more experienced clinician. In general, however, clinician educators have neither received instruction in clinical reasoning nor received training in the ways to teach clinical reasoning. Several other obstacles have been described for teaching clinical reasoning (Box 3.3).

Box 3.3 Proposed obstacles to teaching clinical reasoning

- Focus of the learner on other skill sets (e.g., transesophageal echocardiography);
- Absence of a consensus on the best way to teach clinical reasoning;
- Lack of faculty expertise in instruction in clinical reasoning;
- Inability to assess clinical-reasoning skills;
- Lack of ability to assess efficacy of instruction in clinical reasoning;
- Lack of available time in training.

Assessing clinical reasoning in a written exam is extremely difficult. While it would be easy to write a question regarding the different types of reasoning used in clinical practice or the common types of cognitive errors, it would be much more difficult to write a question that would adequately test the clinical reasoning. This inability to assess clinical-reasoning skills is a fundamental problem in developing a consensus on the best method of teaching the subject. (If the performance of a learner cannot be assessed, how can progress be determined or how can the efficacy of two different educational approaches be compared?) While other specialties cite lack of available time as one of the primary reasons for not providing instruction in clinical reasoning, that limitation is not valid for anesthesia residents – OR rotations provide the perfect setting for instruction in this area. Interestingly the Standardized Oral Examination part of the ABA Applied Examination (previously known as the Part Two exam or "oral boards") presents an opportunity to assess clinical reasoning ("What would you do and why?") of the candidates.

In the absence of studies documenting the efficacy of different ways to teach clinical reasoning, recommendations are limited to the preferences and prejudices of the individual authors. That having been said, authors who write in this area tend to recommend some variation on deliberate practice.[2]

Deliberate Practice

Deliberate practice consists of consolidating a series of small accomplishments to achieve a larger goal. This is accomplished through focused practice with specific feedback regarding areas of failure and with recommendations on how to improve. One of the keys to successful mastery of a subject is the ability to develop a mental model that incorporates a large volume of information into a unified mental structure (i.e., to develop illness scripts). Another key element is challenging the learner with specific, achievable goals; the impression is that the process of confronting an obstacle and finding some way around that obstacle is extremely helpful in mastering the subject.

Anesthesia residency incorporates the elements of deliberate practice outlined in Box 3.4.

The ABA/ACGME Milestones document clearly outlines specific goals of residency training. Presumably the process of resident selection has resulted in trainees being fully committed to successfully completing

Box 3.4 Elements of deliberate practice

- Designed to achieve specific goals;
- Participant is fully devoted to achieving the goals;
- Assessment of performance;
- Recommendations regarding what can be done to improve;
- Practice sessions present constantly expanding challenges.

Box 3.5 Types of medical errors

- **No fault errors:** No clinician could have made the diagnosis (e.g., necessary information was unavailable).
- **System errors:**
  (1) Problems with (a) communication (delay in delivering a critical laboratory result), (b) the organization (lack of availability of a necessary test), and (c) technology (an improperly functioning device);
  (2) Production pressure; or
  (3) Refusal of a payor to authorize a test or treatment.
- **Errors due to knowledge gaps:** The clinician was unaware of the disease or manifestation of the disease.
- **Misinterpretation of diagnostic tests:** The clinician incorrectly believes that the serum calcium value reported was total calcium when it was for ionized calcium.
- **Cognitive errors:** Subconscious errors in thought process; stated to be the cause for the majority of diagnostic errors.

residency. Although some advocates for deliberate practice argue that in some circumstances the student can assess performance, it is generally acknowledged that the deliberate practice is more successful if assessment is provided by an expert in the field. There are two elements of this recommendation. First, assessment needs to be provided to the resident. That subject is discussed in Chapter 20. Second, optimally the assessment needs to be provided by an expert in the field. While this may seem intuitive, it is aligned with the ABA/ACGME requirement that there should be fellowship-trained (or equivalent) anesthesiologists working with residents in specific subspecialty areas. (Example: A cardiac anesthesiologist likely lacks the expertise to provide useful feedback to a resident doing a rotation in an ambulatory surgery environment.) Practice sessions present constantly expanding challenges. This is clearly addressed in the ABA requirement for subspecialty rotations and graduated levels of responsibility.

Errors in Clinical Reasoning

Medical errors have been classified into different types (Box 3.5).

The patient safety movement and the ABA/ACGME Milestones document on systems-based practice attempt to address primarily issues of system errors. Residency training should not only provide enough clinical experience to substantially reduce gaps in knowledge, but should also teach clinical reasoning to reduce the diagnostic errors, that is, cognitive errors.

Diagnostic errors have been described as occurring when all the necessary information was available but the physician made the diagnosis too late, made an incorrect diagnosis, or failed to make the diagnosis altogether. One study reported that in hospitalized patients 17 percent of adverse events were due to problems with diagnoses.[3] Determination of whether a diagnostic error occurred is complex; most errors are recognized only in retrospect and it is nearly impossible to accurately recreate the context in which an error occurred. An assessment of the nature of the error requires a "gold standard" of the accurate diagnosis as well as the factors contributing to this error. Some studies have reported that the most common cause of failure of clinical reasoning is the failure to include the actual diagnosis in the initial differential diagnosis. This failure, in turn, is attributed to the physician's inadequate fund of knowledge.

Common types of cognitive errors:

- **Anchoring**: Placing too much emphasis on the first piece of evidence available with refusal to recognize that this aspect may not be as important as initially anticipated.
- **Blind obedience**: Rigidly adhering to recommendations from "expert" sources (consultants or published material) in the absence of sound reasoning.
- **Diagnostic momentum**: Accepting a previous diagnosis that had been hypothesized by others.

- **Confirmation bias**: Accepting results that favor the initial hypothesis while ignoring those that refute it.
- **Hindsight bias**: Retrospectively applying the knowledge of the outcome when analyzing the clinical scenario that resulted in an error.
- **Premature closure**: Establishing a diagnosis before all information has been accumulated and verified.
- **Search satisficing**: Stopping a search because a diagnosis has been found that fits or is convenient; failing to consider that there may be more than one diagnosis.
- **Posterior probability error**: Taking a shortcut to the patient's usual diagnosis.
- **Outcome bias**: Desiring a certain outcome (or, more likely, desire to avoid a certain outcome) alters judgment.

Some Methods of Teaching Clinical Reasoning

Teaching clinical reasoning while providing clinical care provides the advantage of presenting the information in a "real world" environment in which the presentation may be ambiguous, nuances may be present, and distractions occur. The role of the educator in teaching clinical reasoning varies with the skill level of the learner. For novice learners, the primary expectation is that they develop illness scripts and organize the information in a way that is meaningful to them. For intermediate learners (i.e., those who have had some exposure to the clinical environment but lack a significant number of illness scripts), the primary expectation is that they develop more information to organize their knowledge and that they hone their analytic clinical-reasoning skills. Expert clinicians, those who can rely on nonanalytical reasoning for a large percentage of their patients, need to continue to develop their clinical reasoning by working with other experts who can guide their development.

The unproven hypothesis advanced by some advocates of teaching clinical reasoning is that the most effective way to guide learners is for them to work with a single educator on a consistent basis. One of the problems with current anesthesia education is that, in most environments, a resident rarely spends a significant amount of time with one specific attending anesthesiologist on a recurrent basis. Some element of consistency occurs when residents begin subspecialty rotations (e.g., cardiac anesthesia) and work with a more circumscribed group of attending anesthesiologists.

Pattern-recognition skills generally involve presenting typical presentations of a problem. Developing a problem list is one way to help a learner formulate an illness script. Over time, learners will be able to use an approach that compares or contrasts the presentation of a given patient with the pattern established in their illness scripts.

One way to train individuals for clinical reasoning is to suggest undertaking an analytic review after developing a hypothesis using their "fast" thinking. The analytic review should enumerate those elements of the presentation consistent with their working diagnosis as well as those elements that are inconsistent with that diagnosis. This technique has been shown to not only increase the likelihood of eventually achieving the correct diagnosis in the specific patient under consideration, but also to result in improved diagnostic performance in subsequent cases.

Problem-based learning (PBL) and discussions were attempts to teach critical thinking/clinical reasoning, but disappointing outcomes associated with this method resulted in a dramatic reduction in its use.[4] The poor results have been attributed to the fact that the leader provides no content in this approach; instead the learners were expected to solve the problem as a group. (In effect, there was no expert guiding the learner, that is, a fundamental aspect of deliberate practice was missing.)

Many recommendations for instruction in clinical reasoning in medicine or the other "cognitive" specialties are not valid under the time constraints imposed by a crisis occurring in the OR although they may be efficacious when used retrospectively. One such method is the SNAPPS presentation (Box 3.6).[5] A potential advantage of this technique is that it focuses the learner on the differential diagnosis and areas of uncertainty. This allows the teacher to assess the learner's clinical reasoning.

Another method advocated for teaching clinical reasoning, and that works reasonably well in the OR setting, has been termed the One Minute Preceptor (also sometimes described as the microskills model).[6] The One Minute Preceptor consists of five elements (Box 3.7).

> **Make the learner commit:** Instead of the teacher providing a diagnosis or assessment, the learner is expected to make a commitment to the most likely cause of the problem.

Box 3.6 SNAPPS protocol for teaching clinical reasoning

Summarize the patient (history, physical exam, labs);

Narrow differential diagnosis to the two or three most likely;

Analyze the differential diagnosis by comparing and contrasting;

Probe by asking learner about inconsistencies, concerns, and alternatives;

Plan management;

Select one aspect of case for self-directed learning.

Box 3.7 One Minute Preceptor (microskills method) for teaching clinical reasoning

Make the learner commit;

Obtain evidence from the learner;

Provide general rules;

Reinforce correct thinking/actions;

Remediate errors.

Obtain evidence from the learner: Not only ask the learner to provide evidence that supports the assessment, but also ask the learner why that assessment was proposed as most likely.

Provide general rules: Discuss general rules applicable to the learner's assessment or other items on the differential diagnosis.

Reinforce correct thinking/actions: Provide feedback about the elements of the learner's assessment and reasoning that were correct.

Remediate errors: If the learner's reasoning was incorrect, explain those features in the presentation that were overlooked as well as those elements that were inconsistent with the hypothesis.

Whatever method is used, it is important that the teacher articulate his or her rationale for the diagnosis. This explicitly models the reasoning involved and allows the learners an opportunity to assess the strengths and weaknesses of their thought processes. It is also important that residents be encouraged to find alternative diagnoses rather than simply being allowed to come to an immediate conclusion, even if it is correct. Asking the residents for alternative diagnoses, to describe inconsistencies with their hypothesis, or to ask what the most critical diagnosis could be will all encourage clinical reasoning and

minimize the possibility of confirmation bias such as a posterior probability error or outcome bias.

Although there is no "gold standard" for clinical reasoning, assessment is still an important element of this learning process. The adage that assessment drives learning is probably nowhere truer than for medical students and residents. Because these individuals undoubtedly have a history of successful test taking, if they understand the basis for a test on clinical reasoning, it is reasonable to assume that they will work to acquire the skills necessary to achieve a "good grade." Multiple-choice questions are not well designed to assess clinical reasoning. The questions, especially complex questions, tend to cue the learner to select the correct response. The multiple-choice questions offer the advantage that a wide content area can be evaluated in a short period. Assessing clinical reasoning is extremely difficult; the actual process of clinical reasoning must be inferred from the choices the learner has made but cannot be directly observed.

Teaching Clinical Reasoning to Faculty Members

An essential element to be an expert diagnostician is a vast amount of knowledge organized in a way to provide easy access. This is essential to establish the most common form of nonanalytic reasoning – pattern recognition. Although expertise as a diagnostician is essential to teach clinical reasoning, it is insufficient – faculty need to understand how to teach this skill. Just as few medical schools have courses dedicated to learning clinical reasoning, few faculty members have received instruction on how to teach this subject. If the expectation is that clinical reasoning should be taught during residency, then it is reasonable to expect that faculty will be instructed in how to educate residents in this area. Unfortunately, just as there is no evidence on how to teach clinical reasoning to medical students or residents, there is essentially no documentation of the efficacy of any specific strategy on improving faculty teaching of clinical reasoning. In the best circumstances, faculty development programs in general have been associated with:

- Increased faculty motivation for teaching;
- Increased faculty enthusiasm for teaching;
- Increased faculty self-awareness of teaching skills;
- Stimulation of faculty reflection on teaching objectives; and
- Improved faculty teaching performance.

A review of the literature reveals only two studies reporting on the efficacy of different strategies to teach clinical reasoning to faculty members. One study reports a significant improvement in clinical reasoning (both in terms of the participants' individual skills and in their abilities to teach clinical reasoning to students) following a workshop with Observed Structured Teaching Encounters (OSTEs) that involved using a standardized learner in a simulated scenario. In this situation, the faculty member received feedback based on adherence to some form of standardized, behaviorally based scale. Coaching from a peer, who provides feedback based on observation of the performance of a colleague, has been used successfully in other settings. The second study reports that participants liked and made a commitment to change their teaching practice following a two-hour workshop on teaching clinical reasoning. Based on this dearth of evidence, many authors rely on methods successful for other faculty development programs. In other faculty development programs, outcomes are improved if:

1. Participants practice what is being taught before and after the program;
2. Participants receive feedback on their performance;
3. Sessions include a combination of didactic and interactive components (in the form of small group discussions, etc.); and
4. Courses extend over a period (as opposed to short-term courses, such as weekend workshops).

For those assessing a resident's performance in clinical reasoning, there should be a shared mental model about expectations; there must also be agreement on what constitutes a satisfactory performance. It is probably helpful to provide feedback to faculty members about how their assessments of a resident's performance in clinical reasoning compare with others who evaluated the same resident; this should include both residents whose performance was straightforward as well as those with problematic performance.

In the final analysis, the following points can be made about clinical reasoning.

1. Clinical reasoning may be the most significant thing that is taught in the OR.
2. Failure to establish the correct diagnosis when the requisite information was available or could have been obtained (i.e., failure of clinical reasoning) has been documented in up to 20 percent of autopsy studies and 17 percent of adverse events in hospitalized patients.
3. In other specialties, using real cases has been documented to be more effective in teaching clinical reasoning than cases presented in PBLs.
4. Immediate feedback is important in teaching clinical reasoning.
5. There is no accepted "gold standard" for teaching clinical reasoning, but the One Minute Preceptor (microskills method) and SNAPPS have been used with success in other specialties.
6. There are essentially no studies that report successful instruction of faculty members in ways to assess or teach clinical reasoning to learners.

Selected Readings

T. J. Cleary, S. J. Durning, A. R. Artino Jr. Microanalytic assessment of self-regulated learning during clinical reasoning tasks: Recent developments and next steps. *Acad Med* 2016; 91(11): 1516–21. PubMed PMID: 27191840.

B. Wu, M. Wang, T. A. Grotzer, J. Liu, J. M. Johnson. Visualizing complex processes using a cognitive-mapping tool to support the learning of clinical reasoning. *BM Med Educ* 2016; 16: 216.

References

1. K. G. Shojania, E. C. Burton, K. M. McDonald, L. Goldman. The autopsy as an outcome and performance measure. *Evid Rep Technol Assess* 2002; 202: 1–5.
2. G. Norman. Building on experience – the development of clinical reasoning. *N Engl J Med* 2006; 355: 2251–2.
3. T. A. Brennan, L. L. Leape, N. M. Laird et al. Incidence of adverse events and negligence in hospitalized patients: Results of the Harvard Medical Practice Study. *N Engl J Med* 1991; 324: 370–6.
4. C. Onyon. Problem-based learning: A review of the educational and psychological theory. *Clin Teach* 2012; 9: 22–6.
5. T. M. Wolpaw, D. R. Wolpaw, K. K. Papp. SNAPPS: A learner-centered model for outpatient education. *Acad Med* 2003; 78: 893–8.
6. J. O. Neher, K. C. Gordon, B. Meyer, N. Stevens. A five-step "microskills" model of clinical teaching. *J Am Board Fam Pract* 1992; 5: 419–24.
7. N. Cooper, J. Frain (eds.). *ABC of Clinical Reasoning*. Oxford: Wiley, 2017.

Chapter 4

Curriculum Development

Amy N. DiLorenzo and Randall M. Schell

Introduction

Broadly defined, a curriculum is the collective experiences that learners have to help them reach specific learning goals. It is a framework for the intended goals and objectives, knowledge, experiences, and outcomes of a defined educational experience. The term *curriculum* can be used to describe either the entire course of study for an anesthesiology resident (i.e., from the start of residency training through its conclusion), or a particular course or rotation (e.g., an obstetric anesthesia rotation). A curriculum provides a set structure for the educational program or rotation, and helps both faculty and residents understand the expectations and end goals for the educational experience. Having an organized curriculum in place is helpful to both the residents and the faculty. A benefit to the residents is that their learning experience is commensurate with that of their peers. For example, residents participating in a rotation will be assured that they will have the opportunity for similar experiences based upon the didactics, expectations for procedures, simulation experiences, and educational materials provided. Also, a curriculum helps to convey in advance the expectations for an educational experience and how learning goals may be achieved. Benefits to the faculty include having the knowledge of expectations for resident learning, and having the educational tools available to help residents meet these goals. In addition, curriculum development is a scholarly work product that adds to the developer's academic portfolio. A structured and well-defined curriculum sets expectations appropriately for both the residents and faculty members.

Although all Accreditation Council on Graduate Medical Education (ACGME)–accredited residencies have the same basic expectations as outlined in the program requirements, the specific curricula to meet those expectations are left to the discretion of each individual program. While this provides latitude to develop educational strategies at the local level, it also can provide challenges for program leaders to develop curricula that meet their learners' needs. Medical educators are expected to plan educational experiences; a structured approach to designing curricula can help program directors and other faculty teachers with the process. This chapter outlines expectations for curriculum development for residency programs, basic steps in the curriculum development process, and multiple factors to consider while engaging in the process.

ACGME Requirements

The ACGME Common Requirements[1] and specific requirements for anesthesiology residency programs[2] specify standards for program directors in relation to the development and oversight of curricula.[1]

Key Questions in the Curriculum Development Process

Ralph Tyler wrote *Basic Principles of Curriculum and Instruction* in 1949, but his principles still have relevance today.[2] The book was originally designed as the syllabus for an education course he taught at the University of Chicago. Tyler served as an educational policy adviser to seven US presidents and his contributions to the field of education have had an impact on thousands of educators and students over the years. One of his most famous students was Benjamin Bloom, who developed Bloom's Taxonomy.

---

[1] http://www.acgme.org/Portals/0/PFAssets/ProgramRequirements/CPRs_2017-07-01.pdf (accessed November 18, 2017).

[2] http://www.acgme.org/Portals/0/PFAssets/ProgramRequirements/040_anesthesiology_2017-07-01.pdf?ver=2017-05-17-155314-547 (accessed November 17, 2017).

Tyler outlined four fundamental questions for use when considering the development of new curriculum or modifying an existing curriculum. Table 4.1 illustrates a modified version of the four questions for curriculum development in anesthesiology education.

As part of the preliminary work of designing or modifying existing curricula, faculty will want to consider key questions around the end goals and how to best achieve them (Figure 4.1).

Steps in Curriculum Development

General principles of curriculum development are applicable across specialties. The following discussion outlines five steps necessary for successful curriculum development, as a modified version of Kern and colleagues' model, prevalent in medical education.[3] Figure 4.2 shows a road map of the five steps, illustrating the Latin origin of the word *curriculum*, which originally meant "race" or the "course of a race." However, it should be noted that Kern and colleagues discuss that "curriculum development does not usually proceed in sequence, one step at a time. Rather, it is a dynamic, interactive process that continues and the curriculum evolves, based on evaluation results, changes in resources, targeted learners, and the material requiring mastery." The principles are described here as sequential steps simply for outlining the necessary components of the process in an organized fashion. In this modified model, the problem identification and general needs assessment have been combined with the targeted needs assessment component.

Step 1: Conduct a Needs Assessment

The first step in the curriculum development process is the completion of a targeted needs assessment at the department, division, or rotation level. A needs assessment may serve multiple purposes in the context of curriculum development, and may be prompted by significant changes such as a change in accreditation requirements (e.g., ACGME requirement for

Table 4.1 Curriculum development for anesthesiology residency: Four key questions

1. What do we want the residents to learn during this educational experience?
2. What learning experiences can we provide that will help residents achieve the educational goals?
3. How can these educational experiences be effectively organized?
4. How do we know whether the educational goals have been attained by the residents?

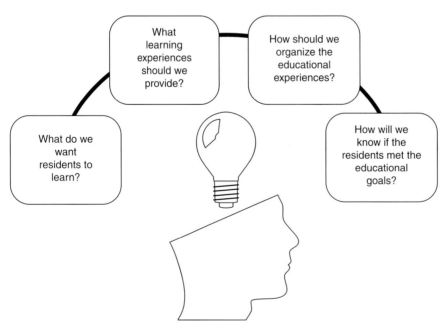

Figure 4.1 Four key questions for curriculum development.

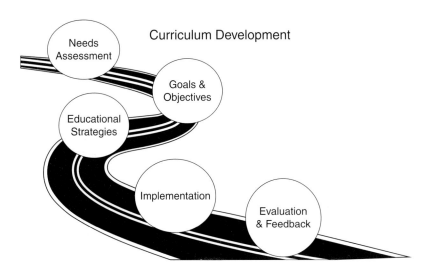

Curriculum Development

Figure 4.2 Curriculum development road map.

simulation), a change in boards requirements (e.g., insertion of the Objective Structured Clinical Exam into the American Board of Anesthesiology [ABA] Certification process), a change in the specialty over time (e.g., the increased use of ultrasound), or a change in the program (e.g., the development of a new rotation such as a perioperative surgical home rotation). Some factors that should be incorporated when performing a needs assessment include:

- Identification of gaps in resident knowledge;
- Identification of gaps in resident procedural skills;
- Identification of areas for improvement in resident attitudes or affective skills; and
- Identification of additional resources needed for teaching (e.g., simulation equipment, textbooks, question banks).

The needs assessment identifies the target learners (e.g., previous experiences), the teachers (e.g., key faculty in the division or service), and the setting(s) (e.g., rotation, clinical locations). The needs assessment process cannot be completed in isolation but should involve key stakeholders in the planned development and delivery of the desired curriculum.[4] It is not only residency program directors who will need and want to engage in the curriculum development process. Associate program directors, division directors, rotation directors, simulation directors, and other faculty teachers and leaders will add expertise to the process of planning educational experiences for residents.

The needs assessment may be conducted by a variety of means including surveys of faculty and residents, focus groups, and in discussions with the program evaluation committee or departmental education committee. Additional mechanisms for conducting the needs assessment are listed in Table 4.2.

Step 2: Develop Goals and Objectives

After the learner group needs have been identified, the curriculum begins to take shape by setting targeted goals and objectives. A goal is the broad educational expectation of the rotation or other educational experience. The objectives are the measurable steps that the resident will take to reach the learning goals. Clearly stated goals and objectives outline the expectations for the learner and are provided to the learner prior to the educational experience. This

Table 4.2 Some examples of methods for conducting a needs assessment

Informal discussions with faculty and/or residents
Formal interviews with faculty and/or residents – recorded and transcribed
Web-based or paper response
Polling through an audience response system
Audits of current resident performance
Audits of current educational experiences that may meet some of the curricular needs
Strategic planning session such as a strengths, weaknesses, opportunities, threat (SWOT) analysis
Program evaluation committee or education committee meetings
Surveys of residency program graduates

guiding document includes both general goals for the experience as well as specific measurable outcomes to direct the educational content, methods of educational delivery, and evaluation techniques that will be employed.[5] Goals and objectives should be structured around the ACGME General Competencies (Table 4.3) and the anesthesiology milestones and corresponding subcompetencies that help to further define the expected experience. It is an expectation of the ACGME that goals and objectives will be developed both for the overall program, as well as for each assignment at each educational level of training.[1] For example, goals and objectives for residents completing their first cardiac anesthesia rotation will be different from the goals and objectives for residents completing their second cardiac anesthesia rotation.

Objectives can be developed in three domains of functioning including the cognitive domain, the psychomotor domain, and the affective (or attitudinal) domain. Objectives in the cognitive domain include the factual knowledge the resident is expected to learn, problem-solving skills, and clinical decision-making skills. Objectives in the psychomotor domain include behavioral skills such as procedural skills (e.g., line placement, transesophageal echocardiography [TEE], regional anesthesia skills) or observable behaviors such as preoperative evaluation or documentation skills. Finally, objectives in the affective, or attitudinal, domain include the resident's expression of attitudes, beliefs, and values. Examples in the affective domain include the demonstration of empathy, the ability to work well with a diverse team, and the ability to effectively manage ethical dilemmas. Most curricula will include objectives in all three (cognitive, psychomotor, and affective) domains of functioning. Suggestions for writing measurable objectives in all domains using active verbs are readily available to educators.[6,7]

Important functions of the goals and objectives include suggesting what learning methods may be appropriate for the curriculum, providing a description of the target learners and the learning environment, and communicating to the residents and faculty what the curriculum addresses and hopes to achieve. Box 4.1 provides an example of goals and objectives for a CA-3 cardiothoracic and vascular anesthesia rotation. This example incorporates the subsequent three steps in the curriculum development process including examples of the educational strategies that will be employed during the rotation, the implementation plan for the rotation, and the evaluation plan for both the rotation and the residents. The goals and objectives are expected to be distributed to residents and faculty in written or electronic form and can communicate the culmination of the curriculum development process.

Step 3: Develop Educational Strategies

Once the goals and objectives are developed, the next step is to develop the most appropriate educational strategies. At this stage, curriculum designers will want to consider what specific learning experiences the residents should have to meet the goals and objectives, and the ways in which that learning content should be made available. The educational strategies should be able to be connected directly back to the measurable objectives in each of the domains (cognitive, psychomotor, and affective).[8] Figure 4.3 provides multiple examples for methods for meeting objectives in each of the three domains. Figure 4.4 illustrates the cyclical nature of learning and how it is supported by each of the three domains.

Additional considerations for development of educational strategies include sequencing, the use of multiple educational methods, and awareness of local resources and needs. A consideration of sequencing of the learning experiences is important. For example, sequencing of rotations, which takes into consideration the progressive acquisition of knowledge and skills over time and experiences. The selected educational strategies should include the use of multiple educational methods to maintain learner interest and motivation, deepen learning, and promote retention of the material. In addition, educational methods should be selected that are locally feasible in terms of available resources. For example, methods requiring the frequent use of standardized patients or high-fidelity simulation might be theoretically ideal, but may be practically restricted in some locations due to limited financial or equipment resources. Future

Table 4.3 ACGME general competencies

Patient care and procedural skills

Medical knowledge

Practice-based learning and improvement

Interpersonal and communication skills

Professionalism

Systems-based practice

Box 4.1 Department of Anesthesiology

Advanced Clinical Cardiothoracic and Vascular Anesthesia Rotation
CA-3

Description of Rotation or Educational Experience

During the CA-3 year, all residents will rotate through an Advanced Clinical Cardiothoracic-Vascular (CTV) rotation for a minimum of one month. Anesthesiology residents will be assigned to the CA-3 rotation after successful completion of eight weeks of CTV anesthesia as CA-1 and CA-2 residents.

The Director of Cardiothoracic Anesthesia is _____.

The Director of TEE training is _____.

At the conclusion of the CA-3 rotation, the resident will be able to:

- Provide safe anesthesia care to adult patients undergoing common cardiac surgical procedures with a minimum of assistance, with graduated responsibility; and
- Provide safe anesthesia care for noncardiac surgery to pediatric patients with congenital heart disease with a minimum of assistance and with graduated responsibility.

Patient Care

Goal

Residents must be able to provide patient care that is compassionate, appropriate, and effective for the treatment of health problems and the promotion of health. Residents are expected to:

Objectives

1. Perform induction of anesthesia;
2. Safely manage the transfer to extracorporeal circulation;
3. Recognize, evaluate, and manage deviations from the normal clinical course;
4. Prepare for the weaning of extracorporeal circulation in cooperation with the surgeon and perfusionist;
5. Communicate patient physiological state to the surgeon and advise on the appropriate pharmacological intervention;
6. Independently resuscitate a patient if necessary; and
7. Perform preoperative assessment of a child with history of congenital heart disease.

Medical Knowledge

Goal

Residents must demonstrate knowledge of cardiac, thoracic, and vascular surgical procedures and the anesthetic options. This will be gained through didactic lectures and independent reading. TEE will be taught intraoperatively by attending anesthesiologists and supplemented by non–operating room resources (e.g., reading TEE studies with attending faculty, use of electronic and conventional texts and TEE simulation).

Residents are expected to:

Objectives

Demonstrate an understanding of:

1. Methods of assessing valvular function or dysfunction including transmitral and pulmonary vein Doppler flow patterns;
2. Knowledge pertinent for insertion of femoral and brachial arterial catheters;
3. The indications for nitric oxide therapy;
4. Surgery for tracheal resection and anesthetic management;
5. Endovascular aortic repair and anesthetic management;
6. Congenital heart disease (to include anesthesia for atrial septal defect [ASD], ventricular septal defect [VSD], transposition of great vessels, Tetralogy of Fallot, coarctation of aorta, and ligation of patent ductus arteriosus);

Box 4.1 *(Continued)*

7. Anesthesia for noncardiac surgery in the child (and adult) with congenital heart disease; and

8. Ventricular assist devices.

Furthermore, residents are expected to:

9. List the indications, contraindications, and limitations of TEE;

10. Insert a TEE transducer under supervision a minimum of five times (should be documented in an activity log); and

11. Demonstrate basic echocardiographic views and cardiac structures to the director or designee (should be documented in an activity log).

Practice-Based Learning and Improvement

Goal

Residents must demonstrate the ability to evaluate published literature on techniques for anesthetic management of cardiac, thoracic, and vascular procedures. Residents are expected to develop skills and habits to be able to:

Competencies

- Identify strengths, deficiencies, and limits in one's knowledge and expertise;
- Set learning and improvement goals;
- Identify and perform appropriate learning activities;
- Locate, appraise, and assimilate evidence from scientific studies related to their patients' health problems; and
- Use information technology to optimize learning.

Residents are expected to:

Objectives

1. Review American College of Cardiology/American Heart Association (ACC/AHA) guidelines on coronary artery bypass grafting; CABG surgery *J Am Coll Cardiol* 2011; 58: e123–210;

2. Review American Society of Echocardiography guidelines on echocardiography (www.asecho.org; accessed November 18, 2017);

3. Review ASA Guidelines on the use of Pulmonary Artery Catheter (www.asahq.org; accessed November 18, 2017); and

4. Review American Society of Echocardiography and the Society of Cardiovascular Anesthesiologists (ASE/SCA) TEE guidelines (www.asecho.org; accessed November18, 2017; 1999 and 2007 – intraoperative TEE, epiaortic and epicardial).

Systems-Based Practice

Goal

Residents must demonstrate an awareness of and responsiveness to the larger context and system of healthcare, as well as the ability to call effectively on other resources in the system to provide optimal healthcare. Residents are expected to:

Competencies

Incorporate considerations of cost awareness and risk-benefit analysis in patient care; and
Advocate for quality patient care and optimal patient care systems.

Objectives

1. Demonstrate an understanding of how a new cardiac surgery service might be added to the existing hospital;

2. Demonstrate an understanding of the absolute and relative costs of cardiac anesthesia interventions and pharmaceuticals;

3. Demonstrate an understanding of the cost of double-lumen tubes and adjuncts;

4. Demonstrate an understanding of the cost of acquisition and repair of fiberoptic bronchoscopes;

5. Demonstrate an understanding of the cost of TEE probes; and
6. Describe the set-up of a TEE service to a hospital administrator.

Professionalism

Goal
Residents must demonstrate a commitment to carrying out professional responsibilities and an adherence to ethical principles. Residents are expected to demonstrate:

Competencies
Compassion, integrity, and respect for others; and
Sensitivity and responsiveness to a diverse patient population, including but not limited to diversity in gender, age, culture, race, religion, disabilities, and sexual orientation.
Residents are expected to:

Objectives
1. Be respectful of the patient's age, gender, culture, and disabilities;
2. Maintain confidentiality;
3. Be appropriately attired with hospital ID displayed; and
4. Be respectful of team members.

Interpersonal and Communication Skills

Goal
Residents must demonstrate interpersonal and communication skills that result in the effective exchange of information and teaming with patients, their families, and professional associates. Residents are expected to:

Competencies
Communicate effectively with patients and families across a broad range of socioeconomic and cultural backgrounds;
Communicate effectively with physicians, other health professionals, and health-related agencies; and
Maintain comprehensive, timely, and legible medical records.

Objectives
1. Maintain a legible intraoperative anesthesia record;
2. Develop consultant-level communication skills in discussing anesthesia-related issues with patients and team members (cardiologists, surgeons, nurses, perfusionists, and anesthesia assistants); and
3. Develop an understanding of the goals of other team members.

Teaching Methods
1. Clinical teaching;
2. Clinical experiences;
3. Performance feedback (verbal and written end-of-month evaluation); and
4. Departmental conferences, subspecialty conferences, podcasts, and discussions.

Assessment Method (Residents)
1. Resident-attending discussions of individual cases will be used to assess patient care, medical knowledge, and systems-based practice;
2. Interpersonal communications skills and professionalism will be assessed by observation and will involve input from team members outside anesthesia;
3. A global evaluation will be submitted to all attending anesthesiologists who had the opportunity to evaluate the resident during each four-week rotation; and
4. A review of the case log will be used to assess practice-based learning.

Assessment Method (Program Evaluation)
1. Resident evaluations of rotation; and
2. Results of resident assessments.

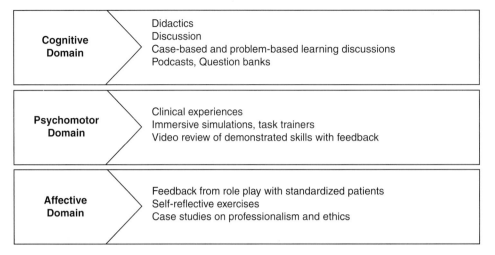

Figure 4.3 Sample methods for achieving educational outcomes.

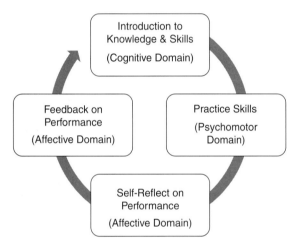

Figure 4.4 Learning cycle with corresponding domains.

needs for resources to support educational methods could be discussed during the strengths, weaknesses, opportunities, and threats (SWOT) analysis or annual program evaluation.

Step 4: Implementation

The implementation step is dedicated to identifying the resources needed to implement the curriculum, obtaining needed support, addressing anticipated barriers, and planning for the roll out of the curriculum. During this step, all practical information about actual implementation of the curriculum is discussed, planned, and addressed so that the plan may become a reality.

Identification of key resources for the curriculum provides a comprehensive and practical look at the

needs to design and implement the plan. Curriculum resources include the following:

- *Personnel* including faculty teachers, administrative support, and standardized patients;
- *Time* including time for faculty to develop educational materials, time to teach and evaluate the learners, time allocated for administrative staff to support faculty efforts, and time dedicated by the learners;
- *Facilities* including space for didactics, equipment for procedures and simulation, clinical sites appropriate for training;
- *Costs* including the direct costs for equipment and educational materials, and indirect costs of faculty time.

Support may need to be sought for one or more of the needed resources from the department chair, program director, division director, or administrative director. A well-planned implementation strategy with a realistic depiction of anticipated costs will be helpful in gaining support from stakeholders and financial decision-makers.

Identification of administrative mechanisms includes practical elements including:

- Designation of an administrative structure for the curriculum to delineate responsibilities (e.g., rotation director, faculty designated to oversee resident evaluations, faculty designated to oversee the didactics);
- A communication plan including how the goals and objectives will be disseminated, how

evaluations will be scheduled, how and when the curriculum development team will communicate about updates and desired curricular changes (e.g., division meetings or monthly education committee meetings); and

- An operations plan including how resident clinical and educational schedules will be prepared, and how data will be collected and analyzed (e.g., evaluation data, procedure log data).

The process of considering and planning resources, support needs, and administrative mechanisms will naturally discuss anticipated barriers to the smooth implementation of the planned curriculum. These barriers should be listed, discussed openly, and addressed in advance if possible. Common barriers include financial and other resources; competing demands on faculty, resident, and administrative support staff time; and at times, attitudes toward change in the department. Not all barriers can be removed, but an open awareness of the issues will help the curriculum development team plan to address and avoid as many as feasible.

Finally, the thoughtful planning and removal of barriers culminates in putting the curriculum into place. A common strategy is to implement the new curriculum first as a pilot and then feedback can be gained to make adjustments before implementing fully.[9] For example, a new curriculum intended for all residents could be piloted first with the experienced CA-3 class to gain their feedback on the effectiveness. Alternately, a cross-section of residents from all training years could pilot the curriculum to gain perspectives from multiple levels of training. Another way to pilot the new curriculum is to implement it for a specified period (e.g., a two-month time frame) to gather opinions and data on the effectiveness and acceptance. After piloting and making adjustments based on feedback, educators may want to consider phasing in the curriculum over time so that adjustments can be made as needed.

Step 5: Evaluation and Feedback

The final step involves both evaluation and feedback for the individual learners, as well as evaluation of the curriculum. This closes the loop in the curriculum development process. Feedback to the resident includes formative feedback during the rotation or educational experience to improve subsequent performance. Formative feedback may be given verbally

(e.g., during a rotation to discuss progress and opportunities for improvement, during a simulation session) and in written form (e.g., in daily evaluations of performance in the operating room). More detail on provision of resident feedback is provided in Chapter 20.

Program curricula are subject to a formalized review and evaluation both throughout the academic year and during the Annual Program Evaluation (APE). Faculty may want to consider a formal evaluation after a pilot of the new or modified curricula to make timely adjustments.[10] This could be accomplished in a variety of ways including surveying the participating residents and faculty or by conducting a focus group with residents. The curriculum development process clearly does not end with Step 5 because the results of evaluations will inform future improvements and changes.

Conclusion

Curriculum development is a dynamic process to craft an educational experience tailored to a specific group of learners. Use of established principles for curriculum design is beneficial to create a high-quality educational experience for the residents. The investment of time in engaging in a practical, systematic, and theoretically sound approach to the development, implementation, evaluation, and continual improvement of curriculum for use in anesthesiology resident education is beneficial to both teachers and learners.

References

1. Accreditation Council for Graduate Medical Education. ACGME Common Program Requirements. 2016. www.acgme.org/What-We-Do/Accreditation/Common-Program-Requirements (accessed November 17, 2017).

2. R. W. Tyler. *Basic Principles of Curriculum and Instruction*. Chicago: University of Chicago Press, 1949.

3. D. E. Korn, P. A. Thomas, M. T. Hughes. *Curriculum Development for Medical Education: A Six Step Approach*, 2nd edn. Baltimore, MD: Johns Hopkins University Press, 2009.

4. J. Grant. Principles of Curriculum Design. In T. Swanwick, ed. *Understanding Medical Education: Evidence, Theory and Practice*. London: John Wiley and Sons, 2010; 1–15.

5. N. N. Khamis, R. M. Satava, S. A. Alnassar et al. A stepwise model for simulation-based curriculum

development for clinical skills, a modification of the six-step approach. *Surg Endosz* 2016; 30: 279–87.

6. D. R. Krathwohl, B. S. Bloom, B. B. Masia, *Taxonomy of educational objectives: Handbook II*. New York: David McKay Co., 1964.

7. A. J. Harrow. *A Taxonomy of the Psychomotor Domain*. New York: David McKay Co., 1972.

8. P. A Thomas, K. E. Kern. From curricular goals to instruction: Choosing methods of instruction. In K. M. Skeff, G. A. Stratos, eds. *Methods for Teaching Medicine*. Philadelphia: ACP Press, American College of Physicians, 2010; 15–47.

9. J. Steinhaeuser, J. F. Chenot, M. Roos et al. Competence-based curriculum development for general practice in Germany: A stepwise peer-based approach instead of reinventing the wheel. *BMC Res Notes* 2013; 6: 314.

10. D. E. Kern, P. A. Thomas. What do leaders need to know about curriculum planning? In L. Pangaro, ed. *Leadership Careers in Medical Education*. Philadelphia: ACP Press, American College of Physicians, 2010.

Chapter 5

Time-Efficient Teaching Strategies in Anesthesia

Manuel Pardo Jr.

Anesthesia clinical teaching often takes place in a time-pressured environment. A common supervision model requires one attending anesthesiologist to oversee care in two operating rooms (ORs) simultaneously. Perioperative efficiency reports typically include "OR entry time" as well as "time from OR entry until skin incision." Resident duty hour restrictions impose other time-based challenges, including the need to limit continuous duty periods and assure a minimum time between duty periods. This may be particularly challenging during rotations (e.g., critical care) with 24-hour in-house call followed by post-call rounds for teaching and transfer of care.

There are other challenges to clinical teaching besides implicit and explicit time pressure. Healthcare systems have become increasingly complex, with the widespread implementation of electronic health records, clinical pathways, and protocols for certain patient populations. There is an ever-increasing focus on quality and patient safety. Finally, the expected knowledge base of an anesthesia trainee has increased over time. These issues are summarized in Table 5.1.

In the face of these challenges, the anesthesia clinical teacher must learn time-efficient strategies for teaching, including the ability to use five- to ten-minute periods for "episodes of teaching." This chapter will

Table 5.1 Challenges in the anesthesia teaching environment

Challenge	Implication for Teaching
Time pressure – Increased focus by healthcare systems on efficiency of care	Working with a learner can increase time spent to complete patient care activities. Instructor should consider ways to provide patient care and teach in a time-efficient manner.
Complexity of healthcare systems – Training experiences often occur in healthcare settings with significant complexity in patients, disease processes, and systems of care	Clinical pathways and protocols need to be explained and followed, increasing the information to be discussed with learner. Electronic health record must be appropriately accessed and managed, which can increase time needed for patient care.
Duty hour limitations – Limitations include an 80-hour work week in the United States (48 hours under the European Working Time Directive), 24-hour limit on continuous duty plus an additional 4 hours for teaching and continuity of care, 8 hours off between work periods (14 hours after a 24-hour duty period)	Limits on duty period length and weekly hours lead to increased handoffs, decreased continuity of patient care, and potentially decreased time for teaching.
Focus on quality and safety of care – Healthcare system has increased focus on quality of care	Increased scrutiny on adequacy of trainee supervision as well as assessment of trainees by competencies and milestones. At the same time, instructors must promote learner autonomy and "conditional independence" in anticipation of independent practice by the resident-level trainee.
Expanded knowledge base – Continual growth in knowledge expected of learners	Vast increase in education resources available to learners, including textbooks (paper or electronic), websites, simulations, etc. Instructors need to help the learner appropriately use education technology to complement patient care experiences. This is particularly important when making suggestions for improving a resident's knowledge base or skills.

focus on the anesthesia resident, whose ultimate goal is the independent practice of anesthesia. The principles also apply to teaching medical students during anesthesia rotations.

The goals of the clinical teacher include providing outstanding patient care and a supportive learning environment for the trainee. A general framework for time-efficient teaching includes the following three-step process: (1) identify the learner's needs, (2) teach rapidly, and (3) have a feedback conversation.[1]

Step 1: Identify the Learner's Needs

By identifying the learner's needs, a teacher can rapidly determine an area of focus for teaching. A teacher should not teach something that the learner already knows, or for which the learner is not developmentally prepared. The range of anesthesia learners includes medical students with very little clinical experience, new anesthesia residents who have completed internship, senior anesthesia residents with increasingly complex patient care experiences, and clinical fellows in a particular anesthesia subspecialty. Although it is tempting to make assumptions based simply on trainee level and experience, there is significant variability, even in learners at the exact same level. The most effective and efficient approach is to (1) ask questions and (2) observe the learner closely.

The initial questions can identify a learner's prior experience with a given clinical situation as well as their perception of their knowledge of that subject. See Table 5.2 for examples of questioning strategies that can be effective. By asking questions, teachers can better determine what learners know – and think they know – about the patients for whom they are providing care.

Table 5.2 Asking questions to identify learner needs during anesthesia care

Stage of Care	Potential Questions to Identify Learner Needs	Possible Learner Needs
Preoperative discussion, initial conversation	Example: Resident scheduled to provide anesthesia for craniotomy. "Where are you in your training? How many of these cases have you done? How have they gone?"	An earlier learner, or one with little clinical experience in a particular area, may benefit from teaching of basic principles of intracranial pressure and effects of anesthetics on cerebral blood flow. A more experienced learner can be queried about more advanced aspects of management such as detection of postoperative complications after craniotomy.
Intraoperative event	Example: Resident is providing anesthesia for extensive posterior spinal fusion. Blood pressure is dropping and motor evoked potential signals have deteriorated. "What is your experience with this procedure? Have you seen this happen before with spinal fusion? What happened, and what did you do? What should we do for this patient now?"	Could discuss what they learned from prior experience, then focus on discussion of potential causes of hypotension (e.g., hemorrhage, venous gas embolism) as well as causes for change in neuromonitoring signals and subsequent approach to management.
Invasive monitoring procedure	Example: Patient needs central line for monitoring or administration of vasopressors. "How many central lines have you performed? What placement techniques have you used?"	Instructor can prepare for different degrees of hands-on assistance and supervision, or an "activated demonstration" of key portions of the procedure. Ultrasound can be used to evaluate vein size and anatomy, which may predict difficulty of procedure and risk of complications such as arterial puncture.
Regional block	Example: Patient would benefit from placement of a thoracic epidural for postoperative analgesia. "How many thoracic epidurals have you done? How many lumbar epidurals? What approaches have you used – midline, paramedian? What has been your success rate in placement? What difficulties have you encountered in the past?"	Instructor can prepare for different degrees of hands-on assistance and supervision, or an "activated demonstration" of key portions of the procedure, such as initial needle insertion point based on anatomic landmarks.

Observing the learner during patient care is another important method to identify the learner's needs. In the OR setting, it is easy to observe a learner during direct patient care activities. However, during clinical rotations such as the preoperative clinic or intensive care unit (ICU), the learner-patient interaction commonly occurs without the presence of the supervising physician. The advantage of direct observation is that the clinical teacher can determine what behaviors and practices should be reinforced, omitted, corrected, or added. In addition, the teacher can ask follow-up questions regarding the thought process used by the learner in the patient care situation. Observations are particularly important during performance of procedures by a learner. Common examples include airway management, line placement, and performance of nerve blocks.

Step 2: Teach Rapidly

After identifying learner needs, the teacher is prepared to teach while personally providing patient care, thereby freeing the resident to concentrate on the learning. One model of rapid clinical teaching that was initially developed in the outpatient medicine setting is called the One Minute Preceptor.[2] This model, which can be adapted as a structure for clinical encounters of various types, consists of the following five steps:

1. **Get a commitment**: Ask the learner a question about an aspect of patient management. The teacher should not express their opinion at this stage.
2. **Probe for supporting evidence**: Ask the learner to explain the rationale for the choices he or she has made.
3. **Teach general rules**: The teacher can explain relevant general principles or concepts that would apply in similar clinical settings.
4. **Reinforce what was done well**: Share positive feedback in a specific manner, based on the explanations given in step 2.
5. **Correct mistakes**: Providing corrective feedback is crucial to improving patient care skills and can serve as the basis for determining a learning plan for the trainee.

See Table 5.3 for a practical example of a One Minute Preceptor teaching interaction.

Another approach to teach rapidly is to use "teaching scripts" to guide the teaching encounter.[3] A teaching script typically includes three to five key teaching points, an appreciation of common errors encountered by learners, and a framework to allow a learner to better remember the concepts. The One Minute Preceptor model is one approach to create a teaching script. With experience, a clinical teacher can develop an extensive number of teaching scripts for a variety of clinical situations. One example is highlighted in Table 5.4.

Procedure skills teaching is an important part of the learning process for the anesthesia trainee. In the surgical literature, three stages of motor-skill acquisition are described, including a cognitive stage, integrative stage, and autonomous stage.[4] Table 5.5 describes these stages using direct laryngoscopy as an example. Providing appropriate procedural teaching involves the same steps of identifying the learner's needs, providing teaching, and having a feedback conversation.

The "activated demonstration" represents another approach to teaching a discrete skill. It is common practice for a teacher to demonstrate a skill while the learner observes; however, a significant downside of this approach is that it is a passive experience for the learner. The concept of an "activated" demonstration indicates that the teacher has made a determination of the learner's relevant knowledge and has chosen a specific learning objective for the demonstration. With an activated demonstration, the teacher provides clear guidance as to what the learner should do during the demonstration, discusses learning points after the demonstration, and shares suggestions for further learning. The activated demonstration can be particularly helpful for a trainee with little clinical experience in anesthesia (e.g., medical student), or for an early-level anesthesia resident attempting a particularly challenging procedure such as thoracic epidural placement. The activated demonstration is not an excuse for the instructor to "steal" a procedure from a trainee who is already capable of performing the procedure in a satisfactory manner under supervision. Table 5.6 provides examples of activated demonstrations in anesthesia care. While these examples illustrate procedure teaching, the activated demonstration can also be used for other patient care situations, such as evaluation of altered mental status in a medically complex patient in the intensive care unit.

Step 3: Have a Feedback Conversation

Providing feedback is a crucial component of time-efficient teaching. Proper feedback should give the learners an understanding of their strengths (what they

Table 5.3 One Minute Preceptor teaching model: Anesthesia example

You are working with a first-year anesthesia resident. A patient with gastroesophageal reflux is undergoing laparoscopic Nissen fundoplication. In the ten minutes after carbon dioxide insufflation, the end-tidal CO_2 increases by 10 mmHg. Ventilator settings have not changed.

Steps	Dialogue between Teacher and Learner
Step 1: Get a commitment	Teacher: Why do you think the CO_2 is increasing? Learner: I think it's from the pneumoperitoneum.
Step 2: Probe for supporting evidence	Teacher: What led you to that conclusion? Learner: It's what I've observed before. Teacher: Could a carbon dioxide embolus present in the same manner? How could you tell these complications apart? What else could cause the increased CO_2?
Step 3: Teach general rules	Based on learner's responses, the teacher can discuss approach to hypercarbia during laparoscopic surgery, including the expected clinical signs and symptoms of other potential causes.
Step 4: Reinforce what was done well	Teacher: You demonstrated a solid understanding of the physiology of CO_2 pneumoperitoneum and the expected pulmonary findings.
Step 5: Correct mistakes	Teacher: I'd suggest you read about the clinical presentation of the complications of laparoscopic surgery including CO_2 embolism and subcutaneous emphysema. I'll give you a reference.

Table 5.4 Example of a teaching script in clinical anesthesia care

Clinical Situation	Key Points	Appreciation of Common Errors	Ways to Create Framework for Learner to Build Illness Script
A patient who had intraoperative pulmonary aspiration of gastric contents is tracheally intubated in the Post Anesthesia Care Unit. You ask the resident to determine whether the patient is ready for extubation. The subsequent teaching interaction is guided by the teaching script.	– Review patient history for baseline cardiac and pulmonary function – Review clinical data for severity of aspiration (impact on oxygenation, ventilation, chest radiograph, if done) – Make sure ventilation mode allows assessment of patient's ability to ventilate spontaneously – Immediate administration of antibiotics is not likely to provide clinical benefit	– Impact of pulmonary complication such as aspiration may be greater in a patient with significant cardiopulmonary disease – Patient with high FiO_2 requirement while intubated may have inadequate oxygenation when extubated due to limitations of supplemental oxygen – If ventilation mode provides too much support (e.g., assist control or high levels of pressure support), may overestimate patient's ability to breathe spontaneously when extubated	– Ask resident about criteria for extubation in the ICU setting, to see if any framework is in place – Consider aspects of pulmonary function affected by aspiration, such as oxygenation, minute ventilation, compliance – For each parameter, ask resident to consider criteria for intubation and mechanical ventilation to promote reflection on extubation criteria

should continue doing) as well as recommendations to improve their skills. The most important aspect of feedback is that it should be a two-way feedback conversation, as opposed to a one-way delivery by the teacher.[5,6] Key elements of effective feedback include establishing a positive learning climate, appropriate content of feedback, and identification of an action plan. (See Chapter 20.) These are summarized in Table 5.7.

Some teaching models, such as the One Minute Preceptor, incorporate feedback as part of the process. In any case, the feedback conversation must be included in any approach to time-efficient teaching. Some teachers are uncomfortable with this aspect of teaching, but following the principles described should allow a conversation that can progress in a positive and engaging manner. An example of a condensed feedback conversation is outlined in Box 5.1.

Table 5.5 Stages of procedure skill learning: Direct laryngoscopy example

Stage	Learner Goal	Learner Performance	Teacher Activities
Cognitive	Understand task, including the clinical context (airway management), relevant anatomy, general approach to procedure using commonly available equipment	Typically erratic, with distinct steps observable	Must be able to break down each step in the process, explain, model, and demonstrate as needed. An intubation training head can be a valuable tool for practice.
Integrative	Comprehend and perform appropriate mechanical (motor) steps in the procedure	Steps are performed more fluidly, with fewer interruptions	Allow learner to practice under supervision, with immediate formative feedback to foster improvement in skill. Video laryngoscopy can enable the teacher to observe the same view as the learner in real time.
Autonomous	Perform the procedure smoothly, rapidly, and efficiently	Continuous and fluid, able to adapt	Continue to provide supervision and feedback as needed, to determine if learner ready for independent practice with the procedure

Table 5.6 Examples of activated demonstration while teaching anesthesia

Situation	Ways to Incorporate an Activated Demonstration during Clinical Teaching
You are working with a medical student on an anesthesia rotation. You would like the student to participate in airway management for a patient requiring tracheal intubation. She has participated in a workshop using an intubation training mannequin.	Use a video laryngoscope for direct laryngoscopy. Guide the laryngoscope through the mouth carefully to avoid dental damage. Allow the student to further manipulate the laryngoscope under your immediate, close guidance to facilitate success without significant prolongation of the procedure.
You are working with an anesthesia resident who is attempting thoracic epidural placement. The resident has performed several lumbar epidurals during a prior rotation, but is having difficulty identifying the epidural space in this patient.	Palpate landmarks to verify proper insertion site. Adjust patient position to see if anatomy improves. If you can reposition the Tuohy needle in the ligamentum flavum, consider allowing the resident to take over and identify the epidural space through loss of resistance. If you identify the epidural space, allow the resident to insert the epidural catheter and proceed with the rest of the procedure.

Table 5.7 Key elements of a feedback conversation

	Guidelines for Feedback
Establishing a positive climate conducive to feedback	– Treat feedback as a conversation – Attitude of teacher is to help the learner improve his or her skills while maintaining a nonjudgmental, supportive, and respectful tone – Understand the emotional impact of feedback, which will depend on the clinical circumstances and the relationship between teacher and learner – Consider where to have the conversation (e.g., in OR during surgery, or in private); the decision will depend on the setting and the content of feedback
Content of feedback	– In general, base feedback on direct observations – Decide timing of feedback based on patient care needs, but as soon as is reasonable – Encourage self-reflection by learner as initial step in conversation – Tailor feedback to the individual, based on the complexity of tasks or events observed, level of training, and nature of performance – Provide specific description of what was done well or ways in which it could have been done better
Action plan	– Learner motivation is a key aspect of the effectiveness of feedback – Help the learner develop an improvement plan – Follow up with learner to review subsequent performance

Box 5.1 Example of a feedback conversation

You observe an anesthesia resident placing a radial arterial line. The resident makes several unsuccessful attempts. You suggest use of an ultrasound probe to guide placement. The ultrasound shows that the needle-insertion site is several millimeters lateral to the artery and the direction of the needle is also too lateral. With appropriate adjustments, the resident successfully places the line. The surgery begins uneventfully. About a half hour later, you return to the OR to discuss the arterial line placement.

Teacher: Can we take a few minutes to discuss the arterial line placement?

Learner: Sure, happy to discuss it.

Teacher: How did you think it went?

Learner: Well, I wish I got into the artery on the first pass.

Teacher: If you had to do it over again, what would you have done differently?

Learner: I would have used ultrasound from the start.

Teacher: How do you think the ultrasound helped you?

Learner: It showed that I was offline.

Teacher: Did the patient have a good pulse to start with?

Learner: Yes.

Teacher: Shall we work on improving your artery palpation skills for those times when the ultrasound is not immediately available?

Learner: How will we do that?

Teacher: Let's palpate the patient's other radial artery, and I'll have you place some dots over the center of the artery with a skin marker, then we'll use the ultrasound to see how precisely you located the artery. By improving those skills, you'll be able to better align your arterial catheter with the course of the artery, which should increase your success rate with arterial lines.

Learner: Great, let's give that a try.

Teacher: I'd also like to mention the parts of the procedure you should continue doing. I noticed that you held the arterial catheter comfortably and securely, and once you saw arterial blood flash back into the catheter, you did a nice job smoothly advancing the catheter. You connected the tubing securely and made sure the dressing would hold everything in place.

Challenges to Time-Efficient Teaching

Following a simple, three-step process can enhance the ability of a teacher to provide outstanding patient care and an engaging experience for a learner. However, there are always challenges to time-efficient teaching. If the clinical schedule includes multiple, short (five- to ten-minute) procedures, the clinical needs of the patient may be of such high intensity that even a five-minute teaching episode is not possible. Examples may include electroconvulsive therapy, or bilateral myringotomy and ear tube placement. In these circumstances, both the teacher and the learner should have reasonable expectations of teaching in such settings. Most of the teaching may occur on the day prior to the procedures during the preoperative case discussion, and the feedback conversation may have to wait until all patients are cared for that day. Fortunately, most surgical procedures of at least an hour in duration should allow several five- to ten-minute intervals in which rapid clinical teaching can occur. In reality, the biggest challenge to time-efficient teaching is an attitude on the part of the teacher that a long period of uninterrupted time is needed for "real" teaching to occur. Once this mental hurdle is overcome, and the teacher and learner embrace these concepts, many teaching opportunities will present themselves even in the busiest of clinical settings.

References

1. D. M. Irby, L. Wilkerson. Teaching when time is limited. *BMJ* 2008; 336: 384–7.

2. J. O. Neher, K. C. Gordon, B. Meyer et al. A five-step "microskills" model of clinical teaching. *J Am Board Fam Pract* 1992; 5: 419–24.

3. D. M. Irby, J. L. Bowen. Time-efficient strategies for learning and performance. *Clin Teacher* 2004; 1: 23–8.

4. R. K. Reznick, H. MacRae. Teaching surgical skills – changes in the wind. *N Engl J Med* 2006; 355: 2664–9.

5. C. E. Johnson, J. L. Keating, D. J. Boud et al. Identifying educator behaviors for high quality verbal feedback in health professions education: Literature review and expert refinement. *BMC Med Educ* 2016; 16: 96.

6. J. Lefroy, C. Watling, P. W. Teunissen et al. Guidelines: The do's, don'ts and don't knows of feedback for clinical education. *Perspect Med Educ* 2015; 4: 284–99.

Chapter

6

Teaching in the Preanesthesia Clinic*

Rebecca M. Gerlach, Jeanna D. Blitz, and BobbieJean Sweitzer

Introduction

Anesthesiologist-led evaluation clinics play an increasingly important role in the perioperative care of patients through streamlining medical testing, improving patient comfort and safety, decreasing cancellations on the day of surgery, and decreasing perioperative morbidity and mortality.[1]

The skills required to be an effective preoperative specialist are diverse and include:

1. Interview and physical examination skills;
2. Medical expertise in a wide variety of diseases;
3. Knowledge in the application of evidence-based practice guidelines;
4. Effective interdisciplinary communication and problem-solving skills; and
5. Administrative skills.

Not all these skills are emphasized during other clinical rotations in traditional anesthesiology training programs. The American Council of Graduate Medical Education (ACGME) mandates that residents must have a minimum two-week rotation in preoperative medicine, however, there is no formal curriculum for that rotation. During this unfortunately inadequate period, the goal is to set expectations for anesthesia residents to become consultants to patients, surgeons, proceduralists, primary care physicians, and specialists. In addition, residents are expected to utilize evidence-based best practices for preoperative assessment, management, and optimization of patients who require anesthesia services. The American Board of Anesthesiology (ABA) and ACGME have published the Anesthesiology Milestone Project,[1] which outlines expectations for

all residents and provides a framework for evaluation. "Patient Care 1, Pre-Anesthetic Patient Evaluation, Assessment, and Preparation" (Figure 6.1) is the milestone most obviously related to resident expectations for performance in the preanesthesia clinic. Other milestones, including "Practice-Based Learning and Improvement 4" (Figure 6.2) and "Interpersonal and Communication Skills 1" (Figure 6.3) are also related to this venue. Select elements of other milestones are also applicable.

Based on the milestones, each resident must be capable of

- Performing a preanesthetic assessment for all patients;
- Serving as a consultant to other healthcare providers;
- Serving as a resource to patients and families; and
- Ensuring effective communication and resolution of conflicts with patients and families.

While this cannot all be achieved during a two-week rotation in the preanesthesia clinic, that experience is the foundation on which other rotations build to meet these objectives. A sample of expectations for rotations of different lengths is provided in Table 6.1.

Though an anesthesiology residency provides the ideal core training needed for preanesthetic care, a focus on teaching clinic-based skills is necessary to ensure providers are adequately trained with both the skills and interest to succeed as perioperative physicians following completion of residency. Worldwide, very few perioperative medicine fellowship programs exist.[2] Links to a selection of fellowship programs existing in the United States and Canada at the time of writing are available in the online content.

A desire to engage with the patient experience is at the core of an effective perioperative specialist. Impressing trainees with the important impact

---

* A sample curriculum for preanesthesia clinic rotation and a list of select perioperative medicine fellowship programs in the United States and Canada are available in the supplemental online content at www.cambridge.org/9781316630389.

Table 6.1 Expectations for rotations of different durations

	2-wk	4-wk	Elective
Obtains medical history	Y	Y	Y
Performs targeted physical examination	Y	Y	Y
Collects data and follows up on testing	Y	Y	Y
Discusses plan with patient and family	Y	Y	Y
Demonstrates knowledge of disease states	Y	Y	Y
Functions as patient advocate	y	Y	Y
Demonstrates awareness of guidelines/protocols	Y	Y	Y
Apply guidelines/protocols		Y	Y
Demonstrates interdisciplinary communication for perioperative planning		Y	Y
Interprets testing and coordinate follow-up appropriately		Y	Y
Performs accurate risk assessment	Y	Y	Y
Incorporates risk assessment into operative planning		Y	Y
Appraises perioperative literature critically		Y	Y
Understands administrative role			Y
Completes quality assessment (QA) and/or quality improvement (QI) project			Y

Has not Achieved Level 1	Level 1	Level 2	Level 3	Level 4	Level 5
	Performs general histories and physical examinations	Identifies disease processes and medical issues relevant to anesthetic care	Identifies disease processes and medical or surgical issues relevant to subspecialty anesthetic care; may need guidance in identifying unusual clinical problems and their implications for anesthesia care	Performs assessment of complex or critically-ill patients without missing major issues that impact anesthesia care with conditional independence	Independently performs comprehensive assessment for all patients
	Identifies clinical issues relevant to anesthetic care with direct supervision	Optimizes preparation of non-complex patients receiving anesthetic care		Optimizes preparation of complex or critically-ill patients with conditional independence	Independently serves as a consultant to other members of the health care team regarding optimal pre-anesthetic preparation
	Identifies the elements and process of informed consent	Obtains informed consent for routine anesthetic care; discusses likely risks, benefits, and alternatives in a straightforward manner; responds appropriately to patient's or surrogate's questions; recognizes when assistance is needed	Optimizes preparation of patients with complex problems or requiring subspecialty anesthesia care with indirect supervision	Obtains appropriate informed consent tailored to subspecialty care or complicated clinical situations with conditional independence	Consistently ensures that informed consent is comprehensive and addresses patient and family needs
			Obtains appropriate informed consent tailored to subspecialty care or complicated clinical situations with indirect supervision		

Figure 6.1 The Anesthesiology Milestone Project. Patient care 1: Preanesthetic patient evaluation, assessment, and preparation.

they have as a perioperative specialist on a patient's experience of their surgery and postoperative outcome provides motivation behind the clinic process. Because much of preanesthetic assessment hinges on multidisciplinary planning and being the "quarterback" for a patient's care, a personal investment in each patient's outcome will elevate the learning experience beyond simply an academic process.

Has not Achieved Level 1	Level 1	Level 2	Level 3	Level 4	Level 5
	Discusses medical plans and responds to questions from patients and their families Acknowledges limits and seeks assistance from supervisor	Explains anesthetic care to patients and their families Teaches basic anesthesia concepts to students and other health care professionals	Effectively explains subspecialty anesthetic care to patients and their families Teaches anesthesia concepts to students and other residents	Explains anesthesia care and risk to patients and their families with conditional independence Teaches anesthesia concepts, including subspecialty care, to students, other residents, and other health professionals	Serves as an expert on anesthesiology to patients, their families, and other health care professionals, (locally or nationally) Participates in community education about anesthesiology

Figure 6.2 The Anesthesiology Milestone Project. Practice-based learning and improvement 4: Education of patient, families, residents, and other health professionals.

Has not Achieved Level 1	Level 1	Level 2	Level 3	Level 4	Level 5
	Demonstrates empathy for patients and their families Communicates routine information in straight forward circumstances with indirect supervision Recognizes situations where communication of information requires the assistance of another individual and asks for help Identifies situations where patient and family conflicts exist and appropriately seeks assistance with resolution Discloses medical errors or complications with direct supervision Recognizes that institutional resources are available to assist with disclosure of medical errors	Ensures that communication of information requiring the assistance of another individual occurs in a timely and effective manner Negotiates simple patient and family conflicts Participates in root cause analysis for issues regarding patients for whom he or she has provided care Discloses medical errors or complications independently as allowed by their institution, if not allowed by their institution demonstrates the ability to disclose medical errors or complications independently, e.g. simulation patient experiences	Communicates challenging information and addresses complex circumstances with indirect supervision Consults appropriate institutional resources with indirect supervision Negotiates and manages patient and family conflicts in complex situations (e.g., psychiatric issues, blood transfusions, cultural factors) with indirect supervision	Communicates challenging information and addresses complex circumstances with conditional independence Consults appropriate institutional resources with conditional independence Negotiates and manages patient and family conflicts in complex situations, including end-of-life issues, with conditional independence	Consistently ensures effective communication and resolution of concerns occurs with patients and/or families Independently negotiates and manages patient and family conflicts in all situations Independently discloses medical errors or medical complications

Figure 6.3 The Anesthesiology Milestone Project. Interpersonal and communication skills 1: Communication with patients and families.

Medical Interview/Physical Examination

The medical history and physical examination form the cornerstones of preanesthetic assessment and determine the selection of appropriate testing, consultation, and perioperative planning. Despite the fundamental importance of this element, anesthesiology residents are seldom observed while taking histories and performing physical examinations and as a result, rarely receive feedback that would allow them to improve their skills. Equally importantly, residents rarely, if ever, are provided an opportunity to see a fully trained, competent anesthesiologist

43

perform a comprehensive history and physical examination, much less articulate their thought processes in arriving at an assessment and plan. When it comes to the preoperative evaluation of patients, the time-honored approach of "see one, do one, teach one" often skips the first step. Modeling expert behaviors can be an effective teaching method.

Throughout medical school, disease-based or systems-based interview skills are taught and evaluated in a checklist-based manner.[3] Because medical students have limited diagnostic and interpretive skills, a successful medical assessment is demonstrated by asking predetermined questions or by performing specific elements of the physical examination. After the acquisition of basic interview techniques during medical school, communication skills improve rapidly during internship and direct the medical interview as experience and pattern recognition grow.[4] Experienced clinicians eschew a checklist-based approach to the medical interview, instead relying on recognition of illness patterns and global assessments (see Chapter 3).[5] This explains why experienced clinicians may not score as well as medical students or inexperienced residents on objective structured clinical evaluations (OSCEs) when performance is judged based on completion of items on a checklist.[6] But global ratings assessments on OSCEs generally improve with increasing clinical experience.[6] Because interview processes become more experiential and less checklist based throughout training, an educator's critique and feedback needs to be targeted at these various stages of clinical training.

Evaluation of competence in preanesthesia consultation is challenging. Even when provided with a standardized tool for evaluation of the same videotaped medical interview, clinicians disagree on judgments of competence.[7] While perhaps not facilitating determinations of competence, a menu-driven evaluation may be a valuable formative tool that helps to ensure uniformity and consistency in the type of feedback provided. Currently, no validated tool exists. The Anesthesiology Milestone Project "Patient Care 1, Pre-Anesthetic Patient Evaluation, Assessment, and Preparation"[1] tool (Figure 6.1) can be used as a basis to provide a comprehensive assessment but is not sufficiently granular for assessment of competence in individual areas such as medical knowledge, problem solving, integration of complex clinical and diagnostic data, interpersonal skills, effective transfer of information, decision-making, or the hundreds of singular

components of doctor-patient and doctor-doctor practices that make up safe and effective medical care.

Structured feedback is a key principle of adult learning in medical education. A standardized tool for evaluation and providing formative feedback can be helpful (Table 6.2).

Videotaping and reviewing the performance of an evaluation, for example, with standardized patients, can provide the opportunity to effectively evaluate history taking and physical examination skills.[8] Competency is assessed both by the actions successfully performed (e.g., eliciting a history of preexisting diseases and previous anesthetic problems, obtaining a smoking history, verifying medication lists) and by what is omitted (e.g., neglecting to gather a detailed history of a relevant reported problem, failing to ask the right questions at the level of the patient's understanding, or overlooking a significant disease in the presence of risk factors). A complete evaluation tool will assess aspects of the patient-physician relationship, medical history taking, anesthesia-focused physical examination, patient education, and completion of preanesthesia records.[9]

It is our belief that evaluation tools are most effective for providing formative feedback and individualized coaching, rather than for scoring or rating clinical competence. Videotaping an interview provides the best way to rate clinical competence, as aspects can be reviewed and played back for the trainee. Given the subjectivity of the evaluation of medical interview performance and the lack of relevance of OSCE-based examination for senior trainees, these techniques need to be further developed for more advanced learners in postgraduate training and tested to demonstrate effectiveness in assessing competency. Instructing, demonstrating, observing, and providing feedback and support will be most effective in shepherding trainees from providers with nascent skills in general medical evaluations of patients into competent, independent practitioners with specific skills necessary to practice anesthesiology.

Medical Expertise

Theories surrounding adult learning have existed since ancient times with a common theme: We learn by doing. The learning that occurs through experience follows "a cyclical process comprising four stages: concrete experience, reflective observation,

Table 6.2 Evaluation of competency in preanesthetic patient assessments

Each component of assessment should be evaluated as Unacceptable (U), Acceptable (A), or Consultant Level (CL)

Component of Patient Assessment	Level of Adequacy in Patient Interaction	Level of Adequacy in Chart Review	Level of Adequacy in Creation of Preanesthesia Medical Record	Level of Adequacy for Day-of-Surgery Anesthesia Team[a]
Identification of planned surgical procedure				
Reason for the planned procedure				
Complete problem list				
Accurate medication list (with doses)				
Accurate allergy list (including reactions)				
Complete past surgeries list				
Accurate pertinent family history				
Accurate pertinent social history				
Menstrual history for females				
Accurate and complete review of systems pertinent to anesthesia				
Documentation of vital signs				
Appropriate cardiac examination				
Appropriate pulmonary examination				
Appropriate neurologic examination				
Application of appropriate risk assessment tools (e.g., STOP-Bang, RCRI, Frailty assessment, Mini-Cog™)[b]				
Appropriate American Society of Anesthesiologists Physical Status (ASA-PS) assignment				
Accurate and complete assessment including risk assessment				
Appropriate diagnostic testing				
Appropriate development and discussion of plan for anesthesia				
Appropriate medication instructions				
Appropriate fasting guidelines				
Appropriate use of consultants				
Appropriate follow-up				

[a] Based on feedback tool embedded in the Anesthesia Record to be completed by the end user, the day-of-surgery anesthesiologist.

[b] STOP-Bang = Sleep apnea assessment tool; RCRI = revised cardiac risk index; Mini-Cog = proprietary instrument designed to detect cognitive impairment in older adults (http://mini-cog.com).

abstract conceptualization and active experimentation."[10] The reflective observation component plays a key role in this process, as without internal reflection and critical appraisal of the data, concrete knowledge acquisition does not reliably occur. The preanesthesia clinic provides ample substrate for experience and experimentation. Without incorporation of internal reflection on previously held beliefs, however, maximal effective learning will not occur.

Increasingly, preanesthesia clinics incorporate a multidisciplinary approach, requiring education and training for physician assistants, advanced practice nurses, hospitalists, surgical and internal medicine trainees in addition to anesthesiology residents. Teaching the required medical content to this diverse group of professionals is challenging. Each group may have gaps in knowledge that do not overlap. (A resident in internal medicine is more likely than a surgery resident to be familiar with guidelines relating to the evaluation of patients with heart disease, but the surgery resident is more likely to be familiar with the anticipated blood loss, and therefore the tolerance for preoperative anemia, with a specific surgical procedure. Neither of those individuals is as likely as an anesthesia resident to be familiar with the physiologic anemia of infancy or how numerous comorbidities, the surgical stress, and physiologic perturbations of anesthesia will combine to impact risk.) The dedicated, individualized training required to identify and address these gaps can be time consuming, making 1:1 faculty teaching and mentoring for each individual not feasible as an isolated teaching approach. Commonly, group training relies on didactic teaching sessions covering vast quantities of information. In the absence of an active or participatory component, learners may not form a deep knowledge of the subject. A learner-focused approach to teaching emphasizes self-directed and active learning, where the learner is responsible for identifying learning needs, creating goals, finding resources, and evaluating outcomes of defined learning activities.[11] This style of learning is applicable to all adult learners, regardless of training and experience. For the anesthesia resident, the curriculum can be developed from a combination of the American Board of Anesthesiology Content Outline[1] and the Anesthesiology Milestones Project.[2]

It would seem that because anesthesiology residents are continually exposed to preanesthetic care through clinical work on all operating-room rotations, experiential and reflective learning would occur in the absence of dedicated training. However, often there is no feedback from experts or supervising faculty for these patient evaluations. With the continued advancement of preoperative medicine and expansion of knowledge (especially regarding guidelines for management of comorbidities such as heart failure, ischemic heart disease, perioperative anticoagulation, and much more) many anesthesiologists are not up to date on best practices. Preoperative medicine has become a specialty practice that requires a level of expertise that an average anesthesiologist may not possess. There is not an expectation that anesthesiologists provide care to critically ill patients in an intensive care unit unless they are trained in critical care. Likewise, we do not expect noncardiac-trained anesthesiologists to provide anesthesia for a heart transplant. And, we certainly would not expect nonspecialty-trained providers to teach novices in these areas of medicine. It is our belief that the same expectation should apply in the preoperative period. Even after a formal rotation in perioperative medicine, however, anesthesiology residents may not perform well on examinations testing basic perioperative concepts.[12,13]

The use of a pretest and posttest surrounding a preanesthesia clinic rotation is an effective way of both gauging the needs of a trainee and providing awareness of their knowledge gaps to inform them of where they should focus their learning. (The concept of test-enhanced learning is discussed in Chapter 18.) Trainees provided with an interactive review of their prerotation test and direction to self-study modules, in addition to didactic teaching, score higher on postrotation tests than with didactic teaching alone.[12] A portion of a self-study module is shown in the appendix to this chapter; a complete example of a curriculum is available in the supplemental material online. This incorporation of active learning and didactic teaching structured into interactive modules is a method to ensure that core concepts, listed in Table 6.2, are covered during the rotation.

In addition to core concepts, a wide variety of diseases and rarer coexisting conditions will be encountered in the preanesthesia clinic. Some conditions (e.g., coronary artery disease [CAD]) are common and likely encountered during the required two-week preanesthesia clinical rotation. However, some (e.g., myasthenia gravis, a family history of atypical pseudocholinesterase) are seen infrequently, but may include those for which an anesthesiologist is the primary resource for directing perioperative management.

---

[1] www.theaba.org/PDFs/BASIC-Exam/Basic-and-Advanced-ContentOutline (accessed November 17, 2017).
[2] www.acgme.org/Portals/0/PDFs/Milestones/AnesthesiologyMilestones.pdf?ver=2015-11-06-120534-217 (accessed November 17, 2017).

Because of the rarity of these conditions, they cannot effectively be taught in a predictable way through clinical experience alone. Involving residents in creating mini-teaching topics, or disease-based "flashcards," can aid in providing education for residents to draw upon when they see patients with these conditions in the future. This technique has the added benefits of teaching residents about available resources while stimulating the spirit of inquiry. Asking a resident to summarize salient features of a disease into a single page, PowerPoint slide, or cue card ensures that they distill complicated aspects of disease into relevant preanesthetic considerations. Rather than settling on an "I don't know" approach, they are trained to develop an understanding of the unfamiliar disease, either through finding a quality review article, searching UpToDate, or using other available summary resources. Subsequent review of "flashcards" that are maintained in a group repository (e.g., on a dedicated website or compiled into a folder) also provides easily digestible learning that can be taught throughout the day while still attending to clinical obligations. The medical expertise required in perioperative medicine is best taught through a combination of techniques that incorporate active learning.

As there is no predicting what types of cases each resident may encounter, providing them with a checklist of experiences to seek may help ensure a complete experience on the rotation. Particularly when clinical work is divided with physician extenders, this provides incentive to actively seek valuable learning experiences. Some essential types of preoperative assessments that should be covered include those listed in Table 6.3.

The preanesthesia clinic often takes on the role of preventative or primary care medicine (e.g., hypertension treatment, lipid level optimization, assessment of thyroid function, initiation of therapy for chronic obstructive pulmonary disease, glucose control). This is especially true for patients scheduled for procedures (e.g., interventional radiology) performed by physicians who do not have admitting privileges, are unaccustomed to seeing patients in advance, and may not understand anything other than rudimentary protocols such as fasting intervals. One of the goals of the preanesthesia clinic is appropriate and efficient use of resources, so being able to assess these conditions and recognize optimal therapies becomes important for avoiding unnecessary referrals to other specialists. As these topics are not traditionally taught during

Table 6.3 Examples of valued experiences in a preanesthesia clinic rotation

Types of Patients

Frail patients

Geriatric patients

Children

Patients for ambulatory surgery procedures

Patients with a history of prior complications related to anesthesia

Patients with extensive comorbidities

Patients with poor health literacy

Patients who are Jehovah Witnesses

Patients with do-not-resuscitate orders

Comorbidities

Coronary artery disease

Heart failure

Diabetes

Obstructive sleep apnea

Pulmonary disease

Hepatic disease

Kidney disease

Neurologic disease

Musculocutaneous disorders

Hematologic disorders

Cancer

Surgical Procedures

Major vascular

Thoracic

Cardiac

Intracranial neurosurgery

Oncologic

Bariatric

Total joint replacement

Extensive spine surgery

intraoperative rotations in anesthesiology, the use of current guidelines becomes an important part of the preanesthesia clinic experience. Frequently, however, anesthesiology trainees may not even know a guideline exists, which guideline to use, or where to find it. Algorithms or tools that are used daily (e.g., American College of Cardiology/American Heart Association [ACC/AHA] cardiac evaluation for noncardiac surgery algorithm[14], the Revised Cardiac Risk Index[15], the STOP-Bang[16] screening for obstructive sleep apnea [OSA]) are best printed and posted on bulletin boards or accessible through computer or smartphone apps. (See Figure 6.4 for an example of resources available on a departmental website.)

The reinforcement of using these tools regularly serves as an educational stratagem. A web resource such as a Wiki or shared folder can be an effective way to compile current relevant guidelines or tools that are frequently used (e.g., American College of Chest Physicians bridging guidelines,[17] OSA screening guidelines, links to the American College of Surgeons National Surgical Quality Improvement Project [ACS NSQIP] risk calculators[18]). Providing easy accessibility permits residents to access the information even when they are on rotations outside of the preanesthesia clinic and reinforces the learning from that rotation. Simply making the guidelines available does not ensure they are interpreted and applied correctly, however. Studies have shown that guidelines fundamental to preanesthesia assessment, such as the ACC/AHA guidelines, are inappropriately applied by anesthesiology residents more than half of the time.[19]14 It is unclear whether this is due to the need for further clarity, inadequate training, or persistence in incorrect practices among faculty that is then passed on to trainees.

Ultimately, a perioperative medicine rotation encourages enthusiasm and future interest in the specialty, whether trainees proceed to pursue it as an area of interest, or simply apply the principles to their daily practice. A journal club focusing on current research or evidence-based practices relevant to care in the preanesthesia clinic provides ongoing education for physician extenders and physicians in the clinic. Educational endeavors and experience working in a preanesthesia clinic demonstrate the dynamic nature of the specialty and the broad focus of anesthesiology practices. A straightforward approach to developing a learning curriculum builds on the following principles:

- Identification of learner needs (i.e., pretest);
- Provision of self-study modules on core concepts;
- Didactic lectures including question-and-answer and case-based examples;
- Problem-based learning (PBL) with active learning and peer teaching;
- Utilization of a checklist of experiences to monitor exposure to a wide range of topics;

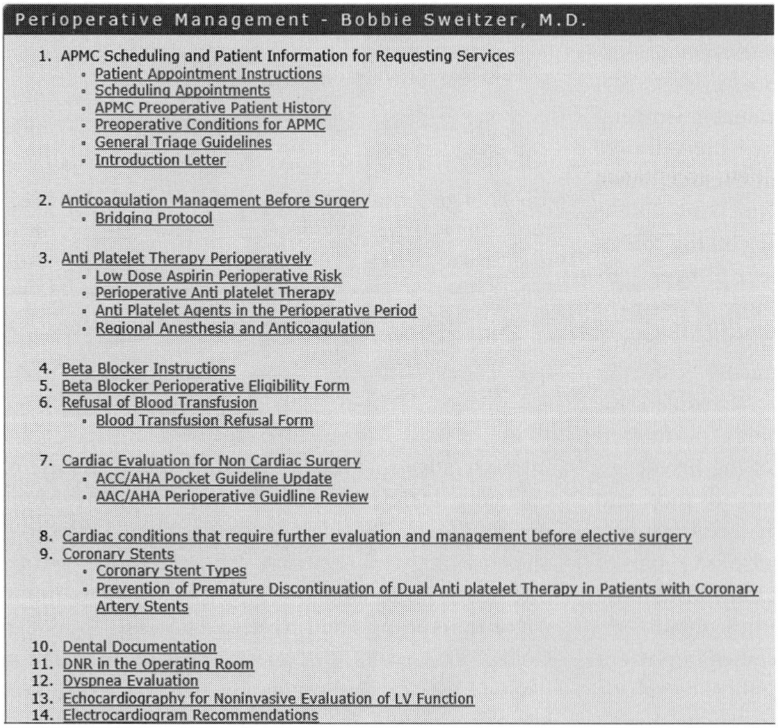
Perioperative Management - Bobbie Sweitzer, M.D.

1. APMC Scheduling and Patient Information for Requesting Services
   - Patient Appointment Instructions
   - Scheduling Appointments
   - APMC Preoperative Patient History
   - Preoperative Conditions for APMC
   - General Triage Guidelines
   - Introduction Letter
2. Anticoagulation Management Before Surgery
   - Bridging Protocol
3. Anti Platelet Therapy Perioperatively
   - Low Dose Aspirin Perioperative Risk
   - Perioperative Anti platelet Therapy
   - Anti Platelet Agents in the Perioperative Period
   - Regional Anesthesia and Anticoagulation
4. Beta Blocker Instructions
5. Beta Blocker Perioperative Eligibility Form
6. Refusal of Blood Transfusion
   - Blood Transfusion Refusal Form
7. Cardiac Evaluation for Non Cardiac Surgery
   - ACC/AHA Pocket Guideline Update
   - AAC/AHA Perioperative Guidline Review
8. Cardiac conditions that require further evaluation and management before elective surgery
9. Coronary Stents
   - Coronary Stent Types
   - Prevention of Premature Discontinuation of Dual Anti platelet Therapy in Patients with Coronary Artery Stents
10. Dental Documentation
11. DNR in the Operating Room
12. Dyspnea Evaluation
13. Echocardiography for Noninvasive Evaluation of LV Function
14. Electrocardiogram Recommendations

Figure 6.4 Examples of online resources available for preanesthetic management of patients.

- Compilation of the most important current guidelines;
- Utilization of decision support tools (e.g., the American Society of Regional Anesthesia (ASRA) app for anticoagulants).[20]

Shared Decision-Making

Once information has been effectively gathered and medical conditions appropriately assessed, a judgment is made regarding the patient's perioperative risk and appropriateness for anesthesia. Often patients do not present in a straightforward manner and do not adhere to guidelines. There may be conflicting priorities that require weighing the evidence. This preoperative decision-making is difficult to teach but may be facilitated by use of a PBL approach. PBL is a well-established method of teaching both critical inquiry and decision-making skills. A preanesthetic clinic provides the ideal venue for PBL or case-based teaching to develop critical thinking skills. Case-based teaching can supplement content areas that trainees may not encounter during their clinic rotation or to discuss challenging scenarios, such as Jehovah Witness patients or ethical decisions surrounding perioperative "do-not-resuscitate" (DNR) orders.

Effective planning and coordination with other anesthesiologists, surgeons, primary care providers, cardiologists, and pulmonologists among others are essential to developing and executing a perioperative plan. The most detailed assessment and investigation is not useful if it does not result in patient acceptance of an implementable plan. For example, a preoperative assessment of glycosylated hemoglobin is only useful if an elevated value prompts a discussion with the surgeon and patient regarding optimal timing for surgery, and a plan for improved glucose management by physicians in the preanesthesia clinic or in conjunction with the primary care team or specialists. Preoperative anemia evaluation for iron deficiency requires a plan for iron supplementation and retesting, with a discussion of the risks and benefits of proceeding with surgery in light of increased risk of blood transfusion versus delaying to increase the hemoglobin. Identification of a patient at risk of postoperative major adverse cardiac events is only helpful to the patient if appropriate risk modification is implemented and a plan for intraoperative and postoperative monitoring and care is arranged.

Communication skills are vitally important in this process. Teaching trainees to assume an advocacy role for the patient's best outcome may place them in direct opposition to the plans of other physicians or even the patient's initial expectations. A limited focus of an anesthesiologist only on the intraoperative period tends to encourage an attitude of "it's not my job." As perioperative specialists and medical professionals, however, it is our job to ensure patients receive the best possible care. Keeping the focus on objective information (e.g., results of tests) and risk-scoring tools (e.g., ACS NSQIP risk calculator[3]) can eliminate opinions or emotions from hindering a scientific, best-practices approach. When communicating with specialists with whom we may disagree, modeling appropriate and clear professional communication supported by facts and evidence is important. In addition to observation of a resident's performance, this can be taught through multidisciplinary simulation exercises involving anesthesiology, surgery, and internal medicine providers, or through simple role play with someone assuming the role of the surgeon who insists the case needs to be done tomorrow despite inadequate preparation. Putting the patient's best interest first should always be the key message of communication. While effective communication skills are hard to teach, modeling good communication teaches the type of behavior trainees need to emulate. The behavior exhibited by the anesthesiologist in this environment constitutes a major element of the hidden curriculum discussed in Chapter 19.

Administration

The first proposal for an outpatient anesthetic clinic was advanced in 1949,[21] and preanesthesia evaluation clinics have been in existence for more than two decades. Despite this history, many anesthesiologists are unaware of essential components of preanesthesia clinic design, such as resident and nursing workflow, patient referral triaging, and the economic underpinning of the clinic.[22] The effective functioning of a clinic is very different from the operating room environment. Anesthesiologists may be unaccustomed to thinking about appointment wait times, patient satisfaction, examination room utilization efficiency, and case cancellation rates. Introducing residents to the function of the clinic during advanced years of training

---

[3] http://riskcalculator.facs.org/RiskCalculator/ (accessed September 17, 2017).

or elective rotations can be an effective way both to develop appropriate expectations of clinic workload and to teach them about hospital administration and economic realities. In hospitals with effective preanesthesia clinics, residents may not appreciate the culture shift that occurred when surgeons began to refer patients to anesthesiologists to prepare them for surgery. An important aspect for surgeon "buy-in" in the establishment of a preanesthesia clinic is the clinical benefit to surgeons for referring their patients. Achieving low case-cancellation rates and minimizing cost of preoperative testing are concrete outcomes that help justify the existence of preanesthesia clinics to hospital administration, particularly in the current cost-containment era.[22-24] Patient-satisfaction scores also become an important metric. Even though the specific details of how to operate a preanesthetic clinic are beyond the scope of what can be achieved in a two-week rotation, simply having trainees work under the direction of an anesthesiologist who is responsible for the administrative functions of a clinic introduces them to the possibility of this specialization after residency.

Involving residents in QA/QI projects provides the opportunity to examine how to deliver care in a timely and cost-effective way.[25] While beyond the scope of a two-week rotation, residents on longer rotations and those choosing to spend elective time in the preanesthesia clinic may become involved in a QA/QI project (see Chapter 22). Additionally, many residents will identify a QA/QI project while in clinic and choose to work on this after completing their rotations. These projects engage the learner in the preanesthesia clinic, fulfill the ACGME requirement for participation in a QA/QI improvement project, and satisfy the need for self-directed learning. They also provide tangible evidence of the results of their engagement in the learning process by having real impact on the functioning of the system in which they work. QA/QI projects that are chosen and designed by the resident are more likely to lead to a personal investment in achieving success. Ensuring that the project has real-life value and avoiding "make-work" type tasks will have both greater educational value and satisfaction as a result.

Conclusion

Training anesthesiology residents to be effective preoperative specialists requires teaching not only *how* we prepare a patient for surgery, but also *why* we do it. Without a focus on improving patient comfort, safety, and overall perioperative outcome, the preanesthesia clinic experience risks becoming another box to be checked in completing residency training. Preoperative specialists must be skilled in all aspects of medical care: effective history taking, examination skills, knowledge of diseases and how to evaluate those diseases, interpreting test results, planning for upcoming events, and communication and coordination. Table 6.4 presents suggestions for how to teach residents in these areas.

Medical knowledge, effective communication, dedication, organizational skills, and excellent interpersonal skills are equally important, but intangible, necessities of being an effective preoperative specialist. Without expertise in *all* these areas, the preanesthesia evaluation process will not maximally benefit patients. Preanesthesia evaluation can play a critical role in a patient's perioperative outcome, including decreasing mortality.[26] The educational process behind training physicians to become perioperative specialists needs to reflect this important role, by incorporating dynamic, engaging modes of education, and ultimately by inspiring learners to proceed to lead the field.

Table 6.4 Content-specific examples of ways to teach in the preanesthesia clinic

Skills	Ways to Teach
History and physical examination	Modeling behavior Direct observation Videotaped exam with feedback
Medical expertise	Pretest to assess areas of weakness Clinical encounters with common conditions "Flashcards" for uncommon conditions Didactic lectures Problem-based learning (PBL) Web-based folders or Wikis
Knowledge of guidelines	Web-based folders or Wikis
Communication/ problem solving	Modeling behavior Direct observation PBL Role play Simulation, videotaping with debriefing
Administration	Modeling behavior Didactic presentations QA/QI projects

References

1. Accreditation Council for Graduate Medical Education and the American Board of Anesthesiology. The Anesthesiology Milestone Project. 2015. www.acgme.org/Portals/0/PDFs/Milestones/ AnesthesiologyMilestones.pdf?ver=2015-11-06-120534-217 (accessed November 18, 2017).

2. A. Gharapetian, F. Chung, D. Wong, J. Wong. Perioperative fellowship curricula in anesthesiology: A systematic review. *Can J Anaesth* 2015; 62: 403–12.

3. E. K. Alexander. Perspective: Moving students beyond an organ-based approach when teaching medical interviewing and physical examination skills. *Acad Med* 2008; 83: 906–9.

4. T. Gude, P. Vaglum, T. Anvik et al. Do physicians improve their communication skills between finishing medical school and completing internship? A nationwide prospective observational cohort study. *Patient Educ Couns* 2009; 76: 207–12.

5. H. G. Schmidt, G. R. Norman, H. P. Boshuizen. A cognitive perspective on medical expertise: Theory and implication [published erratum appears in Acad Med 1992 Apr; 67 (4): 287]. *Acad Med* 1990; 65: 611–21.

6. B. Hodges, G. Regehr, N. McNaughton et al. OSCE checklists do not capture increasing levels of expertise. *Acad Med* 1999; 74: 1129–34.

7. G. L. Noel, J. E. Herbers, M. P. Caplow et al. How well do internal medicine faculty members evaluate the clinical skills of residents? *Ann Intern Med* 1992; 117: 757–65.

8. I. P. Carvalho, V. G. Pais, F. R. Silva et al. Teaching communication skills in clinical settings: Comparing two applications of a comprehensive program with standardized and real patients. *BMC Med Educ* 2014; 14: 92.

9. G. R. de Oliveira Filho, L. Schonhorst. The development and application of an instrument for assessing resident competence during preanesthesia consultation. *Anesth Analg* 2004; 99: 62–9.

10. A. Dionyssopoulos, T. Karalis, E. A. Panitsides. Continuing medical education revisited: Theoretical assumptions and practical implications: A qualitative study. *BMC Med Educ* 2014; 14: 1051.

11. J. A. Spencer, R. K. Jordan. Learner centred approaches in medical education. *BMJ* 1999; 318: 1280–3.

12. E. Hennrikus, C. Candotti, A. Bhardwaj. Teaching perioperative medicine to residents. *JCOM* 2013; 20: 117–21.

13. A. O. Adesanya, G. P. Joshi. Comparison of knowledge of perioperative care in primary care residents versus anesthesiology residents. *Proc (Bayl Univ Med Cent)* 2006; 19: 216–20.

14. L. A. Fleisher, K. E. Fleischmann, A. D. Auerbach et al. 2014 ACC/AHA Guideline on perioperative cardiovascular evaluation and management of patients undergoing noncardiac surgery: A report of the American college of cardiology/American heart association task force on practice guidelines. *J Am Coll Cardiol* 2014; Dec 9; 64(22): e77–137.

15. T. H. Lee, E. R. Marcantonio, C. M. Mangione et al. Derivation and prospective validation of a simple index for prediction of cardiac risk of major noncardiac surgery. *Circulation* 1999; 100: 1043–9.

16. F. Chung, B. Yegneswaran, P. Liao et al. STOP questionnaire: A tool to screen patients for obstructive sleep apnea. *Anesthesiology* 2008; 108: 812–21.

17. J. D. Douketis, A. C. Spyropoulos, F. A. Spencer et al. Perioperative management of antithrombotic therapy: Antithrombotic therapy and prevention of thrombosis, 9th edn.: American College of Chest Physicians evidence-based clinical practice guidelines. *Chest* 2012; 141 (2 Suppl): e326s–50s.

18. American College of Surgeons. New ACS NSQIP Surgical Risk Calculator offers personalized estimates of surgical complications. *Bull Am Coll Surg* 2013; 98: 72–3. http://riskcalculator.facs.org/RiskCalculator/ (accessed September 17, 2017).

19. M. M. Vigoda, B. Sweitzer, N. Miljkovic et al. 2007 American College of Cardiology/American Heart Association (ACC/AHA) Guidelines on perioperative cardiac evaluation are usually incorrectly applied by anesthesiology residents evaluating simulated patients. *Anesth Analg* 2011; 112: 940–9.

20. American Society of Regional Anesthesia. American Society of Regional Anesthesia (ASRA) app for anticoagulants. www.asra.com/page/150/asra-apps (accessed November 18, 2017).

21. J. A. Lee. The anaesthetic out-patient clinic. *Anaesthesia* 1949; 4: 169–74.

22. S. P. Fischer. Development and effectiveness of an anesthesia preoperative evaluation clinic in a teaching hospital. *Anesthesiology* 1996; 85: 196–206.

23. G. S. Murphy, M. L. Ault, H. Y. Wong, J. W. Szokol. The effect of a new NPO policy on operating room utilization. *J Clin Anesth* 2000; 12: 48–51.

24. M. B. Ferschl, A. Tung, B. Sweitzer et al. Preoperative clinic visits reduce operating room cancellations and delays. *Anesthesiology* 2005; 103: 855–9.

25. J. R. Starnes, M. D. McEvoy, J. M. Ehrenfeld et al. Automated case cancellation review system improves systems-based practice. *J Med Syst* 2015; 39: 134.

26. J. D. Blitz, S. M. Kendale, S. K. Jain et al. Preoperative evaluation clinic visit is associated with decreased risk of in-hospital postoperative mortality. *Anesthesiology* 2016; 125: 280–94.

Appendix – Sample Study Module (a sample curriculum for a preanesthesia clinic rotation is available in the supplemental online content at www.cambridge.org/9781316630389)

Case 1: Mr. A (Preassessment)

The patient is a 64-year-old man who is presenting for preoperative testing prior to an incisional hernia repair. He developed a large incisional hernia after having an open partial gastrectomy for stomach cancer four years ago, and it has been bothering him for several years. He has a past medical history (PMH) of obesity, hyperlipidemia, hypertension (HTN), Type 2 diabetes mellitus (DM), nonischemic cardiomyopathy, and compensated systolic heart failure (HF). He had a routine echocardiogram 11 months ago that showed an ejection fraction of 40 percent, moderate left ventricular hypertrophy and no valvular disease. He says that his exercise tolerance is decent, and that he can walk from his house to the street and back to get the mail. He tries to use the stairs at work, which is on the second floor, instead of the elevator, and does not experience shortness of breath or chest pain with this.

- **PMH:** Obesity, HTN, DM, HF, gastric carcinoma.
- **Past surgical history (PSH):** Partial gastrectomy, appendectomy, left knee arthroplasty.
- **Medications:** Aspirin 81 mg, metoprolol tartrate 25 mg BID, lisinopril 20 mg daily, rosuvastatin 40 mg nightly, fish oil.
- **Allergies:** No known drug allergies (NKDA).
- **Social:** He smokes a pack of cigarettes/day and has for 30 years. He used to be a heavy drinker but has not had any alcohol in ten years.
- **Physical exam:**
  - Vital signs: blood pressure: 130/75 mmHg; heart rate: 65 beats per minute; respiratory rate: 14/minute; peripheral capillary oxygen saturation (SpO_2) 99 percent on room air; weight: 85 kg; Height 5'8"
  - Airway: Mallampati 3, good mouth opening, thyromental distance 5 cm, normal dentition
  - Heart: regular rate and rhythm, no murmurs or rubs
  - Lungs: no increased work of breathing, course breath sounds bilaterally.

1. **Which preoperative labs would you order for Mr. A? Check all that apply.**

☐	**A.**	Complete blood count (CBC)
☐	**B.**	Basic metabolic panel (BMP)
☐	**C.**	Prothrombin time/activated partial thromboplastin time/international normalized ratio (PT/aPTT/INR)
☐	**D.**	Hepatic panel
☐	**E.**	None of above
Answer: A, B.		

Don't obtain baseline laboratory studies in patients without significant systemic disease (ASA I/II) undergoing low-risk surgery. There is evidence that many preoperative tests are ordered without indication, abnormal lab tests are rarely acted upon, and abnormal tests are not significantly associated with adverse outcomes.

- Choosing Wisely – American Society of Anesthesiologists. www.choosingwisely.org/societies/american-society-of-anesthesiologists/ (accessed November 17, 2017).
- B. J. Narr, T. R. Hansen, M. A. Warner. Preoperative laboratory screening in healthy Mayo patients: Cost-effective elimination of tests and unchanged outcomes. *Mayo Clin Proc* 1991; 66: 155.

CBC – *Obtaining a preoperative CBC is reasonable in this case.*

- Preoperative anemia has been shown to be associated with increased 30-day mortality for patients undergoing major noncardiac surgery even in the absence of blood loss.
  - G. Fritsch, M. Flamm, D. L. Hepner et al. Abnormal pre-operative tests, pathologic findings of medical history, and their predictive value for perioperative complications. *Acta Anaesthesiol Scand* 2012; 56: 339.
- The American Academy of Family Physicians (AAFP) recommends testing based on conditions that would increase pretest probability of diagnosing anemia (e.g., a chronic inflammatory condition, chronic kidney disease, chronic liver disease, clinical signs, or symptoms of anemia) or for procedures for which significant blood loss is anticipated.
  - M. A. Feeley, S. Collins, P. R. Daniels, et al. American Academy of Family Physicians preoperative testing before noncardiac

surgery: Guidelines and recommendations. *Am Fam Physician* 2013 Mar 15; 87(6): 414–18. www.aafp.org/afp/2013/0315/p414.html (accessed November 17, 2017).

BMP – *Given Mr. A's history of diabetes and use of lisinopril, an angiotensin converting enzyme inhibitor (ACEi), it is reasonable to obtain a BMP in this case.*

- AAFP recommends against routine testing and that findings from the history and physical should drive testing such as chronic kidney disease, HF, complicated diabetes, liver disease, certain medications such as diuretics, ACEi or angiotensin receptor blockers (ARBs).
  - M. A. Feeley, S. Collins, P. R. Daniels et al. American Academy of Family Physicians preoperative testing before noncardiac surgery: Guidelines and recommendations. *Am Fam Physician* 2013 Mar 15; 87(6): 414–18. www.aafp.org/afp/2013/0315/p414.html (accessed November 17, 2017).

Hepatic panel – *There is no clear indication for obtaining a preoperative hepatic panel in this case.*

- Tests of liver function and/or damage are not warranted if the history and physical examination do not suggest liver disease because evidence shows the rate of unexpected abnormalities are very low and the likelihood of altering management even lower.
  - G. W. Smetana, D. S. Macpherson. The case against routine preoperative laboratory testing. *Med Clin North Am* 2003; 87: 7.

Coagulation studies – *There is no clear indication for obtaining a preoperative coagulation panel (PT/PTT/INR) in this case.*

- AAFP recommends tests be reserved for patients with conditions associated with impaired homeostasis (such as liver disease, diseases of hematopoiesis), patients taking anticoagulants, and findings from the history and physical examination that suggest an underlying coagulation disorder (such as spontaneous bruising, excessive surgical bleeding, family history of known heritable coagulopathy).
  - M. A. Feeley, S. Collins, P. R. Daniels et al. American Academy of Family Physicians preoperative testing before noncardiac surgery: Guidelines and recommendations.

Am Fam Physician 2013 Mar 15; 87(6): 414–18. www.aafp.org/afp/2013/0315/p414.html (accessed November 17, 2017).

2. **Which other preoperative tests would you order for Mr. A? Check all that apply.**

☐	**A.**	Electrocardiogram (ECG)
☐	**B.**	Transthoracic echocardiogram
☐	**C.**	Stress test
☐	**D.**	Chest radiograph (CXR)
☐	**E.**	Pulmonary function tests (PFTs)
Answer: A		

ECG – *Preoperative ECG is reasonable in this case, given the patient's history of cardiac disease.* But because he has a functional capacity of greater than 4 metabolic equivalents (METs) without symptoms the utility of an ECG is very low.

- Preoperative resting 12-lead ECG is reasonable for patients with known coronary heart disease or other significant structural heart disease, except for low-risk surgery (IIa)
- Preoperative resting 12-lead ECG may be considered for asymptomatic patients, except for low-risk surgery (IIb)
- Routine preoperative resting 12-lead ECG is not useful for asymptomatic patients undergoing low-risk surgical procedures.
  - 2014 ACC/AHA Guideline on Perioperative Cardiovascular Evaluation and Management of Patients Undergoing Noncardiac Surgery: Executive Summary: A Report of the American College of Cardiology/American Heart Association Task Force on Practice Guidelines. *J Am Coll Cardiol* 2014 Dec 9; 64 (22): e77–137.

PFT/CXR – *While Mr. A has several risk factors for postoperative complications, including an age > 60 years, history of smoking, upper abdominal surgery, HF, and ASA class > II there is no evidence to suggest that preoperative PFTs will predict postoperative pulmonary complications (PPC) or alter management in this case.*

- Risk factors for PPC include age > 60 years, chronic obstructive pulmonary disease (COPD), cigarette use, congestive heart failure, functional dependence, American Society of Anesthesiologists (ASA) classification of II or greater, obstructive sleep apnea, low serum albumin, surgery factors (surgery > three hours, aortic aneurysm repair, thoracic, abdominal, neurologic, head and neck, emergency, or vascular surgery), general anesthesia, impaired sensorium, abnormal findings on chest examination, alcohol use, and weight loss.

- Review did not find evidence showing obesity, asthma, exercise capacity, diabetes, or human immunovirus (HIV) infection were risk factors.
- Important PPC include atelectasis, pneumonia, respiratory failure, and exacerbation of underlying chronic lung disease.
- PPC are equally prevalent and contribute similarly to morbidity, mortality, and length of stay as cardiac complications. PPC may be more likely than cardiac complications to predict long-term mortality after surgery, particularly among older patients.
  - A. Qaseem, V. Snow, N. Fitterman et al. Risk assessment for and strategies to reduce perioperative pulmonary complications for patients undergoing noncardiothoracic surgery: A guideline from the American College of Physicians. *Ann Intern Med* 2006; 144: 575.
- In a study of patients with severe COPD (forced expiratory volume in one second [FEV_1] < 50 percent predicted), preoperative PFTs did not predict the risk of pulmonary complications, whereas length of surgery, ASA class, and type of procedure were all significant predictors.
  - J. A. Brooks-Brunn. Predictors of postoperative pulmonary complications following abdominal surgery. *Chest* 1997; 111: 564.
- In another study, smokers with severe airflow obstruction and an FEV_1 of less than 40 percent of predicted were matched to smokers with a normal FEV_1. Only bronchospasm was more common among those patients with abnormal spirometry. The incidence of postoperative pneumonia, prolonged intubation, prolonged intensive care unit stay, and death were not significantly different between the two groups.

  - D. O. Warner, M. A. Warner, K. P. Offord et al. Airway obstruction and perioperative complications in smokers undergoing abdominal surgery. *Anesthesiology* 1999; 90: 372.
- *Preoperative PFTs and CXR should not be used routinely for predicting risk for PPC.*
  - A. Qaseem, V. Snow, N. Fitterman et al. Risk assessment for and strategies to reduce perioperative pulmonary complications for patients undergoing noncardiothoracic surgery: A guideline from the American College of Physicians. *Ann Intern Med* 2006; 144: 575.
- Subsequent studies have confirmed the value of spirometry and diffusing capacity of the lungs for carbon monoxide (DLCO) in providing an accurate assessment of operative risk for lung resection using thoracotomy. However, the predictive value of FEV_1 and DLCO for PPC is less clear when lobectomy is performed using thoracoscopy, as results have been mixed.
  - R. Zhang, S. M. Lee, C. Wigfield et al. Lung function predicts pulmonary complications regardless of the surgical approach. *Ann Thorac Surg* 2015; 99: 1761.
  - M. F. Berry, N. R. Villamizar-Ortiz, B. C. Tong et al. Pulmonary function tests do not predict pulmonary complications after thoracoscopic lobectomy. *Ann Thorac Surg* 2010; 89: 1044.

Echocardiography – *There is not sufficient evidence that Mr. A needs an updated echo prior to surgery.*

- Class IIa Recommendations
  - It is reasonable for patients with dyspnea of unknown origin to undergo preoperative evaluation of left ventricular function (LV) function. *(Level of Evidence: C)*
  - It is reasonable for patients with HF with worsening dyspnea or other change in clinical status to undergo preoperative evaluation of LV function. *(Level of Evidence: C)*

- Class IIb Recommendations
  - Reassessment of LV function in clinically stable patients with previously documented LV dysfunction may be considered if there has been no assessment within a year. *(Level of Evidence: C)*

- Class III Recommendations
  - Routine preoperative evaluation of LV function is not recommended. *(Level of Evidence: B)*
  - 2014 ACC/AHA Guideline on Perioperative Cardiovascular Evaluation and Management of Patients Undergoing Noncardiac Surgery: Executive Summary: A Report of the American College of Cardiology/American Heart Association Task Force on Practice Guidelines. *J Am Coll Cardiol* 2014 Dec 9; 64 (22): e77–137.

Stress test – *Don't obtain baseline cardiac testing (transthoracic echocardiography/transesophageal echocardiography [TTE/TEE]) or cardiac stress testing in asymptomatic stable patients undergoing low- or moderate-risk noncardiac surgery.*

- Choosing Wisely – American Society of Anesthesiologists. www.choosingwisely.org/ societies/american-society-of-anesthesiologists/ (accessed November 17, 2017).

3. **Which medications would you continue, including on the day of surgery? Check all that apply.**

☐	**A.**	Metoprolol tartrate
☐	**B.**	Lisinopril
☐	**C.**	Rosuvastatin
☐	**D.**	Aspirin
☐	**E.**	None of above

Answer: A, B, C, D

Beta blockers – *Mr. A should continue his metoprolol.*
- Class I Recommendations
  - Beta blockers should be continued in patients undergoing surgery who have been on beta blockers chronically. *(Level of Evidence: B)*
- Class IIa Recommendations
  - It is reasonable for the management of beta blockers after surgery to be guided by clinical circumstances, independent of when the agent was started. *(Level of Evidence: B)*
- Class IIb Recommendations
  - In patients with intermediate- or high-risk myocardial ischemia noted on preoperative risk stratification tests, it may be reasonable

to begin perioperative beta blockers. *(Level of Evidence: C)*
  - In patients with three or more revised cardiac risk index (RCRI) risk factors (e.g., diabetes mellitus, HF, CAD, renal insufficiency, cerebrovascular disease, high-risk surgery), it may be reasonable to begin beta blockers before surgery. *(Level of Evidence: B)*
  - In patients with a compelling long-term indication for beta-blocker therapy but no other RCRI risk factors, initiating beta blockers in the perioperative setting as an approach to reduce perioperative risk is of uncertain benefit. *(Level of Evidence: B)*
  - In patients in whom beta-blocker therapy is initiated, it may be reasonable to begin perioperative beta blockers long enough in advance to assess safety and tolerability, preferably more than one day before surgery. *(Level of Evidence: B)*

- Class III Recommendations
  - Beta-blocker therapy should not be started on the day of surgery. *(Level of Evidence: B)*
  - 2014 ACC/AHA Guideline on Perioperative Cardiovascular Evaluation and Management of Patients Undergoing Noncardiac Surgery: Executive Summary: A Report of the American College of Cardiology/American Heart Association Task Force on Practice Guidelines. *J Am Coll Cardiol* 2014 Dec 9; 64 (22): e77–137.

ACEi – *Mr. A should continue his lisinopril. Patients who continue their ACEi/ARBs have a higher incidence of intraoperative transient hypotension but no difference in other measurable outcomes.*

- Class IIa Recommendations
  - Continuation of ACEi inhibitors or ARBs perioperatively is reasonable. *(Level of Evidence: B)*
  - If ACEi or ARBs are held before surgery, it is reasonable to restart as soon as clinically feasible postoperatively. *(Level of Evidence: C)*
  - 2014 ACC/AHA Guideline on Perioperative Cardiovascular Evaluation and Management of Patients Undergoing Noncardiac Surgery: Executive Summary: A Report of the

American College of Cardiology/American Heart Association Task Force on Practice Guidelines. *J Am Coll Cardiol* 2014 Dec 9; 64 (22): e77–137.

Statins – *Mr. A should continue his Crestor.*

- Class I Recommendations
  - Statins should be continued in patients currently taking statins and scheduled for noncardiac surgery. *(Level of Evidence: B)*
- Class IIa Recommendations
  - Perioperative initiation of statin use is reasonable in patients undergoing vascular surgery. *(Level of Evidence: B)*
- Class IIb Recommendations
  - Perioperative initiation of statins may be considered in patients with clinical indications according to goal-directed medical therapy (GDMT) who are undergoing elevated-risk procedures. *(Level of Evidence: C)*
  - 2014 ACC/AHA Guideline on Perioperative Cardiovascular Evaluation and Management of Patients Undergoing Noncardiac Surgery: Executive Summary: A Report of the American College of Cardiology/American Heart Association Task Force on Practice Guidelines. *J Am Coll Cardiol* 2014 Dec 9; 64 (22): e77–137.

Aspirin – *Mr. A should continue his aspirin.*

- Class I Recommendations: Elective noncardiac surgery should be delayed 30 days after bare metal stent (BMS) implantation and optimally 6 months after drug-eluting stent (DES) implantation.
  - In patients treated with dual antiplatelet therapy (DAPT) after coronary stent implantation who must undergo surgical procedures that mandate the discontinuation of P2Y12 inhibitor therapy, it is recommended that aspirin be continued if possible and the P2Y12 platelet receptor inhibitor be restarted as soon as possible after surgery. *(Level of Evidence: B)*
- Class IIa Recommendations: When noncardiac surgery is required in patients currently taking a P2Y12 inhibitor, a consensus decision among treating clinicians as to the relative risks of surgery and discontinuation or continuation of antiplatelet therapy can be useful. *(Level of Evidence: C)*

- Class IIb Recommendations
  - Elective noncardiac surgery after DES implantation in patients for whom P2Y12 inhibitor therapy will need to be discontinued may be considered after 3 months if the risk of further delay of surgery is greater than the expected risks of stent thrombosis. *(Level of Evidence: C)*
- Class III Recommendations: No Benefit
  - Elective noncardiac surgery should not be performed within 30 days after BMS implantation or within 3 months after DES implantation in patients in whom DAPT will need to be discontinued perioperatively. *(Level of Evidence: B)*
  - 2016 ACC/AHA Guideline Focused Update on Duration of Dual Antiplatelet Therapy in Patients with Coronary Artery Disease. *Circulation.* 2016; 134: e123–e155.

4. **Should Mr. A be referred to his medical doctor for clearance before this surgery?**

☐	**A.**	Yes
☐	**B.**	No

Answer: B

No - Preoperative evaluation by a medical doctor has not been associated with improvement in postoperative outcomes.

Prior studies on the effect of an in-person preoperative evaluation by an internal medicine physician have failed to demonstrate a positive effect on postoperative outcomes. Medical consultation before major elective noncardiac surgery is associated with increased mortality and hospital stay, as well as increases in preoperative pharmacologic interventions and testing. These findings highlight the need to better understand mechanisms by which consultation influences outcomes and to identify efficacious interventions to decrease perioperative risk.

- A. D. Auerbach. Opportunity missed: Medical consultation, resource use, and quality of care of patients undergoing major surgery. *Arch Intern Med* 2007; 167: 2338–44.

By contrast, a structured medical preoperative evaluation in a preoperative evaluation clinic (run either by an anesthesiologist or a hospitalist) may benefit medically complex patients and improve perioperative processes and outcomes.

A preoperative evaluation by a physician not specifically trained in perioperative medicine has been associated with an increased length of stay and increased postoperative mortality; whereas a preevaluation clinic (PEC) run by hospitalists was associated with lower mortality rates at one institution, and attendance at an anesthesiologist-run PEC at another was independently associated with a lower incidence of postoperative mortality in patients undergoing elective surgery. The difference in results among the studies on preoperative assessments by internists, and those of anesthesiologist or hospitalist-directed assessments in a PEC may be due to the perioperativist's ability to improve coordination of care along the entire perioperative continuum, as well as the anesthesiologist's in-depth knowledge of the proposed surgery and anesthetic plans.

- S. Vazirani, A. Lankarani-Fard, L. Liang et al. Perioperative processes and outcomes after implementation of a hospitalist-run preoperative clinic. *J Hosp Med* 2012; 7 (9): 697–701.
- J. D. Blitz, S. M. Kendale, S. K. Jain et al. Preoperative evaluation clinic visit is associated with decreased risk of in-hospital postoperative mortality. *Anesthesiology* 2016 Aug; 125(2): 280–94.

Chapter

7

Teaching in the Operating Room

Edwin A. Bowe

Background

Because residents in anesthesiology spend the preponderance of the time during their training working in the operating room (OR), and because most practicing anesthesiologists spend the vast majority of their time administering or supervising the administration of anesthesia in the OR, it should be evident that this is arguably the most important setting in which clinical teaching is performed. This venue allows (demands) teaching not only of facts (e.g., the proper procedure for checking out an anesthesia machine), but also judgment/clinical reasoning (e.g., "What is the most likely cause of the patient's hypotension and what are the priorities for treating it?"). See Chapter 3 for information on teaching clinical reasoning. The significance of teaching in the OR notwithstanding, there are competing interests for both the learner (e.g., administering the anesthetic, observing the progress of surgery) and the attending anesthesiologist (e.g., providing a safe anesthetic experience, meeting production pressure expectations). This chapter will explore ways to provide an educational experience to the resident in the OR setting.

In his book *Outliers*, Malcolm Gladwell popularized the concept that 10,000 hours of practice are necessary to become a master in most fields. This concept was derived from results of studies on violin students performed by Krampe, Tesch-Romer, and Ericsson in which they determined that the major difference between students who were categorized as "good," "better," or "best" was the number of hours they had spent in practice. As Ericsson points out in his book *Peak*, Gladwell applied the results inappropriately. First, despite having spent an average of 10,000 hours practicing, the "best" students were not yet masters of the violin. Second, the 10,000 hours were an average, so some of the "best" students had spent more than 10,000 hours while others had spent less. Third, the amount of time is not consistent across all fields.

Fourth, the violin students were not simply practicing, but were involved in "deliberate practice" (Box 7.1), which involves individualized training targeting a specific objective.

In 1989 the American Board of Anesthesiology (ABA) increased the duration of residency training from three years ("internship" plus two years) to four years ("internship" plus three years).[1] One of the rationales advanced for the increased duration of training was to be able to increase the number of months spent in critical care medicine (CCM) without diluting the amount of time residents spent in the OR. It was also argued that as the specialty became more complex, more time was needed in the OR and the expanded duration of training permitted that as well. Fast forward to 2017. At this point the ABA mandates more than ten months of training outside the OR setting (two weeks in Preoperative Evaluation Clinic, two weeks in the Postanesthesia Care Unit [PACU], two weeks of Non-OR Anesthesia, four months of CCM, two months Obstetric Anesthesia, three months Pain), of which three months (one month Pain, two months CCM) may be performed in the clinical base year. Based on 36 months of clinical anesthesia training, this leaves a maximum of 29 months of conventional OR anesthesia experience. Assuming an average of 60 hours/week in clinical care (a number that is almost certainly greater than average because data provided by residents include time spent in preoperative assessment of patients, time in lectures, etc.), this leaves less than 7,000 hours

---

Box 7.1 Characteristics of deliberate practice

1. Designed to achieve specific goals;
2. Full attention devoted to practice;
3. Includes assessment of performance – are goals being met, what can be done to improve;
4. Constantly challenged by expanding goals.

of clinical experience in the OR. (This number is further reduced if a program provides training beyond the minimum required for rotations outside of the OR, e.g., PACU, and by any elective time a resident spends on other rotations, e.g., an elective on transesophageal echocardiography.) Stated another way, the maximum amount of time an anesthesia resident spends in the OR is approximately the same amount of time the average "good" violin student spent practicing. Given these constraints, it is imperative that the time residents spend working in the OR provides the maximal educational benefit.

Goals

Working in coordination, the ABA and the Accreditation Council for Graduate Medical Education (ACGME) have defined a framework of milestones to be used in resident evaluations (Box 7.2).[2]

Of these, the OR is uniquely suited for teaching Anesthetic Plan and Conduct (Figure 7.1) and Management of Peri-anesthetic Complications (Figure 7.2).

It can also be reasonably argued that the OR is the best venue for instructing the resident in elements of the Crisis Management milestone (Figure 7.3).

These three milestones could be combined into a single statement of goals for OR rotations that might be phrased as, "At the end of the OR rotations, the successful resident will be able to formulate a plan and provide an anesthetic for complex patients or procedures as well as to identify and manage complications, including those resulting in a crisis." Teaching during an OR rotation should be directed toward achieving this objective. Other milestones that are best taught in the OR (e.g., Technical Skills: Airway Management) are the subjects of other specific chapters in this book.

Box 7.2 The Anesthesiology Milestone Project

Patient Care 1: Preanesthetic patient evaluation, assessment, and preparation.
Patient Care 2: Anesthetic plan and conduct.
Patient Care 3: Peri-procedural pain management.
Patient Care 4: Management of peri-anesthetic complications.
Patient Care 5: Crisis management.
Patient Care 6: Triage and management of the critically ill patient in a nonoperative setting.
Patient Care 7: Acute, chronic, and cancer-related pain consultation and management.
Patient Care 8: Technical skill: airway management.
Patient Care 9: Technical skills: use and interpretation of monitoring and equipment.
Patient Care 10: Technical skills: regional anesthesia.
Medical Knowledge 1: Knowledge of biomedical, clinical, epidemiological, and social-behavioral sciences as outlined in the American Board of Anesthesiology Content Outline.
Systems-based Practice 1: Coordination of patient care within the healthcare system.
Systems-based Practice 2: Patient safety and quality improvement.
Practice-based Learning and Improvement 1: Incorporation of quality improvement and patient safety initiatives into personal practice.
Practice-based Learning and Improvement 2: Analysis of practice to identify areas in need of improvement.
Practice-based Learning and Improvement 3: Self-directed learning.
Practice-based Learning and Improvement 4: Education of patient, families, students, residents, and other health professionals.
Professionalism 1: Responsibility to patients, families, and society.
Professionalism 2: Honesty, integrity, and ethical behavior.
Professionalism 3: Commitment to institution, department, and colleagues.
Professionalism 4: Receiving and giving feedback.
Professionalism 5: Responsibility to maintain personal, emotional, physical, and mental health.
Interpersonal and Communication Skills 1: Communication with patients and families.
Interpersonal and Communication Skills 2: Communication with other professionals.
Interpersonal and Communication Skills 3: Team and leadership skills.

Has not Achieved Level 1	Level 1	Level 2	Level 3	Level 4	Level 5
	Formulates patient care plans that include consideration of underlying clinical conditions, past medical history, and patient, medical, or surgical risk factors Adapts to new settings for delivery of patient care	Formulates anesthetic plans for patients undergoing routine procedures that include consideration of underlying clinical conditions, past medical history, patient, anesthetic, and surgical risk factors, and patient choice Conducts routine anesthetics, including management of commonly encountered physiologic alterations associated with anesthetic care, with indirect supervision Adapts to new settings for delivery of anesthetic care	Formulates anesthetic plans for patients undergoing common subspecialty procedures that include consideration of medical, anesthetic, and surgical risk factors, and that take into consideration a patient's anesthetic preference Conducts subspecialty anesthetics with indirect supervision, but may require direct supervision for more complex procedures and patients	Formulates and tailors anesthetic plans that include consideration of medical, anesthetic, and surgical risk factors and patient preference for patients with complex medical issues undergoing complex procedures with conditional independence Conducts complex anesthetics with conditional independence; may supervise others in the management of complex clinical problems	Independently formulates anesthetic plans that include consideration of medical, anesthetic, and surgical risk factors, as well as patient preference, for complex patients and procedures Conducts complex anesthetic management independently

Figure 7.1 Milestone Patient Care 2. Anesthetic Plan and Conduct. (From the ABA/ACGME "The Anesthesiology Milestone Project.")

Has not Achieved Level 1	Level 1	Level 2	Level 3	Level 4	Level 5
	Performs patient assessments and identifies complications associated with patient care; begins initial management of complications with direct supervision	Performs post-anesthetic assessment to identify complications of anesthetic care; begins initial management of peri-anesthetic complications with direct supervision	Identifies and manages peri-anesthetic complications unique to subspecialty or medically complex patients, and requests appropriate consultations with indirect supervision	Identifies and manages all peri-anesthetic complications with conditional independence	Independently identifies and manages all peri-anesthetic complications

Figure 7.2 Milestone Patient Care 4. Management of Peri-anesthetic Complications. (From the ABA/ACGME "The Anesthesiology Milestone Project.")

Has not Achieved Level 1	Level 1	Level 2	Level 3	Level 4	Level 5
	Recognizes acutely ill or medically deteriorating patients; initiates basic medical care for common acute events; calls for help appropriately	Constructs prioritized differential diagnoses that include the most likely etiologies for acute clinical deterioration; initiates treatment with indirect supervision and seeks direct supervision appropriately	Identifies and manages clinical crises with indirect supervision; may require direct supervision in complex situations	Identifies and manages clinical crises appropriately with conditional independence; assumes increasing responsibility for leadership of crisis response team	Coordinates crisis team response

Figure 7.3 Milestone Patient Care 5. Crisis Management. (From the ABA/ACGME "The Anesthesiology Milestone Project.")

The Operating Room Educational Experience

The educational experience in the OR on any particular day can be seen as being influenced by four different elements.

Assignments

The quality of the resident's educational experience is determined to some degree by case assignment. Multiple factors (e.g., surgical procedure, patient comorbidity, monitoring requirements, experience of the faculty member) have an impact on determining which cases should be assigned to which resident and faculty member combination to maximize the resident's educational experience (Box 7.3).

Ideally each resident should be assigned to cases based on the educational needs and experience of that individual. To accomplish that objective the individual making assignments must have specific knowledge of each resident's status in the program (e.g., the rotations each resident has completed) as well as the resident's prior experiences (e.g., the number of anesthetics provided to patients undergoing cardiac surgery). The former can be provided through access to each resident's rotation schedule. The latter can be addressed by providing the individual(s) making assignments with a regularly updated report of each resident's case log data including how each individual is progressing to achieving the targets of case/procedure numbers established by the ABA.

Effectively making assignments is the first step in determining the learning goals for the resident the following day. Presumably these goals are understood by the faculty member based on the assignment, but especially with a junior faculty member, consideration should be given to having a mentor or the faculty member who makes the assignments briefly discuss learning opportunities provided by the specific cases or patients.

Preoperative Teaching

Teaching in the OR begins with communication between the resident and the faculty member the day before they are assigned to work together. Conventionally the preoperative conversation is used to discuss the patients and procedures for the following day. This permits the resident to develop and describe an anesthetic plan for each case. The faculty member can ask why a specific technique was selected and the resident's perception of the advantages of this technique over others. In essence, this is analogous to the ABA's Standardized Oral Examination part of the Applied Examination (previously known as the Part Two exam or "oral boards") in which the candidates are expected to explain what they are going to do and why. The faculty member can conduct this session in a similar manner by asking how the anesthetic plan would change if certain conditions changed (e.g., "What would you do differently if a preoperative transthoracic echocardiogram revealed that

---

Box 7.3 Some educational factors to consider when making OR assignments

- **Surgical procedure:** Does the procedure offer a unique educational experience (e.g., the learner's first carotid endarterectomy)? Is the procedure a common surgical procedure with which the learner requires more experience (e.g., tonsillectomy and adenoidectomy)?

- **Anesthetic techniques:** Does the procedure use an anesthetic technique with which the resident requires more experience (e.g., mask induction of anesthesia on a child)?

- **Monitoring techniques**: Does the procedure offer the opportunity for a monitoring technique that would be educationally beneficial (e.g., motor-evoked potentials)?

- **Patient comorbidities**: Even if the procedure is mundane, does the patient have a comorbidity that would provide an educational opportunity (e.g., a patient with a left ventricular assist device for a colonoscopy)?

- **Experience of the resident**: How experienced is the resident? (While a laparoscopic appendectomy on a healthy 30-year-old patient may not be as interesting for a third-year resident, it offers an educational experience for a resident in the first or second month of training. If the same procedure is being performed on a woman who is 23 weeks pregnant, the case is probably not appropriate for a beginning resident but does present an excellent educational opportunity for a more experienced resident.)

- **Experience of the faculty member**: Research in other areas has shown that there is an educational benefit to having an educator who recently completed the experience the learner is about to undergo. For that reason, there may be an educational benefit to assigning a new faculty member to work with new residents.

- **Expertise of the faculty member**: Especially if the surgical procedure is complex or if the patient has a serious comorbidity, the educational benefit will likely be increased if a faculty member with specific expertise in the relevant area is assigned to work with the resident (e.g., the educational benefit will probably be increased if a cardiac anesthesiologist, as opposed to an anesthesiologist with expertise in regional anesthesia, supervises a resident anesthetizing a patient with a left ventricular assist device undergoing a colonoscopy).

the patient's heart murmur was due to aortic stenosis instead of being a flow murmur?").

The preoperative discussion also provides an opportunity to determine subjects to be discussed the following day. This establishes the learning goals in the minds of both the faculty member and the resident. If the surgical procedure is something the resident has never done before (e.g., the resident's first carotid endarterectomy) or if the patient has a specific comorbidity (e.g., aortic stenosis), presumably the resident will be told to study those subjects. In this situation, it may be helpful if the faculty member can recommend a specific reference for review. If neither the surgical procedure nor the specific patient seem to offer a fertile topic for discussion, the resident can be instructed to review material not unique to the procedure or the patient. Examples might include the pharmacology of a drug or a class of drugs (e.g., neuromuscular blocking drugs), a monitoring modality (e.g., flow-volume loops and pressure-volume loops available on the anesthesia workstation), or material from the literature (e.g., a recent review article or particularly important article).

The emphasis on OR efficiency creates a situation in which a team of anesthesia providers may not be caring for the patients assigned to them on the prior day. Alternatively, the anesthesia team may be disrupted with the resident and faculty member being split and one reassigned to another room. Even if that occurs and the resident is not doing the case previously assigned or does follow the patient but is no longer working with the attending anesthesiologist assigned the previous day, the resident should have benefitted from the preoperative discussion and the assigned reading.

Intraoperative Anesthetic Management

Intraoperative teaching provides opportunities to instruct the resident not only on the planned events associated with the procedure, but also those situations that are unanticipated. Current theories on excellence in performance for virtually any area, from athletics to medicine, emphasize the importance of developing a "mental model" of the anticipated act. By allowing the resident to anticipate what should occur next, it not only serves as a map for the procedure, it also allows rapid recognition when something aberrant occurs. Arguably the most important element of OR teaching is to facilitate the development of this mental

model by the resident. In its most elementary form, this consists of the routine steps performed prior to induction of general anesthesia (Box 7.4).

Despite the fact that constructing this mental model may seem to be one of the easiest aspects of anesthesia education for a resident, it may be difficult for a new resident if there is variability of sequencing from one attending anesthesiologist to the next. One anesthesiologist may have a specific sequence for applying the monitors (e.g., pulse oximeter first, blood pressure cuff second, electrocardiogram [ECG] last) while another may have a different sequence. The lack of consistency may cause new residents to struggle in developing their own mental model. Observing the resident's performance provides an opportunity to inquire about the reasons why the monitors were applied in a specific sequence. ("I noticed the order in which you applied the monitors. Is there a reason you applied them in that order?") In this circumstance, it may be helpful to explain the rationale for your preferred sequence, for example, "For healthy patients I attach the pulse oximeter first so I can get a measurement with the patient breathing room air; once that value is obtained I begin denitrogenation. I attach the blood pressure cuff second because it takes a finite amount of time for the cuff to cycle and during that time I am applying the ECG leads while denitrogenation is continuing. This sequence is subject to change; if, for example, the patient is hypotensive I will apply

> **Box 7.4 Steps prior to induction of general anesthesia**
>
> - Introduce yourself to the patient.
> - Verify patient identity (name, date of birth, medical record number).
> - Determine the patient's fasting status.
> - Confirm the scheduled procedure with the patient.
> - Review and confirm the preoperative evaluation. Answer the patient's questions.
> - Transport patient to OR.
> - Assist patient's move from stretcher to OR table.
> - Verify appropriate positioning on the table, including application of a restraint.
> - Place monitors and check vital signs.
> - Perform denitrogenation.
> - Perform "time out."

the blood pressure cuff first." While this may seem tedious, it's an important process for residents during the first-month rotation in the OR. The conversation as outlined in the preceding text not only provides the resident with an order of steps, it also gives a rationale for that sequence. Further, consistent with the development of a mental model, it acknowledges that different circumstances may necessitate different responses. Similar instruction, with explanation, can be provided for all phases of the anesthetic from the administration of drugs for induction of general anesthesia to the report ("handoff") given by the resident to the nurses in the PACU.

Instruction involving facts may also be a part of intraoperative teaching (e.g., when an arterial blood gas is obtained, have the resident calculate the arterial oxygen content). That material, however, can be taught in a classroom. Working in the OR allows the resident to put the factual information in a clinical context (e.g., when obtaining an arterial blood gas on a patient with anemia, ask the resident to calculate the cardiac output necessary to maintain a normal oxygen delivery and then ask the resident if it's reasonable to expect the patient to generate that cardiac output).

Teaching can also involve abnormal events, even if they did not occur. For example, "What would you have done if, after you administered propofol but before you administered a neuromuscular blocking drug, you had been unable to ventilate the patient by face mask?" For residents doing their first month in the OR this leads to instruction on simple techniques such tightening down the pressure relief valve, repositioning the patient's jaw, or placing an airway. For more advanced residents this can result in a discussion of the difficult airway algorithm. The complexity of the questions and the depth of the discussion obviously need to be adjusted based on the experience of the resident. The questions can be changed to: "If the patient had become hypotensive following propofol administration for induction, what would you have done? What is the most likely etiology of the hypotension? Which patients are at greatest risk for hypotension following propofol administration? What alternatives to propofol are available? How would you decide which of them to use?" The questions do not necessarily need to have a universally accepted "right" answer. In fact, the scenario may place the resident in a situation that has no single best answer, thereby forcing consideration of multiple alternatives and to weigh the risk of an adverse outcome with the

probability of that outcome. For senior-level residents the intent is to get them to consider alternatives and to explore the consequences of their decisions.

Avoiding duplication of effort improves efficiency as a clinical teacher. A faculty member can utilize existing resources that present material in a way consistent with the brief segments of time commonly available when working with residents in the OR. There are a multitude of books that provide material for questions and answers. *Clinical Cases in Anesthesia* is presented in a question/discussion format similar to how intraoperative teaching may occur. (Example: The chapter on aortic stenosis asks and answers questions regarding the symptoms, long-term prognosis, and etiology of aortic stenosis; methods of calculation and the significance of aortic valve area; the significance of dysrhythmias, and the best method for treatment of hypotension in a patient with aortic stenosis.) *Crisis Management in Anesthesiology* presents select scenarios (e.g., anaphylaxis) and describes in outline form the definition and etiology, presents the manifestations, provides a list of situations that may have a similar presentation, outlines appropriate therapy, and lists complications that may occur as a result of the problem. *Evidence-Based Practice of Anesthesiology* describes the evidence surrounding certain situations (e.g., ideal preoperative hemoglobin concentrations). *Faust's Anesthesiology Review* provides a brief discussion of select issues (e.g., interpretation of the arterial pressure waveform). *Essence of Anesthesia Practice* provides a one-page synopsis of multiple drugs (e.g., atropine), disease states (e.g., amyotrophic lateral sclerosis), and surgical procedures (e.g., laparoscopic cholecystectomy); although convenient because each subject is covered in a single page, the quality of the content varies widely and in many circumstances the treatment of the subject is extremely superficial. Each of these books presents a succinct, organized discussion of well-defined topics that lend themselves well to use in the One Minute Preceptor format (described in more detail in Chapter 3). *Anesthesia and Uncommon Diseases* provides a discussion of diseases arranged by organ system; while each chapter is lengthy, each is also divided into sections (e.g., the chapter on neuromuscular disease has two or three pages devoted to myotonias) that can provide the basis for a brief discussion in the OR. Using a question-and-answer format, *Yao and Artusio's Anesthesiology: Problem-Oriented Patient Management* provides a more comprehensive discussion of various conditions or procedures organized by organ system (e.g., the section on the respiratory system has four chapters, one each on asthma and chronic obstructive pulmonary disease; bronchoscopy, mediastinoscopy, and thoracotomy; aspiration pneumonitis and acute respiratory failure; and lung transplantation) with some chapters in other areas (e.g., pediatric anesthesia); the advantage is that it is more comprehensive but the disadvantage is that the scope of material covered is somewhat limited.

Postoperative Care

For residents who provided the patient's anesthetic in the OR, the postoperative period is generally the time to provide feedback, the topic of Chapter 20.

For residents on a PACU rotation, the postoperative period consists of several different elements, ranging from determining when a patient is ready for discharge home following ambulatory surgery to management of critically ill patients in an intensive care setting. (The latter is covered in Chapter 8.) Although the content is different, the teaching techniques are essentially the same as those employed in the OR. Because anesthesia-related complications are uncommon, most residents will not have experience with the majority of the complications. While factual information can be acquired in the usual manner, simulation with role playing may be the best way to provide educational experience for this subject matter. (Example: Explaining the management and natural course of a corneal abrasion to someone playing the role of a patient or family member.) One fundamental difference is that because a resident working in the PACU is not involved in the continuous monitoring of a patient undergoing an anesthetic, there are fewer concerns about distractions and production pressure. This provides an opportunity to present information in different ways, for example, podcasts/videocasts or other electronic formats. Information on these methods is covered later in this chapter as well as in Chapter 16.

Teaching as a Distraction

Vigilance by the anesthesia provider is obviously one of the keys to a safe anesthetic.[3] One concern is whether teaching in the OR has an adverse effect on vigilance. A study by Weinger et al.[4] measured the response latency to a 1 cm red alarm light located in proximity to a monitor display presenting physiologic parameters. The red light was turned on at random intervals and response latency was determined based on the interval from the time the red light was turned on until a predetermined response from the person performing the anesthetic was recorded. The authors report that response latency was statistically significantly increased in twelve teaching cases versus twelve nonteaching cases throughout the duration of the procedure, but do not provide aggregated data. When looking at five different epochs during the case, response latency was increased only during induction of anesthesia (97 ± 19 vs. 44 ± 12 seconds) and emergence from anesthesia (75 ± 20 vs. 20 ± 2 seconds). Based on the heart rate of the providers, the response latency, and ratings by both the provider and an independent observer, the intervals of induction and emergence were also noted to be the times of greatest workload. The study did not show any difference in response latency in teaching versus nonteaching cases during the maintenance phase (i.e., times of lower workload) of the anesthetic. Further, in the situations studied, the person performing the anesthetic (and the one whose response latency was measured) was the teacher. The situation of the study did not replicate the more common situation in which the learner, not the teacher, is performing the anesthetic. Accordingly, the data suggest that the impact of teaching on vigilance is minimized during periods of decreased workload, that is, during the maintenance phase of an uncomplicated anesthetic. The implication is that the maintenance phase is the ideal time for teaching.

An Anesthesia Patient Safety Foundation (APSF) workshop in 2016 addressed the issue of distractions in the OR. Using an anonymous audience response system, participants in the conference overwhelmingly (95 percent) recognized that distractions in the anesthesia work environment may jeopardize patient safety. (Interestingly the electronic medical record and the electronic anesthesia record were identified as constituting some of the distractions.) The majority (65 percent) of participants did not favor prohibitions on the nonclinical use of personal electronic devices or reading in the OR; 86 percent of participants believed that a zero-tolerance policy regarding the use of personal electronic devices or reading in the OR was too restrictive. In general, clinical use of personal electronic devices and reading were described as acceptable. Because teaching activities involve clinically relevant material, presumably these activities would be viewed as acceptable, that is, not compromising patient safety or the quality of patient care. The attendees were not asked to address the form that teaching would take.[3]

Delivery of Material

Box 7.5 presents some examples of teaching methods that could be used in the OR.

Question-and-answer sessions: Probably the way most of us were taught in the OR during our training, this consists of the educator asking a series of questions and then probing the learner for deeper comprehension of the subject matter.

Advantage:
- Allows the teacher to customize the experience for each individual learner.

Disadvantage:
- Requires the physical presence of the faculty member in the room during all learning.

Article review: As described earlier in this chapter, the preoperative phone call provides an opportunity to assign an article for review. The expectation would be that the resident would read the article in advance and the article can be discussed during the day. On

occasion, however, things do not go according to plan and different cases may be added to the room. In those circumstances, it may be appropriate to provide an article for the resident to review during the anesthetic.

Advantages:
- The resident should be learning even in the absence of the faculty member.
- The interaction between the resident and faculty member should be occurring at a higher level, that is, analogous to the "flipped classroom."
- The resident has something tangible relating to the teaching that occurred.

Disadvantage:
- There may be a greater potential for the resident to be distracted if reading the article during the anesthetic.

Question-and-answer handout: A sheet of questions can be given to the resident. The questions could be short answer or multiple choice. Several sources exist for multiple-choice questions. Some textbooks provide questions and answers but the quality of the answers in certain textbooks has been suspect. The American Society of Anesthesiologists also produces Anesthesiology Continuing Education and Self-Education and Evaluation programs annually consisting of 200 items, each of which consists of a question, the answer, a discussion, and references. (Care must be taken to avoid violation of copyright law in using items from other sources.) The resident would be expected to complete the answers to the questions while the faculty member was out of the room. This permits the resident to participate in the educational activity at times of diminished workload. When the faculty member returns, the resident's answers can be discussed. The same thing can be done electronically (e.g., e-mail a copy of the question sheet to the resident and have the resident complete the form and return it electronically).

Advantages:
- Some learning could be occurring while the attending was out of the room.
- The discussion between the resident and the faculty member tends to occur on a higher level.
- The resident has something tangible relating to the learning that occurred that day. (If the electronic approach is used, this can be easily stored by the resident.)

Box 7.5 Presentation of teaching material

Different ways to present teaching material to a resident anesthetizing a patient undergoing resection of a carcinoid tumor.

- Question-and-answer session. (Example: Ask a series of questions regarding carcinoid syndrome.)
- Article review. (Example: Give the resident an article on the anesthetic implications of carcinoid syndrome and return later for a discussion.)
- Question-and-answer handout. (Example: Give the resident a handout containing a series of questions similar to those that would be presented verbally in the first example.)
- Video. (Example: Have the resident watch a videocast on the anesthetic management of patients with carcinoid syndrome.)
- E-learning experience. (Example: Develop an interactive program that guides the resident through content related to anesthetic management of patients with carcinoid syndrome.)

Disadvantages:

- Questions are scripted in advance and are not individualized to the resident.
- It is possible that the resident will use online resources to answer the questions, in which case the information will not reflect the resident's knowledge but learning will still be occurring.
- There is a potential for the resident to be distracted by answering the questions, by looking up answers online, or both.

Videocasts: The resident can be provided access to a videocast and then asked questions based on the content (i.e., analogous to the "flipped classroom" in didactic presentations). Adding an audio element (i.e., a videocast with a narrative as opposed to a simple series of slides with all the content appearing on the slides) seems to be a bad idea. The audio would likely interfere with other conversations in the OR as well as any audible alarms. Conversely, the audio may be difficult to hear due to noise or ongoing conversations.

Advantages:

- Some learning could be occurring while the attending was out of the room.
- The discussion between the resident and the attending would be expected to occur at a higher level.

Disadvantages:

- The use of a videocast by the resident may be perceived by OR staff as being less likely to be associated with patient care and learning.
- Once a video is started it may be less likely to be paused than to put down a piece of paper or stop entering answers on a computer or tablet, thereby making a video more distracting.
- Audio in the video is more likely to be distracting to the resident and to others in the room.
- Creating a video is relatively labor intensive.

Interactive e-learning experience: There are several authoring programs that allow creation of an e-learning experience. The most sophisticated of these programs allow the creator to produce a branched experience in which each user has a unique experience and is directed through the interaction based on answers to questions (see Chapter 16). This is as close to the 1:1 faculty teaching experience as can be delivered without requiring physical attendance of the faculty member during the teaching session. An e-learning experience typically presents some material to the learner who then must answer a question. Envision a circumstance in which the e-learning experience presents a patient with carcinoid syndrome who develops intraoperative hypotension. The resident is then asked to select from several drug choices for the treatment of the hypotension. If the resident selects an agent with beta-adrenergic effects, the resident is taken to another screen that describes the reported association between the administration of beta agonists and worsening hypotension caused by increased release of vasoactive substances from the tumor. The resident can then be returned either to the original question or a different question from which agents with significant beta agonist effects have been removed. This process is repeated until the resident answers the question correctly, at which point a more detailed discussion of the management of hypotension in a patient with a carcinoid tumor is presented. In 2017 the Adobe's Captivate program is probably the most robust program for authoring e-learning projects. The ability to create complex branching projects with detailed reporting occurs at the cost of significant complexity (which requires a substantial time investment on the part of the faculty member to learn the program or a substantial departmental cost to hire someone to do the authoring). In addition, the program is expensive. (Some universities have an arrangement with Adobe allowing use of Captivate by faculty members, so the acquisition cost may not be a consideration.) At the other end of the spectrum is Google's suite of programs, Google for Education, which also allows authoring e-learning projects. Google's programs are easier to learn, but have limitations compared to Captivate. Access to Google's programs is currently free for those institutions that have signed up for Google's "G Suite for Education" program. Once the resident completes the e-learning project, the faculty member can be notified electronically. The initial responses of the resident can be used as the basis for an individualized discussion and an evaluation to assure comprehension of the material by the resident.

Advantages:

- Some learning could be occurring while the attending was out of the room.
- The script is adjusted for the performance of the resident, permitting individualized learning.
- Subsequent discussion between the resident and the faculty member tends to occur on a higher level.

Disadvantages:

- Creation of the content is time consuming.
- The resident may use online resources to answer the questions, so the responses may not reflect the resident's knowledge.
- The e-learning project may distract the resident from patient care.

Suggestions for New Faculty Members

Few residents receive instruction in how to teach during their training (see Chapter 21). Upon completion of training it seems that most programs assume that if residents can do a case, they can teach other residents to do the same case. While it may well be accurate that the new graduate can direct someone on how to perform the anesthetic, that does not guarantee the person will be an effective teacher. But, as noted in the preceding text, work in other areas has demonstrated that teaching/learning is enhanced if the teacher has recently completed the training the learner is currently undergoing. While new faculty members are adapting to the role of teacher, they are also preparing for the ABA Applied Examination. This makes it even more important that they are efficient in their teaching. Following are some suggestions that may be helpful for the first few years as a faculty member:

1. Develop certain areas of instruction that can be used in almost any circumstance. Examples would include discussions of the pharmacology of commonly used anesthetic agents (e.g., fentanyl, midazolam), monitoring techniques (e.g., nerve stimulator, capnography), physiology (oxygen consumption/oxygen delivery, assessment of renal function), or the anesthesia machine (e.g., vaporizer function, circuits, and valves).

2. Use relevant articles from the recent anesthesia literature. A review article may be discussed in terms of the applicability to practice. In addition to applicability to practice, an original research article may also be discussed in terms of an assessment of methodology (e.g., were the exclusion criteria too stringent, was the research methodology appropriate, how many patients were lost to follow-up, is the statistical analysis appropriate). This not only instructs the resident in the specific field in which the research was

conducted, but also initiates a discussion of appropriate research methods (see Chapter 23).

Even an attending anesthesiologist with a full-time clinical appointment is unlikely to work in the OR more than 228 days in a year. If a residency training program has a total of twelve residents/year, and if the new attending anesthesiologist worked only with first-year residents and worked with each of them an equal number of days during the year, the attending anesthesiologist would work with each first-year residents approximately 19 times during the year. (Obviously the frequency is reduced if the number of residents in the program is increased or if the faculty member worked with more than just first-year residents.) Effectively that means that the attending anesthesiologist needs to have material prepared for only 19 different days. If the new faculty member selects one article from the literature each month, by the end of the first year that will provide twelve of the 19 subjects necessary to have a different topic for each resident every day. Adding just one article/month over several years will result in a substantial repository of material that can be used for intraoperative teaching.

There is value associated with keeping track of what material is covered with each individual resident. Presumably most faculty members have a body of material they want to cover with every resident. At the same time, there is a desire to avoid going over the same material with a resident twice. Keeping some form of "log" to track material that has been presented facilitates both of these processes. A table (Figure 7.4) with the name of each resident and the title of each section of content allows the faculty member to be certain that the topic of discussion is not being duplicated and to select uncovered material that is most relevant for the upcoming patients/cases.

While the tracking function can be accomplished by use of a spreadsheet, there are multiple applications that include a notebook function that permits inclusion of not only the table, but also the educational material. This facilitates electronic distribution of the material to the residents while making it easy to add or delete material.

As the potential for creating robust electronic notebooks has increased it's now possible to have a separate section for each resident or for each section of content (Figure 7.5). Handouts, copies of articles, or quizzes can be created once and distributed to a resident for discussion.

Another alternative is to use file sharing/storage/collaboration software such as Dropbox. With this technique the faculty member can store all relevant material (handouts, quizzes, articles) in a primary folder and create separate folders for each resident. Residents are given access to their folders and material can be copied from the primary folder to the folder for each resident as appropriate.

Summary

OR rotations are arguably the most important part of residency training because most residents will spend the majority of their time in the OR after completing training. The ABA/ACGME Milestone project outlines goals related to intraoperative learning. Adherence to elements of "deliberate practice" (specific goals, assessment of performance with feedback that emphasizes areas for improvement, constantly challenging the learner) should increase the efficacy of intraoperative education. The OR educational experience begins when assignments are made; those assignments determine what the resident should learn the next day. The preoperative call from the resident to the attending should not be used solely to discuss the anesthetic management of patients the following day, but should be used to establish teaching/learning goals. Materials provided at this time can make the educational experience more effective the following day. Teaching in the OR can take many forms, from 1:1 question-and-answer sessions to handouts with questions, to e-learning activities. Methods that allow learning to occur without requiring the presence of the attending anesthesiologist may be most efficient. Multiple sources can provide the basis for mini-lectures in the OR; others provide questions that can be used for resident education. Developing a "portfolio," and tracking the educational experiences provided to each resident can minimize duplication of effort and make certain that all the necessary information is covered.

References

1. J. E. Havidich, G. R. Haynes, J. G. Reves. The effect of lengthening anesthesiology residency on subspecialty education. *Anesth Analg* 2004; 99: 844–56.

2. Accreditation Council for Graduate Medical Education and the American Board of Anesthesiology. The Anesthesiology Milestone Project. 2015.

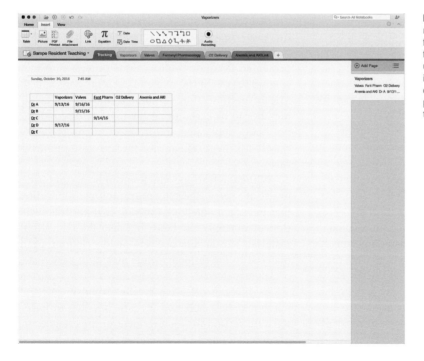

Figure 7.4 Sample Microsoft OneNote notebook showing tracking of material for each resident. Note that each subject for discussion has its own tab. Content used for teaching each subject may be inserted in the relevant tab to facilitate distribution to the resident during preoperative discussion the night before the case or during the day.

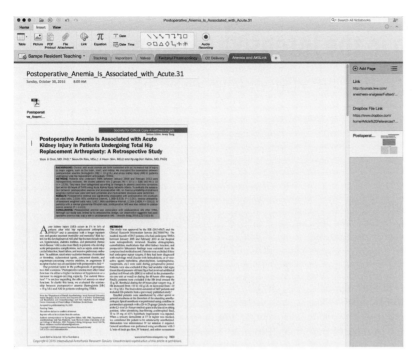

Figure 7.5 Sample OneNote notebook showing article for distribution/review.

www.acgme.org/Portals/0/PDFs/Milestones/
AnesthesiologyMilestones.pdf. (accessed November
18, 2017).

3. B. J. Thomas. Distractions in the operating room: An
anesthesia professional's liability? *APSF Newsletter*
2017; 31: 59–61.

4. M. B. Weinger, S. B. Reddy, J. M. Slagle. Multiple
measures of anesthesia workload during teaching and
nonteaching cases. *Anesth Analg* 2004; 98: 1419–25.

Chapter

8

Teaching in the Intensive Care Unit
Creating an Effective Educational Experience

Gary R. Stier

Introduction

Teaching within the intensive care unit (ICU) environment is challenging, both for the learner and the teacher. The dynamics of patient care, expanding clinical workloads, documentation requirements, frequent interruptions, and the depth of knowledge required in caring for critically ill patients present serious obstacles to effective education. Moreover, instructors may lack sufficient knowledge of how best to deliver a quality teaching experience to achieve the desired outcomes. Education within the ICU environment is most successful when appropriate content is included within a well-designed curriculum that integrates relevant teaching theory with educational methods that engage the learner, creating enthusiasm and motivation for learning. Effective role modeling, feedback, and teacher self-reflection complete the necessary components of a successful learning experience (Figure 8.1). This discussion will review the relevant educational methods and tools necessary for creating an effective and rewarding teaching experience within the ICU.

Establishing Expectations for Learning

Preparation and Learning Objectives

Teaching effectiveness begins with clearly detailed learning goals and objectives aligned to the educational level of the learner. The creation of an organized framework is necessary to guide the learner and to communicate clear expectations for the intended educational outcomes. Learning objectives should describe the specific knowledge, skills, and attitudes to be demonstrated at the conclusion of the learning experience. The inability to define educational objectives is one of the primary reasons underlying an unsuccessful learning experience. Three frameworks are particularly useful as a reference in the development of learning objectives for the ICU:

1. The Accreditation Council for Graduate Medical Education (ACGME) educational objectives for the six general competencies (www.acgme.org/Portals/0/PFAssets/ProgramRequirements/CPRs_2017-07-01.pdf; accessed November 3, 2017);
2. The Anesthesiology Milestone Project (www.acgme.org/Portals/0/PDFs/Milestones/AnesthesiologyMilestones.pdf; accessed November 3, 2017);
3. Bloom's Taxonomy of Educational Objectives.[1]

The integration of these three outlines provides an organized and detailed road map for developing meaningful educational objectives (Table 8.1).

The ACGME has identified six core competencies (or attributes) that trainees should demonstrate upon completion of residency training. The six competencies include:

- Patient care;
- Medical knowledge;
- Interpersonal and communication skills;
- Professionalism;
- Practice-based learning and improvement; and
- Systems-based practice.

Generic learning objectives have been developed for each of these six competencies; these objectives can be utilized as an excellent starting point in customizing teaching outcomes specific to the ICU. The ACGME Anesthesiology Milestone Project is an additional framework that can be applied in organizing the educational objective outcomes into developmental stages appropriate to each level of learner (i.e., Post Graduate Year 1, PGY-1; to Post Graduate Year 4, PGY-4). The Anesthesiology Milestone Project (jointly developed by the ABA and the ACGME) categories particularly applicable to the ICU experience are outlined in Table 8.1. Finally, Bloom's Taxonomy of Educational Objectives is a complementary framework for classifying educational objectives into a hierarchical

Table 8.1 Format for developing learning objectives for the ICU

1. Begin with the ACGME's six general competencies framework, as outlined in the common program requirements
2. Customize the generic goals and objectives within each general competency to reflect ICU-relevant subject matter, focusing on:
   a. American Board of Anesthesiology (ABA) content outline topics for critical care
   b. ABA In-Training Examination (ITE) keywords relevant to critical care
3. Clearly specify the goals and objectives expected for each level of learner, incorporating the ACGME Anesthesiology Milestones most relevant to the ICU, such as:
   a. Patient Care (PC)
      i. PC-5: Crisis Management
      ii. PC-6: Triage and Management of the Critically III Patient in a Nonoperative Setting
      iii. PC-8: Technical Skills: Airway Management
      iv. PC-9: Technical Skills: Use and Interpretation of Monitoring and Equipment
   b. System-Based Practice (SBP)
      i. SBP-1: Coordination of Patient Care within the Healthcare System
   c. Medical Knowledge (MK)
      i. MK-1: Knowledge of biomedical, clinical, epidemiological, and social-behavioral sciences
   d. Practiced-Based Learning and Improvement (PBL&I)
      i. PBL&I-3: Self-Directed Learning
   e. Professionalism (P)
      i. P-4: Receiving and Giving Feedback
   f. Interpersonal and Communication (IC)
      i. IC-2: Communication with Other Professionals
      ii. IC-3: Team and Leadership Skills
4. Ensure that the objectives within each of the ACGME competency categories address the cognitive, psychomotor, and affective domains, where applicable
5. Arrange the goals and objectives within each competency category to reflect increasing complexity and cognitive ability, as described in Bloom's Taxonomy.

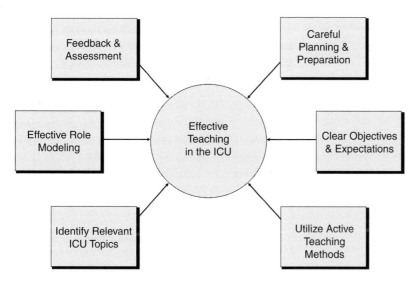

Figure 8.1 Components of effective teaching in the ICU.

structure representing different levels of learners. It is useful for further organizing, and later assessing, learning outcomes within the appropriate ACGME competency categories. Bloom's Taxonomy focuses upon educational outcomes in the context of three key domains: cognitive (knowledge), psychomotor (skills), and affective (attitudes and behaviors). The cognitive and psychomotor domains are best aligned with the ACGME *patient care and medical knowledge* core competencies; the affective domain associates best with the *interpersonal communication and professionalism* competencies. Within each of the domains, the specific objectives are arranged in order of increasing complexity, as appropriate for the different levels of learners. With respect to the cognitive (knowledge) domain, Bloom organized the educational objectives into six categories (in order):

- Knowledge;
- Comprehension;
- Application;
- Analysis;
- Synthesis; and
- Evaluation.

Each category represents incrementally higher-order thinking and is dependent upon the cognitive level that precedes it. Specifically, the learner must first possess the knowledge before it can be used to understand, apply, analyze, and then fully evaluate a particular clinical condition. In this context, the learning objectives should first identify the particular medical conditions with which the learner should be familiar during the rotation, defining the expectation that the learner must subsequently demonstrate an understanding of the disorder through actions, including timeliness of response, work up, management decisions, and in the assessment of the results. The objectives should be clearly outlined for each level of learner. For example, consider a patient with septic shock; appropriate learning objectives include:

- Ability to demonstrate an awareness of the signs and symptoms of septic shock;
- The capacity to develop a differential diagnosis of possible infectious sources;
- Evidence of an understanding of septic shock management by subsequent medical decision-making; and
- The ability to assess the response to treatment using appropriate tests.

In this example, each of these objectives is arranged to assess incrementally higher-order thinking skills, as recommended by Bloom. The PGY-1 trainee might only be expected to demonstrate the knowledge of the signs and symptoms of septic shock, while a PGY-4 trainee would be expected to demonstrate all the aforementioned objectives.

Educational objectives directed at the psycho-motor (procedural skills) domain should plainly identify, define, and outline the specific proficiencies that the learner is expected to demonstrate; explain the situations under which the skills are expected to occur; and describe the criteria for acceptable performance of the intended skills.

Learning objectives focusing on the affective domain might include statements, such as:

- Demonstrates respect for others.
- Exhibits attention to the particular topics being taught.
- Displays active participation and engagement in group discussions.
- Shows evidence of self-directed learning.
- Models effective communication skills and professionalism during interactions with team members, staff, and families.
- Prioritizes time effectively to meet the needs of the patient and care team.

Learning objectives can be distributed to the residents in advance of the rotation as a paper copy, an e-mail, or by providing a link to a departmental wiki or other online site. Ideally, the ICU rotation director meets with each resident prior to the start of the rotation to ensure that the objectives are understood.

It is essential that the expectations align with the composition of the team, level of training, and previous ICU experiences. Delineating the roles and responsibilities of each ICU member is important and should specify the expectations regarding knowledge, presentation style, technical skills, and assessment methods. Failure to achieve the desired learning outcomes is often related to:

- A lack of clear objectives and expectations;
- Focusing on recounting data and facts rather than on the development of problem-solving skills and attitudes;
- Inability to actively engage the learner in the learning process;
- Teaching that targets the incorrect level of learner; or
- A lack of personalized attention directed to the learner.

A well-designed teaching curriculum with clearly articulated objectives will avoid these pitfalls.

Teaching in the Intensive Care Unit: How to Teach

Active Teaching Methods

Once the learning objectives and expectations have been developed, attainment of the intended educational outcomes is facilitated using effective teaching methods demonstrated to maximize learner growth. A variety of teaching theories focused upon adult learning have been promoted over the years and can serve to inform the teacher. Educational theories of particular relevance include Malcolm Knowles Andragogy Learning Theory and David Kolb's Experiential Learning Cycle.[2,3] A common theme is the emphasis placed upon the importance of *active learning*, in which the learner develops new concepts and paradigms that integrate past and current experiences, that is, develops and refines illness scripts (see Chapter 3); inspires a desire to test the theories in new situations; and promotes a willingness and motivation for self-directed learning. Examples of active learning opportunities encountered in the ICU include the indications for, and performance of, an awake intubation or placement of a pulmonary artery catheter and the performance of a bedside ultrasound to investigate a patient with worsening hypoxia.

The integration of active teaching techniques more effectively enhances student engagement, requiring the learner to "process information, participate in problem-solving, and defend clinical decisions." In this context, less emphasis is placed upon the teacher as the source of knowledge, while more emphasis is directed toward student self-direction and autonomy. In essence, the teacher's role is more appropriately viewed as a facilitator of learning through the incorporation of teaching methods that stimulate the student's motivation to learn, involve the student in conversations, and identify optimal learning opportunities. The core elements of active learning focus upon student activity and commitment to the learning process, in contrast to the traditional lecture format where students passively receive information delivered by the instructor (e.g., didactic lectures, bedside teaching).

The ICU environment provides many opportunities in which active teaching methods can be utilized: clinical rounds, teaching conferences, journal club, small group discussions, and simulation learning activities. Examples of active teaching methods are outlined in Table 8.2.

The One Minute Preceptor, in particular, is a well-described and effective active teaching tool that can be utilized to engage the learner during clinical teaching rounds. The One Minute Preceptor, originally described in 1992,[4] is a five-step "microskills" model of clinical teaching around which teacher-student conversations can be built. In this method, the preceptor listens to the case presentation and avoids interruptions. When the learner finishes the presentation of history, physical examination, and data, the preceptor begins the teaching encounter using the five steps outlined in Table 8.2. Box 8.1 provides an example of a One Minute Preceptor dialogue:

As illustrated, the One Minute Preceptor is a useful technique in which to structure short clinical teaching encounters that actively engage the student in a nonthreatening environment. Moreover, this method promotes ownership of clinical problems, allows the learner and teacher to identify knowledge gaps, focuses upon learning, and has been demonstrated to improve key teaching behaviors.

Other useful active teaching techniques include the SNAPPS technique[5] and the "flipped classroom" (see Chapter 15) method (Table 8.2). The SNAPPS approach is similar to the One Minute Preceptor method, engaging the learner in an interactive discussion with the preceptor. The flipped classroom format facilitates learner-preceptor interaction and can be easily integrated into the more traditional didactic teaching conference format. This technique assigns required reading or video material for the learner to review out of class, typically the day prior to the teaching conference; on the day of the scheduled conference, the educational time is used for student-focused activities such as an interactive problem-based learning question-and-answer session. The flipped classroom format actively engages the learners and probes the learner's understanding of the topic.

Teaching in the Intensive Care Unit: What to Teach

The ICU environment provides excellent opportunities for the learner to broaden abilities in all three domains of Bloom's educational objectives: cognitive, psychomotor, and affective. Knowledge is gained through a variety of experiences:

- Clinical rounds and bedside teaching;
- Problem-centered formal teaching conference;

Table 8.2 Active teaching methods

Active Teaching Methods	Method Description	Benefits
Clinical Teaching Rounds		
One Minute Preceptor[4]	Clinical rounding teaching method is composed of 5 steps: (1) Get a commitment (i.e., What is going on?); (2) Probe for supporting evidence; (3) Teach a general principle; (4) Reinforce what is done well; (5) Give guidance about errors and omissions	Time-efficient; focuses on learning; engages the student during rounds; promotes ownership of clinical problems
SNAPPS[5] **S**ummarize **N**arrow **A**nalyze **P**robe **P**lan **S**elect	Learner-centered model consists of 6 steps: (1) **S**ummarize the history and findings (2) **N**arrow the differential (3) **A**nalyze the differential (4) **P**robe the student with questions (5) **P**lan management (6) **S**elect a case-related issue for self-directed learning. The teacher enters the discussion at step 4	Emphasizes organized communication and stimulates discussion of the differential diagnosis and management. The discussion can involve the entire group
Chart-Stimulated Recall	The learner presents an assigned patient, detailing the diagnosis and medical treatment plan	Challenges the student to defend the work up, evaluation, diagnosis, and treatment plan
Didactic Teaching Conferences		
Flipped Classroom	Assigned reading/learning activity occurs prior to formal educational activity. Subsequent discussion occurs over the assigned material	Promotes self-directed learning; focuses on higher level of cognitive skills; more time spent applying what was learned to patient care
Audience Response Systems (Clickers)	Topic-focused multiple-choice questions are presented to the learners using slide presentation format and the audience responds anonymously using the "clickers" for their answers	Promotes enthusiasm and engagement; challenges knowledge level; safe environment
Problem-Based Learning	Case presentation followed by an active discussion regarding diagnosis and management	Strengthens critical thinking skills, such as applying knowledge to a real setting, analyzing problems and developing solutions, evaluating reasoning processes or actions
Simulation Training		
Mannequins, Task Trainers, Real-Life Volunteer Models	Instructor-led teaching of procedures/clinical scenarios/team building exercises utilizing mannequins or volunteers	Opportunity to learn and practice procedural skills in a safe, protected, educational environment
Crisis Management	Simulated clinical crisis management scenarios are presented within a group setting utilizing mannequins, computer-based tools	Teaches communication skills, team leadership, and medical knowledge

- Web-based resources that include self-directed learning modules, webcasts, podcasts, and video-enhanced programs, for example,
  - Society of Critical Care Medicine Learn ICU (www.learnicu.org/; accessed November 3, 2017);
  - UpToDate (www.uptodate.com/; accessed November 3, 2017);
  - Anesoft Corporation (http://anesoft.com/; accessed November 3, 2017);
  - OpenAnesthesia (www.openanesthesia.org; accessed November 3, 2017);
  - MedEdPortal (www.mededportal.org; accessed November 3, 2017);
  - Medscape Critical Care (www.medscape.com/criticalcare; accessed November 3, 2017);

Box 8.1 Example of teaching using One Minute Preceptor

Learner: *"The patient is an 82-year-old male with a history of dementia, diabetes, and cardiovascular disease who presented to the emergency department from a skilled nursing facility with a two-day history of altered mental status, fever, and tachypnea."*

Preceptor: **Get a commitment**: *"What do you think is going on?"*

Learner: *"I think the most likely diagnosis is infection, probably pneumonia."*

Preceptor: **Probe for supporting evidence:** *"Why do you think it is pneumonia? Are there any other possibilities?"*

Learner: *"Pneumonia is likely as the patient is tachypneic and febrile. The patient could have another source of infection, such as urinary tract infection, deep venous thrombosis, pulmonary embolus, or a neurologic infection."*

Preceptor: **Teach general rules**: *"The patient has an indwelling urinary drainage catheter, so the most likely source of infection should be the urinary tract; as such, it is most appropriate to start with a urinalysis and urine culture, as well as blood cultures."*

Preceptor: **Reinforce what was right**: *"Your presentation was organized and focused on infection as the likely diagnosis of the altered mental status."*

Preceptor: **Correct mistakes and discuss next steps**: *"You should have included the presence of a chronic urinary catheter in your presentation and stated that this was a likely source of infection and altered mental status in the patient."*

- An assigned reading bibliography of high-value peer-reviewed publications; and
- Educational materials available from professional societies focused on critical care medicine, for example,
  - Society of Critical Care Medicine (www.sccm.org; accessed November 3, 2017);
  - European Society of Critical Care Medicine (www.esicm.org; accessed November 3, 2017);
  - American College of Chest Physicians (www.chestnet.org; accessed November 3, 2017);
  - Society of Critical Care Anesthesiologists (https://socca.org; accessed November 3, 2017).

In particular, the Society of Critical Care Anesthesiologists publishes an *ICU Residents Guide* (https://socca.org/residents-guide; accessed November 3, 2017), which is a concise handbook of important critical care topics encountered on the ICU rotation. Particular focus should be centered upon ICU-related topics included within the ABA Content Outline (www.theaba.org/PDFs/BASIC-Exam/Basic-and-Advanced-ContentOutline; accessed November 3, 2017) and the ABA ITE keyword list (Tables 8.3 and 8.4).

Once identified, these topics should be listed in the "Patient Care" and "Medical Knowledge" sections of the learning objectives for the rotation.

The ACGME Anesthesiology Milestones can be utilized as a reference in organizing the topics by educational level. For example, the PGY-1 resident should be expected to acquire the medical knowledge of common medical and surgical problems encountered within the ICU (Milestone Level 1), whereas the PGY-3 resident should be anticipated to demonstrate knowledge of the more complex medical and surgical disorders presenting in critically ill patients (Milestone Level 3).

The ICU provides a unique setting in which to develop psychomotor (procedural) skills. Technical proficiencies include airway management and tracheal intubation in the non-operating-room setting, placement of invasive arterial and central venous catheters, lumbar puncture, point-of-care ultrasound (POCUS), paracentesis, and thoracentesis among others (Table 8.5).

These skills can be taught in a variety of ways: teacher demonstration, direct supervision, web-based procedural videos, and simulation training using mannequins or task trainers. Procedural videos – for example, Procedures Consult[1] – are excellent resources in which to review critical care techniques, particularly invasive vascular procedures, such as placement of arterial and central venous lines. *The New England Journal of Medicine* website includes a robust video library covering relevant procedures performed in the critical care environment.[2] These videos are 10–15-minute tutorials that review every step in performing the particular procedure. In addition to using POCUS to assist in guiding the placement of invasive vascular lines (e.g., including central

---

[1] www.proceduresconsult.com/medical-procedures/anesthesia-specialty.aspx (accessed November 3, 2017).
[2] www.nejm.org/multimedia/medical-videos (accessed November 3, 2017).

Table 8.3 Critical care: What to learn

ABA In-Training Content Outline-Critical Care Topics
Trauma
Evaluation of the trauma patient
Hemorrhagic shock
Mass casualty: crisis management and teamwork
Burn management
Biological warfare
Shock States
Etiology and classification
Pathophysiology
Septic shock and life-threatening infection
Systemic inflammatory response syndrome (SIRS)
Multiple organ dysfunction syndrome (MODS)
Poisoning and Drug Overdose
Near-drowning
Infection Control
General and universal precautions
Needle stick injury
Catheter sepsis
Nosocomial infections
Antibiotics: antibacterial, antifungal, antiviral, antiparasitic
Antibiotics: antimicrobial resistance
Ventilator Management
Types of ventilation strategies
Volume-controlled ventilation
Pressure-controlled ventilation
Positive End-Expiratory Pressure (PEEP) therapy
Inspired oxygen concentration
Tidal volume
Pressure-Support Weaning

venous and arterial catheters), POCUS has other applications in the ICU including volume assessment and determination of lung pathology (pneumothorax, pneumonia, etc.). POCUS can be taught utilizing web-based videos, teacher demonstrations, and didactic lectures. Simulation training (see Chapter 17) is a particularly effective learner-focused active teaching exercise that facilitates learning in all three of the educational domains (knowledge, skills, attitudes). Simulation utilizes a variety of devices, including task trainers, high-fidelity whole-body mannequins, simulated patients, and computer-simulation software.

Simulation training is particularly useful in teaching ICU-related technical skills, such as airway management (see Chapter 10), vascular access, bronchoscopy, and POCUS (see Chapter 13). The high-fidelity human simulator challenges the learner to integrate cognitive, psychomotor, and affective skills in a non-threatening educational environment. Simulation scenarios focused on crisis management, such as cardiac arrest, acute respiratory failure, anaphylaxis, septic shock, multiple trauma, surgical airway, and cardiac dysrhythmias are relevant scenarios applicable to the critical care experience. The post simulation scenario debriefing session provides an interactive educational opportunity to review the learner's actions and provide teaching. In comparison to traditional didactic teaching sessions, simulation training has been demonstrated to be more engaging for the learner.

The ICU setting is an excellent venue in which to cultivate affective skills, including interpersonal and communication proficiencies, professionalism, and team leadership. Frequent interactions with other healthcare professionals (e.g., respiratory therapists, nurses, dietitians, physical therapists) challenge the learner to develop healthy and appropriate interpersonal and communication skills that reinforce the team model of care. In the ICU setting, the student can learn that the delivery of efficient and safe care is enhanced by including staff in management decisions and in formulating care plans. Transfers-of-care (handoffs) offer valuable opportunities to refine communication skills; indeed, ineffective handoff processes have been associated with medical errors and patient harm.[6] A variety of formal handoff methods and programs have been promoted and can serve as a guide to developing an ICU-specific transfer-of-care process.[7] Another tool demonstrated to improve communication among staff is the Agency for Healthcare Research and Quality (AHRQ) TeamSTEPPS® (Strategy and Tools to Enhance Performance and Patient Safety) method,[3] an evidence-based collaboration and communication program aimed at optimizing team performance within a healthcare delivery system. The TeamSTEPPS framework is comprised of five key principles: team structure, leadership, situation monitoring, mutual support, and communication. The TeamSTEPPS method has been demonstrated to improve patient care through better communication, enhanced problem solving, and by the implementation of a culture of safety within the ICU.[8]

---

[3] www.ahrq.gov/teamstepps/index.html (accessed November 3, 2017).

Table 8.4 Critical care: What to learn. Examples from the 2016 ABA ITE published keywords

ABA ITE 2016 ICU-Related Keywords	
Difficult airway – Predictors	Hetastarch – Complications
Subclavian vein anatomy	Hetastarch – Coagulation effects
Central venous pressure (CVP) waveform and pathology	Fresh frozen plasma: Indications
Septic shock: Metabolic effects	Cardiovascular effects: Vasopressin
Goal-directed therapy: Sepsis	Dexmedetomidine: Central nervous system (CNS) effects
Intravenous fluids and sepsis	Pericardial effusion – Imaging
Catheter-related sepsis: Prevention	Hypothermia after cardiac arrest
Low mixed venous O_2 – Differential diagnosis	Organ donor: Diabetes insipidus
Mixed venous oxygenation – Determinants	Diabetic ketoacidosis: Treatment
Pulmonary capillary wedge pressure: Accurate measurement	Serotonin syndrome: Clinical findings
Pulmonary compliance – Measurement	Syndrome of inappropriate antidiuretic hormone secretion (SIADH): Diagnosis
Pulmonary vascular resistance – Calculation	Hyponatremia – Causes
Pulmonary embolus: Diagnostic tests	Hyponatremia – Differential diagnosis
Relationship of alveolar ventilation to $PaCO_2$	Serum osmolality: Components
Hypercarbia-systemic effects	Contrast dye: Nephrotoxicity
Weaning from mechanical ventilation: Management	Hyperbaric oxygen: Indications
Transfusion-related acute lung injury (TRALI)	Needlestick injury: Postexposure Prophylaxis
Colloid administration: Complications	

Professionalism (see Chapter 19) is an additional affective skill frequently challenged in the high-intensity environment of the ICU. Multitasking of clinical duties, responding to the many staff questions directed to the learner during a shift in the ICU, arranging for needed tests and imaging studies, and obtaining subspecialty consultations create stress that can test an individual's patience. Preceptor role modeling, combined with formal didactic teaching focused upon communication and professionalism skills provide the learner with useful tools to further develop these competencies. Leadership is an additional skill that can be developed during the ICU experience. Taking ownership of a patient's medical care plan, decision-making, and managing critical events are instances in which the learner can develop essential team leadership abilities. Finally, simulation (especially interdisciplinary simulation) is an excellent tool in which to cultivate all three affective skills – communication, professionalism, and team leadership – in one teaching exercise. These abilities can be evaluated as part of simulation scenarios, further reinforcing the value of simulation training within a well-rounded ICU curriculum.

Role Modeling

Effective role modeling is a key element of a successful teaching effort. Observing the way the instructor appropriately interacts and communicates with allied healthcare professionals is an essential part of clinical teaching, particularly as it contributes to the development of professionalism and communication skills in the learner. Family conferences, in particular, offer a setting in which preceptor role modeling can be demonstrated. During these meetings, clearly verbalizing expectations, being respectful and compassionate, demonstrating good listening skills, and allowing enough time for questions are characteristics of an effective role model. Throughout the daily work routine, a positive role model exhibits an enthusiasm for teaching, excellent reasoning skills, leadership, organizational abilities, and the prioritization of clinical needs. Within the ICU setting, role modeling becomes one of the more powerful measures of transmitting values, attitudes and patterns of thought, and behavior to students. Indeed, instructor role modeling may be more educationally effective than traditional didactic lectures

Table 8.5 ICU-related skills

Procedure	Use
Arterial catheter	• Hemodynamic monitoring • Arterial blood gases • Arterial lactate levels
Central venous catheter (CVP catheter, pulmonary artery catheter)	• Hemodynamic monitoring • Venous blood gases (MVO_2) • Central venous access
Lumbar puncture	• Diagnosis of CNS infections • Diagnosis of subarachnoid hemorrhage
Tracheal intubation • Awake flexible fiberoptic • Awake direct laryngoscopy • Intravenous induction	• Respiratory failure • Altered mental status
Percutaneous tracheostomy	• Prolonged tracheal intubation • Emergency airway
Ultrasound • Vascular • POCUS	• Vascular access • Cardiac evaluation (function, effusion, valve morphology, volume)
Ventilator management	• Respiratory failure • Ventilator weaning
Intraosseous line	• Emergency intravenous access
Thoracentesis and thoracostomy tube	• Therapeutic pleural fluid drainage • Pleural fluid diagnostic tests • Pneumothorax
Paracentesis	• Therapeutic • Diagnostic
Thoracic epidural catheter	• Pain management (e.g., rib fractures)

focused on professionalism. Instructors who demonstrate good role-modeling attributes can have a profound and lasting impact on the learner, greatly enhancing teaching effectiveness.

Feedback and Assessment

Learner Feedback

Timely feedback is imperative for the educational growth of the learner. The intent of feedback should be to inspire self-reflection and generate motivation to learn. Feedback can be provided following the case presentation, subsequent to ICU rounds, or later in a more confidential setting. For feedback to be most effective, it is crucial to ensure that the student first understands the stated objectives and the intended outcomes of the rotation. Feedback should review the observed learner behaviors and be specific rather than using generalizations. The conversation should include a discussion of what the learner did well, and how the learner might improve.

Learner Assessment

In evaluating learner performance, it is important to assess whether the goals and objectives of the course were achieved. Meaningful assessment should evaluate growth within the domains of knowledge, skills, and attitudes. With respect to knowledge, performance on pre- and postrotation quizzes, standardized tests, and bedside discussions should be considered. Although written examinations are an appropriate component of the evaluation process, they do not assess higher cognitive skills and cannot predict whether the learner has become clinically competent and can exercise safe clinical judgment. In this setting, Miller's learning pyramid[9] provides a very simple assessment framework for evaluating learner performance within the context of the stated objectives. In utilizing Miller's assessment framework, knowledge forms the foundation with competence, formation, and action (in that order) completing the pyramid (Figure 8.2).

The lower two levels of the Miller Pyramid reflect cognition, while the upper two levels reflect behavior. Learner performance is assessed by how the knowledge is applied to inform and influence clinical decisions (including the indications for procedures) and in communication with team members and patient families. The Miller Pyramid shares similarities with Bloom's Taxonomy for developing learning objectives in the cognitive domain (Figure 8.2). In both models, lower-order skills, such as knowledge, must be mastered before higher-order skills (concepts, pattern recognition, analyzing, performing) can be achieved. The assessment process should incorporate these frameworks, ensuring that the achievement of the specific skills is aligned with the level of learner. Chart-stimulated recall (CSR) is a particularly useful exercise in which to evaluate the student's higher cognitive capabilities, as illustrated by both Miller's pyramid and Bloom's cognitive domains. CSR utilizes a medical chart or clinical presentation from which the students must defend the workup, evaluation, diagnosis, and treatment of selected cases; thus, CSR is useful for assessing clinical reasoning and judgment.

In evaluating growth within the psychomotor domain, technical skills can be assessed utilizing procedural checklists, personal observation, and simulation. With respect to the affective domain, communication and professionalism can be evaluated using the 360-degree evaluation format, personal observation, peer evaluations, and discussions with ancillary staff who worked with the learner. The objective structured clinical examination (OSCE) and simulation training exercises are useful tools in which to simultaneously evaluate all three educational domains of knowledge, skills, and attitudes within the clinical scenario. The evaluation process should be customized to consider the varied educational levels – from the PGY-1 to the PGY-5 training level. For anesthesiology residents, incorporating the Anesthesiology Milestone Project framework into the evaluation process will ensure that the learning expectations and outcomes at each stage of development are clearly aligned with the appropriate level of learner.

Teacher Self-Assessment

Clinicians do not become teachers by virtue of their medical expertise alone; rather teaching effectiveness depends upon the institution of a personal program of continual professional development and self-evaluation. Instructor self-assessment is crucial in maximizing teaching effectiveness and for professional growth. In this regard, the Dundee 3-Circle outcomes model is a useful framework for self-assessment that describes three categories of teaching outcomes that should be applied in the clinical environment:[10]

1. Tasks of the teacher;
2. Approach to teaching;
3. Professionalism.

The *tasks of the teacher* include activities such as planning bedside teaching, multidisciplinary rounds, small group lectures, time management,

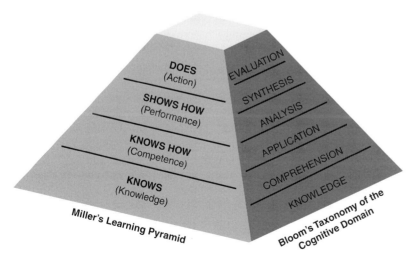

Figure 8.2 Frameworks for learner assessment: Miller's Pyramid and Bloom's Taxonomy of the cognitive domain.

family conferences, and providing learner feedback and assessment. ICU bedside rounding is a particularly effective venue for cultivating teaching skills. Interactions with the patient and bedside nurse teach professionalism and communication skills. The performance of a focused physical examination, discussion of diagnostic tests, and formulation of the differential diagnosis and management plans teach higher cognitive learning skills, essential to growth within the patient care and medical knowledge competencies. The *approach to teaching* involves the incorporation of evidence-based learning theory into effective teaching methods, integrating evidence-based medicine into daily care plans, enthusiasm for teaching, and role modeling. Teacher *professionalism* includes behaviors such as welcoming feedback from learners, self-reflection of strengths and weaknesses, mentoring, and ongoing professional development activities.[10] Assessing teaching effectiveness utilizing this organized structure will provide a solid foundation to improve teaching success.

Program Assessment

An assessment of the effectiveness of the ICU curriculum and educational experience is necessary to ensure that the learner has the best opportunity to achieve the desired outcome. Methods used to assess effectiveness include:

- Formal written or web-based surveys;
- Resident verbal feedback;
- 360-degree evaluations;
- Anonymous suggestion boxes; and
- The results of written knowledge tests.

A regular review of the teaching curriculum, utilizing a variety of assessment tools, is vital to ensure that the ICU experience remains educationally relevant, creates learner enthusiasm and motivation for learning, and promotes professional growth.

Summary

The creation of an effective ICU teaching program requires careful planning and preparation to deliver a curriculum that results in learner enthusiasm and motivation for self-directed learning and professional growth. The integration of relevant adult learning theories into effective teaching methods that target the three domains of learning provide the necessary structure upon which to develop a successful teaching experience. Effective role modeling, timely learner feedback and assessment, and teacher self-evaluation complete the program. If this curriculum framework is implemented, the intended educational teaching and learner outcomes will be achieved and the benefits will be realized in the quality of the clinical care that is delivered.

References

1. B. S. Bloom. *Taxonomy of Educational Objectives: The Classification of Educational Goals.* Handbook I Cognitive Domain. Longman, NY: Longman, 1956.

2. M. S. Knowles. *The Modern Practice of Adult Education: From Pedagogy to Andragogy.* Englewood Cliffs, NJ: Cambridge Adult Education, 1980.

3. D. A. Kolb. *Experiential Learning: Experience as the Source of Learning and Development.* Englewood *Cliffs,* NJ: Prentice-Hall, 1984.

4. J. Neher, K. C. Gordon, B. Meyer et al. A five-step "microskills" model of clinical teaching. *J Am Board Fam Pract* 1992; 5: 419–24.

5. J. M. Pascoe, J. Nixon, V. J. Lang. Maximizing teaching on the wards: Review and application of the one-minute preceptor and SNAPPS models. *J Hosp Med* 2015; 10: 125–30.

6. A. J. Starmer, N. D. Spector, R. Srivastava et al. Changes in medical errors after implementation of a handoff program. *N Engl J Med* 2014; 371: 1803–12.

7. A. J. Starmer, J. K. O'Toole, G. Rosenbluth et al. Development, implementation, and dissemination of the I-PASS handoff curriculum: A multisite educational intervention to improve patient handoffs. *Acad Med* 2014; 89: 876–84.

8. L. Thomas, C. Galla. Building a culture of safety through team training and engagement. *BMJ Qual Saf* 2013; 22: 425–34.

9. G. E. Miller. The assessment of clinical skills/competence/performance. *Acad Med* 1990; 63: S63–7.

10. S. Ramani and S. Leinster. AMEE Guide no. 34: Teaching in the clinical environment. *Med Teacher* 2008; 30: 347–64.

Chapter

9

Pain Medicine Education in Anesthesiology Training

Matthew Reed, Naileshni Singh, and Jordan Newmark

Introduction

Anesthesiology and pain medicine encompass four key areas of endeavor including patient care, education, research, and practice administration.[1] A strong educational component is essential to ensure the development of skilled clinicians equipped to pursue the other three areas. As a subspecialty of anesthesiology, pain medicine garners learners from varied backgrounds and specialties. Providing the best learning experience for such a heterogeneous group of professionals is challenging but presents a significant opportunity and responsibility.

Educational Goals

In 1999 the Accreditation Council for Graduate Medical Educations (ACGME) introduced the concept of six core competencies (patient care, medical knowledge, professionalism, interpersonal communication, system-based practice, and practice-based learning and improvement). In 2015, these competencies were transitioned into an outcome-based assessment in which competencies are assigned to measurable and observable developmental steps known as educational milestones (Figure 9.1).[1][2]

Implementation of milestones is left to individual programs that are beginning to develop educational programs that meet competency goals. For example, Rebel et al. describe a curriculum using simulated clinical examinations and technical tasks scored by faculty using checklists as the basis for milestone teaching and assessment.[3]

Additional milestones for fellowship training in pain medicine were published in 2015 and are divided amongst the six core competencies: six in patient care, three in medical knowledge, four in systems-based practice, four in practice-based learning, four in

professionalism, and three in interpersonal and communication skills.[2] Through use of the milestones, individual programs or institutions are tasked with ensuring that each trainee achieves the specified competencies. Additionally, practice guidelines, such as those provided by governing bodies or credentialing organizations, may serve as objectives in assessing individuals and may be used in the development of learning tools.

The core competencies of pain management for resident-level training have been developed as four broad domains (see Table 9.1) by Fishman et al.[4]

The first domain focuses primarily on acquisition of the knowledge base necessary for practice. The second and third domains focus on clinical application of that knowledge, and the fourth domain focuses on integration of the competencies mastered in the first three domains in multidisciplinary settings.

Traditional Teaching Methods

While there has been little research into appropriate teaching practices in pain medicine, the basic methodologies used for undergraduate and graduate medical education can be adapted to pain medicine. Research on the teaching of pain medicine is sparse and fragmented at the level of undergraduate medical education.[5] The application of evidence-based learning methodologies should promote mastery of the core competencies of pain medicine.

Traditional teaching methods include varied implementations of didactic lectures, problem-based learning (PBL), and Socratic teaching. Didactic lecturing, where the "expert" delivers large amounts of information in a systematic manner, is a mainstay of undergraduate and graduate medical education. The medical education community's continued reliance

---

[1] www.acgme.org/Portals/0/PDFs/Milestones/ AnesthesiologyMilestones.pdf (accessed November 4, 2017).

[2] www.acgme.org/Portals/0/PDFs/Milestones/ PainMedicineMilestones.pdf (accessed November 3, 2017).

Has not Achieved Level 1	Level 1	Level 2	Level 3	Level 4	Level 5
	Performs targeted history and physical examination for patients with pain, including the use of common pain scales

Initiates non-interventional, routine therapy for common pain problems with indirect supervision | Diagnoses common acute and chronic pain syndromes; evaluates efficacy of current medication regiment

Implements non-interventional pain treatment plans with indirect supervision

Performs simple interventional pain procedures (e.g., trigger point injections, scar injections, lumbar interlaminar epidural steroid injection [ESI], intravenous [IV] regional blocks) with direct supervision

Identifies structures seen on ultrasound and basic fluoroscopy | Formulates differential diagnoses of acute and chronic pain syndromes; identifies appropriate diagnostic evaluation

Participates in complex procedures (e.g., thoracic ESI, medial branch blocks, radiofrequency procedures, sympathetic blocks) for alleviating acute, chronic, or cancer-related pain, under direct supervision

Prescribes initial therapy for pain medication, and adjusts ongoing medication regimen with indirect supervision; uses ultrasound and fluoroscopy with direct supervision | Acts as consultant for acute pain management to junior residents and other health care providers with conditional independence

Consults with non-anesthesiologist specialists regarding pain management as appropriate

Recognizes treatment failures and obtains appropriate consultations, including with a pain medicine specialist | Participates in coordination of care for patients with complex pain problems

Serves as a consultant to other members of the health care team regarding initial evaluation and management of the patient with acute, chronic, or cancer-related pain |

Figure 9.1 Patient Care 7: Acute, chronic, and cancer-related pain consultation and management. (From the ABA / ACGME "The Anesthesiology Milestone Project .")

Table 9.1 Domains of pain management

1.	Multidimensional nature of pain: What is pain?
2.	Pain assessment and measurement: How is pain recognized?
3.	Management of pain: How is pain relieved?
4.	Clinical conditions: How does context influence pain management?

Source: Adapted from Fishman et al. (2013).[4]

on this modality over the decades speaks to its efficiency and cost-effectiveness in disseminating large amounts of information to a maximum number of learners. One expert lecturer can reach many learners. Through teleconferencing and online streaming of didactic sessions, technologic advances allow even greater numbers of learners to be reached now than in years past. This efficiency in disseminating information, however, is contrasted by decreased levels of engagement among learners. Didactic lecture sessions are traditionally viewed as exercises in passive rather than active learning. Passively learned medical knowledge is not retained as well and may not be incorporated into clinical practice.[6] Technological advances including audience response systems where participants can offer answers to questions posed by

the lecturer (see Chapter 15), or e-learning (either synchronous or asynchronous) that allows participants to ask questions of their own (see Chapter 16) show some promise in addressing concerns of learner engagement and information retention.[7]

Despite its limitations, didactic lecturing remains the most commonly used tool to disseminate the fundamental concepts of pain medicine to new trainees. Didactic lecturing is best suited to promote mastery of the first domain of core competencies in pain medicine. Because these individuals do not typically have a consistent knowledge base related to pain medicine, didactic lecturing is frequently used in an effort to establish foundational knowledge.

PBL was developed as an alternative to the passive learning associated with didactic lecturing. (See Chapter 15 for a more detailed discussion of PBL.) In an attempt to make medical education more interesting and relevant for students, Howard Barrows described[6] dividing a class into small groups each of which was given a problem, or "PBL scenario," to complete along with needed resources to assist them. Group members must engage in self-directed learning before cooperating with each other to apply their newly acquired knowledge. Barrow's four key educational objectives for PBL are outlined in Table 9.2.[8]

Table 9.2 Barrow's educational objectives for problem-based learning[8]

1. Structuring of knowledge for use in clinical context.
2. Development of effective clinical-reasoning process.
3. Development of effective self-directed learning skills.
4. Increased motivation for learning.

Table 9.3 Comparison of didactic lecturing and problem-based learning

	Didactic Lecturing	Problem-Based Learning
Resource Utilization	Low	High
Group Size	Large	Small
Knowledge Acquisition	Equivalent	Equivalent
Knowledge Retention	+	++
Social and Cognitive Performance Improvement	-	++

Increased number of plus signs (+) indicates more evidence of benefit.

Source: Adapted from Neville (2009). [6]

Knowledge-based assessments of PBL-based curricula show little difference from traditional curricula, but there appear to be some improvements in knowledge retention and social and cognitive performance.[6] See Table 9.3 for additional comparisons[6] between a traditional lecture and a PBL session.

Improvements in the social and cognitive performance areas of medical practice are key to mastery of the pain management core competencies involving the patient-doctor interaction and interdisciplinary collaboration.

The PBL format was rapidly incorporated by medical schools such that today few medical students are likely to have graduated without experiencing some form of PBL. Graduate medical education programs have also incorporated many components of PBL, but there is little published research detailing these efforts and no research describing the use of PBL in pain medicine. Based on the documented advantages in social and cognitive performance that have been achieved in conjunction with use of PBL, it is logical to incorporate this mode of teaching in the area of pain management.

The third traditional teaching method ubiquitously utilized in residency and fellowship training programs is the Socratic method. Socrates was known for leading his listeners through a series of questions designed to create doubt about their core assumptions on a given topic.[9] Once in this state of doubt or confusion, known as aporia, the listeners became more receptive or curious to learn new truths. The closest application of this in medicine is the practice of "pimping." Pimping was first described in 1989 by Brancati in an article for the *Journal of the American Medical Association* where he described "pimping" as senior physicians asking junior trainees difficult questions in rapid succession to establish the power hierarchy of a team.[10] While written tongue-in-cheek, the article highlighted the abuses many medical students have experienced at the hands of senior physicians purporting to use the Socratic method. The key difference between "pimping" and the Socratic method primarily lies in the questioner's intent. Practitioners of the Socratic method create a safe learning environment where the understanding of the learner can be explored for the purpose of direction rather than humiliation or evaluation (Table 9.4).[11]

Use of the Socratic method is applicable to acquisition of any of the pain medicine core competencies. It provides a more granular opportunity to reinforce concepts and skills taught during didactic lecturing or PBL sessions.

Didactic lecturing, PBL, and Socratic questioning as described in the preceding text form the basis of traditional teaching methods in anesthesiology education. The implementation of these methodologies is diverse. With duty hour restrictions, resident time in clinical and educational activities has decreased.[12] To accommodate these changes, residency and fellowship programs have embraced different forms of self-directed learning to replace lost didactic lecturing time while reserving face-to-face time for active learning activities. One form of self-directed learning, blended learning, refers to the incorporation of educational tools such as videocasts, podcasts, and online assessments to augment formal didactic or PBL sessions. Outcomes research for blended learning shows that knowledge acquisition is comparable with traditional didactic lecturing, but is dependent on the quality of the learning tool and the engagement of the learner with that tool.[13] A related educational approach is the "flipped classroom" (see Chapter 15) in which the study of basic facts occurs independently, before face-to-face interactions where the

Table 9.4 The Socratic method versus pimping

Technique	Socratic Method	Pimping
Goals	• Respectful codiscovery • Instruct at individual learner level • Elucidate gaps in knowledge for learner benefit • Encourage critical reasoning	• Humiliation • Establish power hierarchy • Knowledge assessment for grade assignment • Encourage rote memorization
Types of Questions	• Focused on conceptual understanding	• Focused on esoteric trivia

Source: Adapted from Oh and Reamy (2014).[11]

focus is on higher-level integration of knowledge.[14] These asynchronous educational approaches are well suited to pain medicine education where learners are frequently at multiple sites with varying schedules making it difficult to schedule formal group didactic opportunities. With much of the foundational-level fact-based learning taking place outside of formal sessions, more time and attention can be focused on ensuring that face-to-face encounters are engaging and high quality.

While didactic lecturing and PBL sessions primarily occur outside of direct patient care settings, Socratic questioning is well suited to use during clinical care. Even the best-planned PBL sessions are unlikely to rival the level of engagement between a trainee and an attending anesthesiologist providing care at the bedside of an actual patient. Not only are highly relevant clinical topics more easily conceptualized at the bedside, clinical teaching also provides opportunities to demonstrate physical examination skills, teach professionalism, and appropriately model the doctor-patient relationship.[15] Including patients in the educational process has been shown to improve patient perceptions of their care.[16]

Demonstration of procedural techniques and assessment of trainee proficiency have also traditionally been performed at the bedside, largely out of necessity given the lack of alternative options for teaching and assessing these skills. Advanced simulation technologies such as web tutorials/instruction, computer simulations, standardized patients (SPs), and advanced mannequin simulations offer potential improvements in patient safety and more rapid trainee skill acquisition for a host of interventional procedures and emergency situations, such as cardiac arrest or sedation-related respiratory distress (see Chapter 17). These high- and low-fidelity technologies are promising and will be discussed further, but basic instruction on the doctor-patient interaction and physical examination skill acquisition is often achieved with direct bedside patient interaction.

Simulation and Immersive Learning in Pain Medicine

According to the Society for Simulation in Healthcare (SSH), simulation is defined as "the imitation or representation of one act or system by another. Healthcare simulations can be said to have four main purposes – education, assessment, research and health system integration in facilitating patient safety."[17] The use of simulation for pain medicine education is emerging as a novel and exciting teaching technique.[18] Additionally, it allows for performance comparisons between learners given the consistent nature of each scenario, which does not occur in real-world clinical settings. Because of this, the ACGME allows training programs to use simulation performance data during clinical competency committee reviews. Thus, here we will provide an overview of the use of simulation in its current state as well as its potential future use for pain medicine education.

Pain simulation modalities are often characterized by their level of fidelity. Low-fidelity simulators include anatomical models and task trainers. These instruments are useful when teaching pain-related procedural skills. One example includes the use of lumbar puncture trainers, which decrease patient discomfort, may increase comfort for the learner, and facilitate developing an accurate approach and consistent technique.[19] For ultrasound skills related to pain medicine, the utilization of "phantom" technology is becoming more popular.[20,21] Phantom task trainers are made of durable, elastomeric rubber that provides clear imaging of structures, haptic feedback, and resistance to needle-related damage. A 3D virtual human back, developed from computed tomographic and magnetic resonance images, has been developed; the device allows adjustments to the level of difficulty.[22] The use of fluoroscopy is common to allow for safe needle placement during interventional pain procedures. Several fluoroscopic compatible, pain-related task trainers exist, including the comprehensive AR351 Adam, Rouilly Pain Relief Manikin.[3][22] The AR351 allows trainees to practice lumbar sympathetic, splanchnic, trigeminal ganglion, celiac, and superior hypogastric nerve blocks; epidural and facet joint injections at cervical, thoracic and lumbar levels; and sacroiliac joint injections. The device includes a spine that is x-ray compatible therefore allowing radiographic confirmation of needle placement.

A higher level of fidelity beyond task trainers can be found with the use of virtual-reality technologies. Virtual patients (VPs) are computer-based, interactive, simulated patients. Pain medicine immersive learning experiences using VP technology have recently been described for both educational and research purposes.[23,24] It has several advantages over the use of live, SP actors due to lower cost and time for SP training, increased consistency during the interaction, and greater availability for access and scheduling of sessions. The use of VPs will likely increase in the future as simulation methods related to pain medicine continue to expand.

The highest level of fidelity is achieved with the use of SPs. SP-based immersive learning experiences in pain medicine are gaining popularity, particularly for communication skills, difficult conversations, and interdisciplinary team training. Plymale et al. describe a successful, SP-based cancer pain simulation that allowed medical students to enhance their assessment and management skills within this context.[18] Other SP-based pain-related simulations for residents and fellows include discussing procedural complications or errors with patients and their family, ethical decision-making regarding do not resuscitate/do not intubate orders, and managing patient opioid prescriptions when unexpected urine drug-test results are obtained.[25,26]

The process of debriefing, as well as providing feedback to participants after an immersive learning exercise is crucial for maximizing its benefits. *Feedback* and *debriefing* are terms commonly used interchangeably, however as described by Sawyer et al., they are

two distinct constructs.[27] Feedback is a unidirectional process by which data and assessment regarding performance is provided to the participant in an effort to allow for future improvement.[27] In contrast, debriefing is an "interactive, bidirectional, and reflective discussion or conversation [which] involves some level of facilitation or guidance (either by a facilitator or the learners) to assist the reflective process."[27] (See Chapter 17 for a discussion on debriefing and simulation.)

Assessment of Learning in Pain Medicine

Assessment of skills acquisition in pain medicine and anesthesiology depends on the goal of providing formative and summative critique. Formative assessments are those that improve the learning process while summative assessments are typically high stakes and serve to advance the learner to the next level if particular criteria are met. Summative assessments are those required by governing bodies in certification or recertification in anesthesiology, pain medicine, or other fields.[28] Typically the criteria for advancement are well delineated in summative assessments, rigorously tested, and standardized.

The ABA has a content outline[4] available for practicing pain providers that may help inform assessment tools for licensed practitioners such as those enrolled in Maintenance of Certification in Anesthesiology (MOCA) or MOCA Pain Medicine. Additionally, groups like the American Society of Regional Anesthesia and Pain Medicine (ASRA) have practice guidelines[5] relevant to measuring competencies using tools such as the local anesthetic toxicity checklist.[29] Local and state medical boards often publish best practices that can be developed into assessment tools that are relevant to daily clinical care.[30]

For residents and fellows, the ACGME has recognized several different modalities that are effective in the assessment of learning. Simulation-based education, direct observation of patient encounters, and audit of medical records have been recognized as

---

3 www.adam-rouilly.co.uk/productdetails.aspx?pid=2788&cid=403 (accessed November 3, 2017).

4 www.theaba.org/PDFs/Pain-Medicine/PMContent Outline (accessed November 3, 2017).
5 www.asra.com/advisory-guidelines (accessed November 3, 2017).

having the highest level of evidence for assessment of learning.[31] But each core competency may have specific assessment modalities that are better suited to evaluating achievement of objectives.[32] For example, assessment of medical knowledge may be suited to an examination using multiple-choice answers, which has been commonly undertaken by anesthesiology governing boards and validated as an effective modality. Patient care can be assessed using direct observation, objective structured clinical examinations (OSCEs), peer review, SPs (who may also be able to participate by reviewing the learner), chart review, simulation with structured debriefing, checklists for technical and nontechnical skills, or case-based oral examinations. Practice-based learning may be assessed using portfolios and chart reviews or even patient feedback. Skills in professionalism and communication may be challenging to assess due to the complexity of the trait and the multitude of factors believed to encompass these "soft competencies."[33] However, achievement in communication skills and professionalism may be determined through the use of evaluation instruments that focus on leadership, teamwork, and patient care such as the Non-Technical Skills Scale (NOTECHS) or Anaesthetists' Non-Technical Skills (ANTS).[34-36] More typically, direct observation by supervisors, peers, and ancillary staff comprise assessments of professionalism. Competencies are also interdependent and, by using one tool or activity, multiple skill sets can be gauged.

Frequent evaluations of learners will reflect a better measure of competency and will provide greater fidelity for skill acquisition; the achievement of competency can evolve at a different rate within each individual.[37] Due to the fluidity of competency achievement, metrics will need to be retooled to keep pace with the learner's and instructor's goals. But while the focus of learning is often on the individual, the competency of clinical teams is likely more relevant for patient care. The concept of collective competence, or the skills that a team may possess to provide safe and effective care, is equally as pertinent to patient care as individual learning in a complex healthcare system.[38] Assessment tools in this domain, such as NOTECHS, Global Rating Scale, or Clinical Teamwork Scale, may focus more on teamwork and leadership.[39]

The difficulties in creating and implementing assessment metrics are numerous. Observation of one encounter, regardless of the competency or ability being assessed, may not reflect the entirety of the learner's capabilities. Many tools may not be generalizable to a particular setting, learner, or objective and may not be sensitive for the construct intended. Tools that have been developed internally will likely not have undergone the statistical analysis necessary to document validity or reliability. In addition to reliability and validity, assessments will need to be acceptable to the learner and teacher, have an educational impact, and be feasible.[40] The complexity and unpredictability of workplace assessments cannot be standardized for each trainee. These issues make any one evaluation tool or time-point inadequate for assessment (see Chapter 20). Instead, assessments should be planned with identified times, frequently completed across multiple clinical settings, and involve many well-trained raters.

The use of raters to evaluate learning experiences is also problematic. Most raters are simply peers, supervisors, or other individuals not specifically trained in evaluation and who may not be familiar with the evaluation metric or the goals of the assessment tool. Raters use their own experiences to provide context to evaluate learners, but this may not accurately reflect whether a competency is achieved.[41] Evaluators should be trained in the construct they are employing so results are more reproducible between assessments.[31] Providing education and instruction for these individuals will help reduce bias and increase interrater reliability. Receiving formative feedback from trainees may facilitate retraining of novice raters into expert raters. Additionally, the use of multiple raters may mitigate dangers of this type of evaluation because "hawks" and "doves" can be identified with appropriate adjustments made in the final calculation.[42]

While many assessment tools are suitable for an artificial learning environment, the goal of educators is to develop and implement learning programs that lead to improved patient care, quality, and safety.[43] In pain medicine, the objective is to master challenging clinical situations, such as difficult patient conversations, and be an expert interventionalist. ASRA has used simulation to validate a training and assessment tool for the treatment of local anesthetic toxicity.[20] This example illustrates that validation testing of assessment tools in pain medicine needs to be done to meet the competency challenges for providers. Other examples include use of modified Delphi techniques and calculating interrater reliability or intraclass correlations to evaluate in-house assessments; however, this may not be applicable to other situations due to the lack of robust validity and reliability testing. There are a myriad of challenges in evaluating pain medicine competencies and skills at the prelicensure, graduate, and practicing provider levels.

Summary

Pain medicine encompasses patient care, education (of patients and learners), research, and practice administration. A strong clinical background is an essential foundation for skilled clinicians equipped to pursue the other three areas. Through the Anesthesiology Milestones Project, the ACGME has stipulated minimal goals of resident education in pain management. While didactic lectures (the "sage on the stage") may be provided to a maximum number of learners at minimal cost, this passive learning technique may not result in optimum learning and changes in practice. The use of technology (e.g., videocasts) magnifies the ability to reach a greater number of learners, but may not result in any improvement in knowledge acquisition in the absence of more active learning. Use of PBLs, which present an opportunity for more active learning, have not been demonstrated to be associated with increased acquisition of foundational knowledge, but have documented advantages in social and cognitive performance – two areas that are critical in pain management. Properly applied, the Socratic method (as opposed to "pimping") may be effective in stimulating active learning. The use of simulation, in the form of task trainers, VPs, and SPs, presents an opportunity not only for resident education, but also for assessment of performance. Assessment of knowledge through standardized testing is widely accepted. Other tools for the assessment of the other domains of pain medicine have not been developed and validated.

References

1. A. J. Schwartz. Education: An essential leg for anesthesiology's four-legged stool! *Anesthesiology* 2010; 112: 3–5.

2. J. E. Tetzlaff. Assessment of competency in anesthesiology. *Anesthesiology* 2007; 106: 812–25.

3. A. Rebel, A. N. DiLorenzo, R. Y. Fragneto et al. A competitive objective structured clinical examination event to generate an objective assessment of anesthesiology resident skills development. *A A Case Rep* 2016; 6: 313–19.

4. S. M. Fishman, H. M. Young, E. Lucas Arwood et al. Core competencies for pain management: Results of an interprofessional consensus summit. *Pain Med* 2013; 14: 971–81.

5. L. Mezei, B. B. Murinson. Johns Hopkins Pain Curriculum Development Team: Pain education in North American medical schools. *J Pain* 2011; 12: 1199–208.

6. A. J. Neville. Problem-based learning and medical education forty years on: A review of its effects on knowledge and clinical performance. *Med Princ Pract* 2009; 18: 1–9.

7. A. Pradhan, D. Sparano, C. V. Ananth. The influence of an audience response system on knowledge retention: An application to resident education. *Am J Obstet Gynecol* 2005; 193: 1827–30.

8. G. Chilkoti, M. Mohta, R. Wadhwa, A. K. Saxena. Problem-based learning research in anesthesia teaching: Current status and future perspective. *Anesthesiol Res Pract* 2014; 2014: 263948.

9. A. Kost, F. M. Chen. Socrates was not a pimp: Changing the paradigm of questioning in medical education. *Acad Med* 2015; 90: 20–4.

10. F. L. Brancati. The art of pimping. *JAMA* 1989; 262: 89–90.

11. R. C. Oh, B. V. Reamy. The Socratic method and pimping: Optimizing the use of stress and fear in instruction. *Virtual Mentor* 2014; 16: 182–6.

12. S. V. Desai, L. Feldman, L. Brown et al. Effect of the 2011 vs. 2003 duty hour regulation-compliant models on sleep duration, trainee education, and continuity of patient care among internal medicine house staff: A randomized trial. *JAMA Intern Med* 2013; 173: 649–55.

13. J. Kannan, V. Kurup. Blended learning in anesthesia education: Current state and future model. *Curr Opin Anaesthesiol* 2012; 25: 692–8.

14. V. Kurup, D. Hersey. The changing landscape of anesthesia education: Is flipped classroom the answer? *Curr Opin Anaesthesiol* 2013; 26: 726–31.

15. S. Ramani. Twelve tips to improve bedside teaching. *Med Teach* 2003; 25: 112–15.

16. L. S. Lehmann, F. L. Brancati, M. C. Chen et al. The effect of bedside case presentations on patients' perceptions of their medical care. *N Engl J Med* 1997; 336: 1150–5.

17. D. F. Carter. Man-made man: Anesthesiological medical human simulator. *J Assoc Adv Med Instrum* 1969; 3: 80–6.

18. M. A. Plymale, P. A. Sloan, M. Johnson et al. Cancer pain education: The use of a structured clinical instruction module to enhance learning among medical students. *J Pain Symptom Manage* 2000; 20: 4–11.

19. H. Chen, R. Kim, D. Perret et al. Improving trainee competency and comfort level with needle driving using simulation training. *Pain Med* 2016; 17: 670–4.

20. Y. H. Kim. Ultrasound phantoms to protect patients from novices. *Korean J Pain* 2016; 29: 73–7.

21. A. K. Brascher, J. A. Blunk, K. Bauer et al. Comprehensive curriculum for phantom-based training of ultrasound-guided intercostal nerve and stellate ganglion blocks. *Pain Med* 2014; 15: 1647–56.

22. N. Vaughan, V. N. Dubey, M. Y. Wee, R. Isaacs. A review of epidural simulators: Where are we today? *Med Eng Phys* 2013; 35: 1235–50.

23. L. D. Wandner, M. W. Heft, B. C. Lok et al. The impact of patients' gender, race, and age on health care professionals' pain management decisions: An online survey using virtual human technology. *Int J Nurs Stud* 2014; 51: 726–33.

24. J. Boissoneault, J. M. Mundt, E. J. Bartley et al. Assessment of the influence of demographic and professional characteristics on health care providers' pain management decisions using virtual humans. *J Dent Educ* 2016; 80: 578–87.

25. B. C. Hoelzer, S. M. Moeschler, D. P. Seamans. Using simulation and standardized patients to teach vital skills to pain medicine fellows. *Pain Med* 2015; 16: 680–91.

26. G. J. Brenner, J. L. Newmark, D. Raemer. Curriculum and cases for pain medicine crisis resource management education. *Anesth Analg* 2013; 116: 107–10.

27. T. Sawyer, W. Eppich, M. Brett-Fleegler et al. More than one way to debrief: A critical review of healthcare simulation debriefing methods. *Simul Healthc* 2016; 11: 209–17.

28. J. R. Boulet. Summative assessment in medicine: The promise of simulation for high-stakes evaluation. *Acad Emerg Med* 2008; 15: 1017–24.

29. J. M. Neal, R. L. Hsiung, M. F. Mulroy et al. ASRA checklist improves trainee performance during a simulated episode of local anesthetic systemic toxicity. *Reg Anesth Pain Med* 2012; 37: 8–15.

30. S. M. Fishman. *Responsible Opioid Prescribing: A Clinician's Guide.* Federation of State Medical Boards. Washington, DC: Waterford Life Sciences; 2014.

31. S. R. Swing, S. G. Clyman, E. S. Holmboe, R. G. Williams. Advancing resident assessment in graduate medical education. *J Grad Med Educ* 2009; 1: 278–86.

32. J. R. Boulet, D. Murray. Review article: Assessment in anesthesiology education. *Can J Anaesth* 2012; 59: 182–92.

33. R. R. Gaiser. The teaching of professionalism during residency: Why it is failing and a suggestion to improve its success. *Anesth Analg* 2009; 108: 948–54.

34. A. Mishra, K. Catchpole, P. McCulloch. The Oxford NOTECHS System: Reliability and validity of a tool for measuring teamwork behaviour in the operating theatre. *Qual Saf Health Care* 2009; 18: 104–8.

35. G. Fletcher, R. Flin, P. McGeorge et al. Anaesthetists' Non-Technical Skills (ANTS): Evaluation of a behavioural marker system. *Br J Anaesth* 2003; 90: 580–8.

36. A. M. Cyna, M. I. Andrew, S. G. Tan. Communication skills for the anaesthetist. *Anaesthesia* 2009; 64: 658–65.

37. F. Semeraro, L. Signore, E. L. Cerchiari. Retention of CPR performance in anaesthetists. *Resuscitation* 2006; 68: 101–8.

38. L. Lingard. Paradoxical truths and persistent myths: Reframing the team competence conversation. *J Contin Educ Health Prof* 2016; 36(Suppl 1): S19–21.

39. D. N. Onwochei, S. Halpern, M. Balki. Teamwork assessment tools in obstetric emergencies: A systematic review. *Simul Healthc* 2016; 12(3): 165–76.

40. C. P. van der Vleuten, L. W. Schuwirth. Assessing professional competence: From methods to programmes. *Med Educ* 2005; 39: 309–17.

41. M. J. Govaerts, L. W. Schuwirth, C. P. Van der Vleuten, A. M. Muijtjens. Workplace-based assessment: Effects of rater expertise. *Adv Health Sci Educ Theory Pract* 2011; 16: 151–65.

42. M. Feldman, E. H. Lazzara, A. A. Vanderbilt, D. Diazgranados. Rater training to support high-stakes simulation-based assessments. *J Continuing Educ Health Prof* 2012; 32: 279–86.

43. I. Bartman, S. Smee, M. Roy. A method for identifying extreme OSCE examiners. *Clin Teach* 2013; 10: 27–31.

44. S. Griswold, S. Ponnuru, A. Nishisaki et al. The emerging role of simulation education to achieve patient safety: Translating deliberate practice and debriefing to save lives. *Pediatr Clin North Am* 2012; 59: 1329–40.

Chapter 10

A Foundation for Teaching Airway Management

Marc Hassid, J. Scott Walton, John J. Schaefer III, and Stephen F. Dierdorf

Introduction

Airway management is the scaffolding upon which the whole practice of anaesthesia is built. Consequently, education in airway skills must occupy a central place in anaesthetic management, since it is within the realms of respiratory management that the penalties for misadventure are greatest.

R. A. Mason, *British Journal of Anaesthesia*
1998; 81: 305

The importance of airway management cannot be overemphasized. The adverse consequences of airway mismanagement were brought into sharp focus by the seminal article by Caplan et al. published in 1990 that analyzed poor patient outcomes reported to the American Society of Anesthesiologists (ASA) Closed Claims Study.[1] In this analysis, respiratory events accounted for 34 percent of all reported injuries and 85 percent of the respiratory cases resulted in death or permanent neurologic injury. The authors concluded that 72 percent of those adverse events, especially inadequate ventilation and esophageal intubation, could have been prevented with better respiratory monitoring. Prevention of complications from difficult tracheal intubation, however, would require more than just improved monitoring alone. In 1993, the ASA Task Force on Management of the Difficult Airway published *Practice Guidelines for Management of the Difficult Airway*.[2] These guidelines were updated in 2003 and 2013.[3,4] Comparing the time period of 1970–89 to the time period of 1990–2007, there was a decrease in the percentage of closed claims for esophageal intubation and inadequate oxygenation/ventilation, but an increase in the percentage of claims for difficult ventilation and aspiration.[5] Management of the patient with a difficult airway, consequently, remains a high priority. Despite the emphasis on airway management by the ASA and many anesthesiologists, a standardized, comprehensive airway management education curriculum for anesthesiology residents has

not been achieved. Surveys of anesthesiology residencies published in 1995 and 2003 indicated that only 27 to 33 percent of responding programs had formal rotations in management of the difficult airway.[6,7] A similar survey published in 2011 indicated that 49 percent of programs had a formal airway rotation (Figure 10.1).[8]

Although there is a trend to more programs incorporating formal airway management rotations into their curriculum, the rate of progress has been surprisingly slow. The educational quality of the programs varies widely. In 1995, of eight techniques queried, more than half the programs indicated that for three of the techniques the only instruction provided was by lecture and there was no hands-on experience with the techniques in either models or patients. By 2009, 75 percent of programs still did not use some form of task trainer in instruction during the difficult airway rotation. In 1995, most rotations were 1.5 weeks or less in duration; by 2009 in more than 80 percent of the programs the duration of the difficult airway rotation was one month or longer.

Better respiratory monitoring has decreased the incidence of some adverse events (e.g., unrecognized esophageal intubation, inadequate ventilation). It is unlikely that any further significant decreases in the incidence of adverse events from airway management will occur until better education and training in airway management is incorporated into anesthesiology residencies.[9]

The obstacles to implementation of a comprehensive airway management educational program are significant. The first impediment is the vague, nonspecific airway management requirement by the Accreditation Council for Graduate Medical Education (ACGME). The current (2016) revision of the ACGME Requirements for Graduate Medical Education in Anesthesiology[1] are nebulous and offer

---

[1] www.acgme.org/Portals/0/PFAssets/ProgramRequirements/CPRs_2017-07-01.pdf; (accessed November 3, 2017).

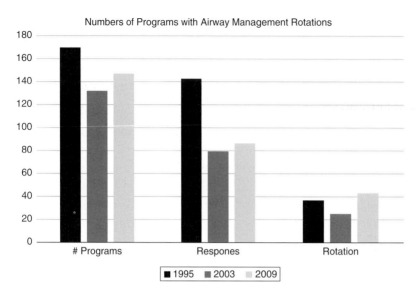

Numbers of Programs with Airway Management Rotations

Figure 10.1 Number of training programs with specific training in difficult airway management (data from references 6, 7, 8). Note that data from 2011 include residency training programs in Canada.

no guidance on how to teach airway management.[10] (According to section IV.A.5.a).(2).(l).(i) "Residents … must achieve competence in the delivery of anesthetic care to … patients whose peri-operative care requires specialized techniques, including a broad spectrum of airway management techniques, to include laryngeal masks, fiberoptic intubation, and lung isolation techniques such as double lumen endotracheal tube placement and endobronchial blockers.") Other impediments include lack of opportunities for residents to manage difficult airways and production pressure that interferes with clinical instruction. Many training programs rely on basic airway management techniques and sporadic "hit or miss" clinical opportunities. The absence of an ACGME requirement to quantify experience with airway management techniques impedes the ability of residency program directors to track resident progress with these skills. The experience of trainees is, therefore, inconsistent, and objective evaluation of their competence for independent practice is difficult. There is a critical need for clear definitions of competence and published, well-defined procedural learning curves.

The development of new airway devices over the past 20 years has expanded the airway management armamentarium and increased the complexity of airway education. No single device, however, guarantees a safe airway for all patients under all circumstances. Anesthesia trainees need to be thoroughly educated in the use of different types of airway devices and understand the strengths and weaknesses of each device.[11] The trainee must also develop an integrative approach to airway management that permits a rapid change to an alternative technique if the primary airway technique fails. The framework for *clinical judgment* in airway management should be built on the ASA Guidelines for Management of the Difficult Airway.

How Can Airway Management Be Taught?

Each training program must develop its own system. The first task for the program director is to identify and recruit faculty with airway management skills and a passion for teaching those skills. Airway management skill levels vary greatly among faculty, and it is important that the use of different airway devices be taught by faculty experienced with each device.

This chapter should serve as a foundation on which an instructional program can be built. The first section of the chapter provides information about the risks of poor or failed airway management. The trainee must have a thorough understanding of the devastating consequences of inadequate ventilation and oxygenation. The next four sections discuss the stages of skill acquisition, the role of simulation, respiratory anatomy and physiology, and preoperative airway assessment. The final sections review different airway devices and management techniques. The template for how to teach their use is similar for all airway devices and techniques:

1. The trainees should receive didactic instruction on the device structure and the theory of how it should work. This can be accomplished with a traditional lecture format or online instructional programs.

2. The trainees should be instructed with a task trainer (mannequin) on proper insertion technique. This should be done one on one or in small groups so that each trainee masters the device on the task trainer. The instructor must carefully monitor the trainee to ensure quality performance.

3. After the trainees have mastered use of the device with the task trainer, instruction can proceed to a high-fidelity human patient simulator. The purpose of this phase is to allow the trainee to experience in real time successful use and the consequences of device failure (e.g., severe hypoxemia).

4. After the trainees become proficient with the device in the high-fidelity simulator, they can begin to use the device in patients with normal airways. This phase is suitable for noninvasive devices used in the normal course of intraoperative management (e.g., bag-mask ventilation, pharyngeal airways, supraglottic airways, direct laryngoscopes, videolaryngoscopes, and flexible fiberoptic laryngoscopes). Invasive airway techniques will require practice with a simulator, animal models, or human cadavers.

Educational Models for Skill Acquisition

As accreditation bodies have moved toward competence-based outcomes of learning, the Dreyfus model for skill acquisition has become popular with medical educators (Figure 10.2).[12]

Dreyfus described five levels of skill acquisition: novice, advanced beginner, competence, proficiency, and expertise.[13] A modification of the Dreyfus model can be readily adapted to learning airway management skills (Table 10.1).

The desired achievement level depends on what is expected of the practitioner in practice. The advanced beginner level might be expected of the senior medical student and competence or proficiency expected of emergency medicine physicians and critical care physicians. Anesthesiology residents should be proficient or expert with several airway devices and techniques by the end of their residency. The educator needs to know a target range for number of uses of a device by each resident that will result in proficiency. Learning tables or curves for different techniques can be determined by analyzing multiple published studies (Table 10.2).

The resident must, however, receive high-quality instruction and supervision in all teaching phases to correctly employ the device or technique. Some residents and anesthesiologists will become proficient faster than others as a result of differences in prior experience or learning abilities. Qualities that are characteristic of physician experts include persistence, focus, and thoroughly honest self-assessment.[14] The most direct question to ask oneself when an airway technique fails is: "Did the device fail because of

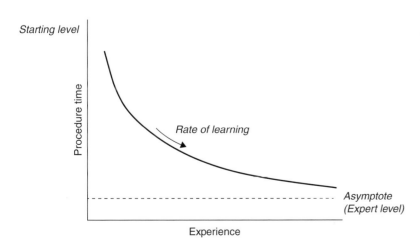

Figure 10.2 Theoretical learning curve for skill acquisition. The trainee becomes proficient when he or she approximates the asymptote of the curve.

Table 10.1 Dreyfus stages of adult skill acquisition modified for airway management skills[12]

Novice	Acquires basic rules of device use with a task trainer.
Advanced beginner	Starts to use the device in normal patients.
Competence	Can use the device in normal patients without supervision.
Proficiency	Can use the device in many patients with abnormal airways and can modify the initial technique or employ an alternate technique when the primary technique fails
Expertise	Mastery of many airway management techniques and devices and can apply them for successful management of many different airway anomalies.

Table 10.2 Benchmarks for acquisition of airway skills based on number of uses*

	AB	C	P	Reference #
Bag-Mask-Ventilation	5	15	25	94
Supraglottic Airway	5	20	40	95–97
Videolaryngoscopy	5	10	30	49–51, 53–57
Direct Laryngoscopy	5	20	50	44, 98–100
Fiberoptic Intubation	5	10	30	61, 62, 64
Transtracheal Jet Ventilation**	2	5	10	
Cricothyrotomy**	2	5	10	

AB = advanced beginner; C = competent (~85 percent success)***; P = proficient (~95 percent success)***

Competency and proficiency should be individualized for each technique

  * Best evidence summary of published studies, may not be definitive.

 ** Experience obtained with task trainers, cadavers, and/or animal models.

*** Competence and proficiency are not well defined by research.

design limitations or patient characteristics *or* was it my failure to use the device correctly?"

There are three important principles for teaching airway management:

1. If the instructor can see the same airway image at the same time the trainee sees it, the instructor can provide more effective teaching of device use. Teaching with airway devices with video capabilities (e.g., videobronchoscope, videolaryngoscope) improves the quality of teaching and shortens the time required to achieve a specific skill level.[15]

2. The best initial experience for management of the difficult airway is management of the normal airway. Trainees familiar with the use of a device for management of the normal airway would be anticipated to be more likely to successfully employ that device for the management of a difficult airway.

3. Procedural logs for residents with information about device and technique use will help the educator track each resident's progress. Procedure logs can be used to construct learning curves

for individual residents and groups of residents. The procedural log should focus on performance end points as well as the number of procedures. Specific data to include in the procedural log should include number of attempts at the procedure, when the attempt was successful, and a subjective proficiency grade as determined by the instructor (Table 10.3). Analysis of data obtained from the procedure logs can be used to improve the quality of the educational process.[16,17]

Teaching the teachers is a critical part of a successful airway education program and the positive influence of high-quality teaching with task trainers, simulators, and patients must be recognized. Anesthesiology faculty members have different airway experiences and different skills. A standardized airway management education program, however, requires that each of the teaching faculty be thoroughly familiar with the theory and practical application of the different devices and techniques to be taught.

Table 10.3 Airway device procedure log

Device: _____ Date: _____

Device attempt number (resident specific): _____

Patient Airway: Normal   Abnormal

If abnormal, describe: _____

Resident: _____

Insertion attempts: _____

Time to ventilation (CO_2 appears on capnography): _____

Proficiency grade: N   AB   C   P   E

Proficiency grade is a subjective grade by the instructor:

N = novice;

AB = advanced beginner;

C = competent;

P = proficient;

E = expert.

Role of Simulation for Airway Instruction

The rudiments of an airway device can be initially taught with the aid of task trainers (mannequins). These task trainers allow the trainee to acquire basic skills for the device. Some task trainers are specific for a unique device and others can be used for multiple devices. After the initial instruction period, the trainee can practice with the task trainer for as much time as it takes to master the basic skills. It is important, however, for the instructor to carefully guide the trainee with the task trainer. The goal is for the trainee to have *perfect (deliberate) practice*. Imperfect practice will lead to poor performance. Deliberate practice must be intense and focused on continual skill improvement. High-quality simulation-based education with *deliberate practice* has been shown to be better than traditional clinical education for the acquisition of many skills.[18] Some of the problems with current task trainers include lack of complete task/skill fidelity, variability in task trainer fidelity, and a lack of validated curricula and performance assessment. Future improvements in the fidelity of task trainers may permit a more analytic evaluation of airway skills.[19] After trainees demonstrate acquisition of the necessary basic skills on a task trainer, they can begin to use the device in patients with normal airways under close supervision by a faculty member.

High-fidelity simulation has been developed to introduce the influence of time and changes in the clinical situation on airway management. The trainee must understand that once a patient becomes apneic, ventilation must be restored within a short period. Dynamic simulation allows the instructor to mimic clinical situations and allows the trainee to employ different airway management techniques without the risk of injury to a patient. Dynamic exercises help the trainee develop critical judgment and integrate different airway management methods in a logical manner.[20]

Simulation programs based on the ASA Guidelines for Management of the Difficult Airway can be developed to teach the four different scenarios that typically occur during the administration of anesthesia (Table 10.4).

Functional Airway Anatomy and Physiology

For purposes of airway management, the anatomic upper airway extends from the nares and mouth to

Table 10.4 The four scenarios presented in the ASA difficult airway guidelines

1. Can ventilate, cannot intubate

2. Cannot ventilate, cannot intubate – supraglottic device for ventilation

3. Cannot ventilate, cannot intubate – subglottic technique required for ventilation

4. Preoperative airway examination predictive of difficult ventilation and intubation – awake intubation required

the tracheal carina. This includes the nasopharynx, oropharynx, hypopharynx, larynx, subglottis, and trachea. These are the structures that are encountered during placement of airway devices and tracheal tubes.[21]

The upper airway is a complex organ that performs mastication, swallowing, breathing, and phonation while preventing aspiration.[22] A high grade of neuromuscular coordination is required to permit these functions to occur in a coordinated fashion.[23]

Induction of anesthesia or sedation causes a decrease in pharyngeal muscle activity and subsequent displacement of the soft palate, epiglottis, and tongue against the posterior pharyngeal wall, thereby decreasing the size of the upper airway lumen and causing upper airway obstruction.[24] (See Figure 10.3.) This can be demonstrated with a fiberoptic examination of the upper airway in an anesthetized patient.

Head extension and opening of the mouth with anterior displacement of the mandible (Esmarch-Heiberg maneuver, triple airway maneuver, jaw thrust) opens the airway and relieves the obstruction.[25]

The most important aspects of physiology that the trainee must understand are the rapidity with which arterial oxygen desaturation occurs after the onset of apnea, the importance of denitrogenation, and the

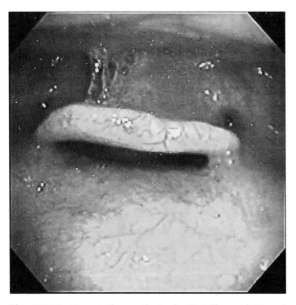

Figure 10.3 Airway in the anesthetized patient. The epiglottis and soft palate have relaxed against the posterior pharyngeal wall and have obstructed the upper airway.

effect of patient positioning on denitrogenation (e.g., denitrogenation of the morbidly obese patient in the semiupright position).[26,27] Young children, obese patients, and pregnant patients at term desaturate more quickly than lean adults (Table 10.5).

Denitrogenation increases the interval of apnea prior to hypoxemia. Once arterial oxygen saturation decreases to 90 percent, a rapid, non-linear desaturation occurs despite denitrogenation. Requesting assistance with airway management should occur as soon as the "cannot ventilate, cannot intubate" event is recognized, even if the oxygen saturation is 100 percent.

Preoperative Airway Assessment

Trainees should be instructed to answer the following questions during the preoperative airway assessment:

1. Will mask ventilation be difficult?
2. If ventilation becomes difficult, will a supraglottic device be likely to work?
3. Will intubation be difficult?
4. If ventilation and intubation become impossible, will a subglottic device be likely to work?
5. Will the patient's current clinical condition allow adequate time for difficult airway techniques?
6. If the patient is in a nonoperating room site, should the airway be managed in the operating room?
7. Will the patient's mental status (e.g., disorientation) affect the ability to perform an awake intubation?

Standard elements of the preanesthetic airway examination include mouth opening, upper lip bite test, neck mobility, thyromental distance, interdental distance, condition of the teeth, and Mallampati scoring. The Mallampati exam is a test of mouth opening and may be indicative of the ability to displace the tongue with a laryngoscope blade.[28] Many attempts have been made to develop a preoperative airway assessment method that accurately predicts difficult airway management. None of the proposed assessment methods, however, has proven to be completely reliable.[29] In a study of 1,502 patients, Langeron reported a 5 percent incidence (75 patients) of difficult mask ventilation; however, only 1 patient was impossible to ventilate. Of the 75 patients with difficult mask ventilation, only 17 percent were predicted from the preoperative exam.[30] Kheterpal in a study of 22,660 patients reported a difficult mask ventilation

Table 10.5 Time to arterial oxygen saturation of 90 percent after apnea (minutes) [26,27,101–103]

Age	No Denitrogenation	Denitrogenation
1 month	0.25	1.5–1.9
8 years	0.47	3.1–3.9
18 years	0.74	5.1
Lean adult	1	7–8
Obese adult (supine)	< 1	2.7
Obese (semiupright)	< 1	3.6
Pregnant woman	0.26	4

incidence of 1.4 percent and an impossible mask ventilation incidence of 0.16 percent.[31]

Teaching airway assessment should encompass the breadth of airway assessment yet focus on the modalities with highest predictive value. Trainees will benefit from bedside teaching that emphasizes predictors of straightforward and difficult airways. The imperfect predictive value of airway assessment, however, serves as a rationale for routine, well-formed plans for unanticipated difficult airway management.

Airway Devices and Techniques

In the next sections of this chapter, different types of devices and airway management techniques are discussed and important information pertaining to each one is presented. This information provides the foundation for the development of comprehensive instruction of airway devices and techniques.

Pharyngeal Airways

After deep sedation or general anesthesia, relaxation of the pharyngeal muscles causes the tongue, soft palate, and epiglottis to relax and obstruct the upper airway. Nasopharyngeal and oropharyngeal airways (OPAs) are designed to push the base of the tongue and epiglottis anteriorly, thereby opening the airway. Although many different types of oropharyngeal airways have been used, the classic design of the Guedel OPA has proven to be the most useful. Proper sizing of the OPA is important as improper sizing may aggravate airway obstruction. An OPA that is too small can push the tongue posteriorly and obstruct the airway. An OPA that is too long can deflect the epiglottis into the glottic inlet and cause airway obstruction.[32] Most adults will require a 9 cm or 10 cm OPA. The wide variation in the size of children requires a readily available supply of many different OPA sizes.

Optimal bag-mask ventilation should be stressed after induction of anesthesia as it maximizes oxygenation and will increase the time to hypoxia after apnea begins. Two-person ventilation is a very effective ventilation technique that is often overlooked.[33] One person inserts an OPA and elevates the mandible with two hands (triple airway maneuver, jaw thrust) while maintaining a tight fit of the mask on the face. This maneuver opens the upper airway and seals the face-mask to the face. The second person compresses the reservoir bag and manually ventilates the patient (Figure 10.4). Alternatively, one person can employ the two-handed technique and use the anesthesia ventilator to provide mechanical ventilation.

Supraglottic Airways

The invention of the laryngeal mask airway (LMA®) by Brain provided a new method for airway management.[34] Since the LMA was introduced into clinical practice in the United Kingdom (1988) and the United States (1991), many types of supraglottic airways (SGA) have been developed (Table 10.6). New models of SGAs are continually being introduced into clinical practice.

The thousands of articles about SGA use that have been published since Brain's initial report are a testament to the success of the basic design. Although the SGA is relatively simple in concept, proper insertion technique of the different types is critical for successful application to a wide variety of patients. Despite the wide variety SGA models available, the fundamentals of insertion and use for all SGAs are similar (Table 10.7).[35]

A
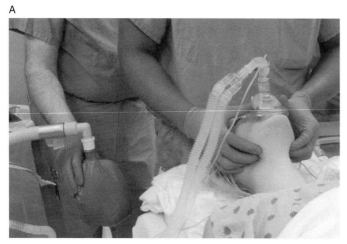

B
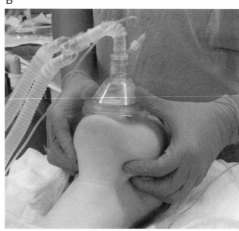

Figure 10.4 Two-person ventilation after induction of anesthesia. (A) Insertion of an oral airway and two-handed jaw thrust in preparation for two-person ventilation. (B) Second person is providing manual ventilation as the first maintains an open airway.

Evidence suggests that there is a short-term and a long-term learning curve. Proficiency with SGA insertion can be achieved within 50 to 75 uses, although competence can be achieved with as few as 10 uses.[36] The degree of expertise, however, required for anesthesiologists for diverse applications may require several hundred uses. [37] Fiberoptic examination through the SGA after it has been positioned provides valuable information for the trainee concerning correct position and potential malposition (Figure 10.5). Such information can help the trainee manage SGA placement problems.

Introduction of a tracheal tube through an SGA is an important strategy in management of a difficult airway. The SGA may be useful after failed intubation to maintain or establish ventilation. Once ventilation is established, the SGA can be used as a conduit for tracheal intubation. Although blind advancement of a tracheal tube through the SGA can be attempted, fiberscopic guidance of a tracheal tube (with or without an intubation catheter) is more reliable and demonstrated in the video found at this website: www.youtube.com/watch?v=o_ShiJed3Es.[38] Intubation through an SGA has a high failure rate when performed by an inexperienced anesthesiologist. Training, however, increases the likelihood of success.

The intubating LMA (ILMA) is a useful device for management of the difficult airway as it serves two functions. It can be used as an SGA for ventilation and as a conduit for tracheal intubation. The design

features that permit tracheal intubation include a wide-bore, anatomically curved airway tube and a hinged epiglottic elevating bar (Figure 10.6).

As the tracheal tube passes through the airway tube, the tracheal tube deflects the elevating bar upward and moves the epiglottis out of the way of the advancing tracheal tube. The ILMA will accommodate an 8.0 mm tracheal tube. The tracheal tube can be passed blindly through the airway tube and into the trachea. The first attempt of blind tracheal tube passage is, however, not always successful. Fiberscopic guidance of the tracheal tube through the glottis and into the trachea is more reliable.[39]

There are several SGAs (e.g., combitube, laryngeal tube) that are not widely used by anesthesiologists in the operating room, but are commonly used by healthcare providers for prehospital resuscitation.[40] It is, however, incumbent on the anesthesiologists to be familiar with these devices. The overall success of prehospital resuscitation is poor and the choice of airway management techniques is controversial.[41]

Conventional Laryngoscopy

Although there have been many modifications of laryngoscope blades, conventional rigid direct laryngoscopy has changed little over the past 80 years. Successful tracheal intubation using direct laryngoscopy requires line of sight. Human anatomy precludes line-of-sight visualization of the larynx without airway manipulation. The rigid laryngoscope

Table 10.6 Examples of supraglottic airways

Laryngeal Mask Airway	
Reusable	
Classic	
ProSeal	
Flexible	
Single Use	
Protector	
Unique Evo	
Fastrach (ILMA)	
Supreme	
I-Gel	
Ambu	
AuraOnce	
Aura-i	
AuraGain	
Aura40	
Air-Q	
Air-Q	
Air-Q Blocker	
Laryngeal Tube	
Combitube	
Reusable Laryngeal Masks	
LMA®	LMA® Classic™
	LMA® ProSeal™
	LMA® Flexible™
Single Use Laryngeal Masks	
LMA®	LMA® Protector™
	LMA® unique Evo™
	LMA® Fastrach™ (ILMA)
	LMA® Supreme™
i-gel™	i-gel™ supraglottic airway
Ambu®	AuraGain™
	Aura-i™
	AuraOnce™
	AuraFlex™
	AuraStraight™
	Aura40™
air-Q®	air-Q™
	air-Q blocker™
Laryngeal Tubes	
Combitube®	Combitube™
Ambu®	King-LT-D™
	King LTS-D™

Table 10.7 Instruction program for supraglottic airway

Task Trainer
1. Instruction of insertion technique by faculty.
2. Trainee practice with SGA.
3. Fiberscopic examination of SGA placement.
4. Practice tracheal intubation through SGA.
a. Fiberscopic assistance.
b. Blind with intubating LMA.
Patient (Lean, Normal Airway Anatomy)
1. Insertion demonstration by faculty.
2. Fiberscopic examination of position after faculty insertion.
3. Trainee insertion followed by fiberscopic examination.
4. After competence with SGA in adults, SGA insertion in children.

A
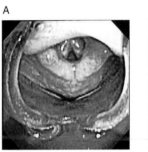
B
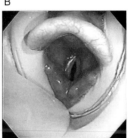
C
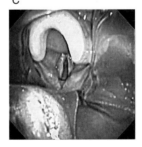

Figure 10.5 Fiberoptic views through different LMAs in normal position. (A) Unique™ (single use) LMA, (B) Proseal™ LMA, (C) Supreme™ LMA.

blade provides direct visualization of the laryngeal inlet by displacing the tongue into the submandibular space. The incidence of difficulty with conventional laryngoscopy is much higher than normally assumed. Minor difficulty occurs in more than one-third of surgical patients and moderate to severe difficulty occurs in 8–13 percent of intubations.[42,43] Although many of the difficulties can be overcome, the risk of injury to the upper airway increases as

A

B

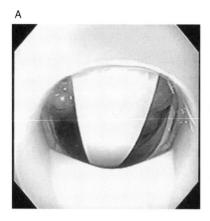
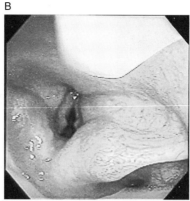

Figure 10.6 Fiberoptic views through an intubating LMA. (A) Epiglottic elevating bar. (B) The tracheal tube has deflected the elevating bar and has pushed the epiglottis out of the way of the advancing tracheal tube.

Table 10.8 Instruction program for direct laryngoscopy

Task Trainer

1. Review of upper airway anatomy.
2. Review of proper patient positioning.
3. Demonstration of laryngoscopy with C-MAC® videolaryngoscope by instructor.
4. Trainee practice with videolaryngoscope, conventional laryngoscope with curved and straight blades.

Operating Room Patient (Lean, Normal Airway)

1. Trainee intubations (10) with C-MAC® videolaryngoscope.
2. Trainee intubations (10) with conventional laryngoscope with Macintosh blade.
3. Trainee intubation (10) with conventional laryngoscope with Miller blade.

more force is exerted by the laryngoscope blade on upper airway tissue to obtain direct line of sight to the laryngeal inlet.

Direct laryngoscopy is a skill that every anesthesiologist must master and any provider delivering emergency patient care must be competent (Table 10.8).

Proficiency with direct laryngoscopy requires more attempts than is generally assumed and most likely exceeds 50 successful intubations.[44,45] The technical nature of tracheal intubation is such that some trainees will achieve competence with fewer attempts than other trainees. All trainees should complete an instructional course that requires repeated, successful intubation of a task trainer prior to attempting to intubate patients. Emphasis should be placed on proper positioning of the patient and correct technique to

avoid excessive force and soft tissue trauma during laryngoscopy. A comparison between how experienced and inexperienced laryngoscopists manipulate the laryngoscope has shown a difference. Experienced laryngoscopists hold the laryngoscope closer to the junction of the handle and blade (Figure 10.7A), whereas, inexperienced laryngoscopists hold the laryngoscope by the handle (Figure 10.7B).

The technique used by novices is more likely to result in a lever action on the upper teeth, thereby increasing the risk of patient injury.[46] Instruction in proper laryngoscope grip in the initial phases of teaching will improve performance.

Several introducers (airway exchange catheter, AEC) and stylets have been developed to assist with tracheal intubation (Table 10.9).[47]

Stylets are placed inside the tracheal tube and manipulated to guide the tracheal tube into the larynx (Figure 10.8).

Introducers are devices of small diameter that are designed to be passed through the glottis and into the trachea when glottic exposure is poor and a tracheal tube cannot be directly inserted (Figure 10.9).

After passage of an introducer into the trachea, the tracheal tube is threaded over the introducer. Introducers may be used with a laryngoscope or an SGA. Some introducers are hollow to accommodate a flexible fiberoptic scope. Hollow introducers may be fitted with a 15-mm connector that can be attached to an anesthesia breathing circuit for the delivery of oxygen. Positive pressure ventilation through a long narrow tube, however, is not always easy. AECs can be used for a staged extubation in patients when the ability to tolerate extubation is questionable (Figure 10.10). Introducers and AECs

A

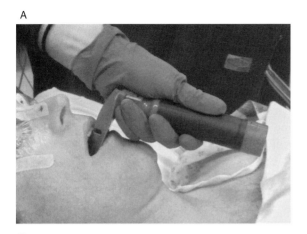

B

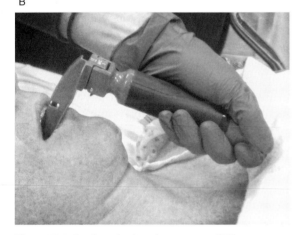

Figure 10.7 Hand grip for direct laryngoscopy. (A) The experienced laryngoscopist grips the laryngoscope at the junction of the handle and the blade. (B) The inexperienced laryngoscopist grips the laryngoscope higher up the handle. This grip increases the likelihood of pressure and leverage on the teeth.

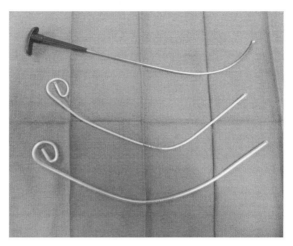

Figure 10.8 Tracheal tube stylets. (A) The stylet at the top is a rigid stylet to be used with the GlideScope® (Verathon). (B) The bottom two stylets are malleable adult and pediatric stylets (Teleflex, Ireland).

Table 10.9 Examples of tracheal tube introducers

Frova Intubating Introducer* (www.cookmedical.com/products/cc_caefii_webds; accessed November 5, 201/)
Cook® Airway Exchange Catheter* (www.cookmedical.com/products/cc_cae_webds/; accessed November 5, 2017)
Arndt Airway Exchange Catheter* (www.cookmedical.com/products/cc_caelma_webds/; accessed November 5, 2017)
Aintree Intubation Catheter* (www.cookmedical.com/products/cc_caeaic_webds/; accessed November 5, 2017)
Eschmann-Style Bougie**(www.sharn.com/bougies/p/TrachealTubeIntroducer/; accessed November 5, 2017)
Malleable Intubating S-Guide**(www.sharn.com/bougies/p/TrachealTubeIntroducer/; accessed November 5, 2017)
InterGuide Tracheal Tube Introducer Bougie***(www.intersurgical.com/products/airway-management/interguide-tracheal-tube-introducer-bougiel; accessed November 5, 2017)

 * Cook Medical (Bloomington, IN) (www.cookmedical.com; accessed November 5 2017)
 ** Sharn Anesthesia, Inc. (Tampa, FL) (www.sharn.com; accessed November 5, 2017)
 *** Intersurgical Ltd. (Berkshire, UK) (www.intersurgical.com; accessed November 5, 2017)

can cause airway trauma such as bronchial rupture and pneumothorax.[48]

Trainees should practice the use of introducers and exchange catheters on task trainers until they are completely familiar with the technique. Tracheal tube exchange with an introducer should not be performed by the inexperienced laryngoscopist in a patient with a difficult airway.

Videolaryngoscopy

The major difficulty with conventional, direct laryngoscopy is that it requires line of sight for the laryngoscopist to see the glottis. Early indirect intubating laryngoscopes relied on fiberoptic bundles attached to a rigid laryngoscope blade. These devices, however, achieved only limited success. The development of miniature imaging devices (charge-coupled devices, CCDs) allowed manufacturers to introduce a new type of indirect laryngoscope: videolaryngoscopes. Although the GlideScope was the first videolaryngoscope to gain widespread use, others quickly became available (Table 10.10) (Figure 10.11).[49]

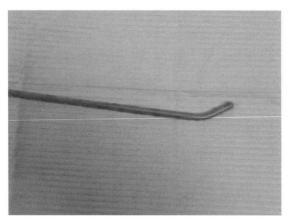

Figure 10.9 Bougie. Note the curved distal end to facilitate passage into an anteriorly directed glottis inlet. The bougie serves as a guide for passage of an endotracheal tube (SunMed, Largo, FL 33773).

A

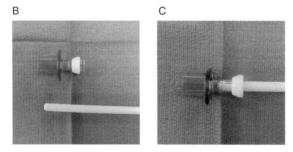

B   C

Figure 10.10 Airway exchange catheter (Cook Medical, Bloomington, IN 47404). (A) Distal hollow end of AEC, (B) Proximal end of AEC with unattached 15 mm connector, (C) Proximal end of AEC with 15 mm connector attached.

Two basic designs of videolaryngoscopes have evolved. One type has an open blade requiring the use of a styleted tracheal tube. The second type has a channel or tunnel that accommodates the tracheal tube and guides the tube into the larynx.

Many articles have been published about the use of videolaryngoscopes in patients with normal and difficult airways. Experienced anesthesiologists have similar intubation performance with videolaryngoscopes and traditional laryngoscopes in patients with normal airways. In patients where direct laryngoscopy has failed, compared with a repeat attempt with a conventional laryngoscope and blade the time to intubation is shorter and the rate of success is > 90 percent with a videolaryngoscope.[50–52] Inexperienced laryngscopists have a higher rate of successful intubation of patients with normal airways with a videolaryngoscope.[53,54]

The videolaryngoscope, however, is a very useful tool for teaching clinical laryngoscopy. When instructing trainees with no experience with laryngoscopy in patients, the instructor can demonstrate upper airway anatomy and landmarks for tracheal intubation. The trainee can then perform several intubations with the videolaryngoscope and then progress to conventional laryngoscopes.

The technique for videolaryngoscopy is different than the technique for direct laryngoscopy. It is important to keep the videolaryngoscope blade in the midline and place the tip of the blade proximal in the vallecula. Once the blade is positioned, a slight radial deviation of the laryngoscopist's left wrist will rotate the glottic inlet posteriorly. If the blade of the videolaryngoscope is inserted too deeply into the vallecula, the glottis is pushed caudad making passage of the tracheal tube more difficult (Video 10.1).

The hyperangulation of most videolarygnoscope blades permits a good view of the glottis. Passage of a tracheal tube, however, can be difficult and a stylet is usually required to guide the tracheal tube into the glottic opening.

Videolaryngoscopes provide a wide-angle view of the hypopharynx and improved visualization of the glottis in patients with pharyngeal pathology, such as tonsillar hypertrophy, posttonsillectomy bleeding or a tonsillar abscess (Video 10.2).

Which videolaryngoscope is the best is a subject of considerable debate. There are several commercially available videolaryngoscopes. The C-MAC and GlideScope are the most popular. The C-MAC seems to be the preferred videolaryngoscope for both experienced and novice laryngoscopists.[55–57] As described in the preceding text, the standard curved blade for the C-MAC is very similar to the standard Macintosh blade and is very convenient for tracheal intubation of a wide variety of patients. A stylet is very rarely

Table 10.10 Videolaryngoscopes

GlideScope® (https://verathon.com/glidescope/, accessed November 5, 2017) (Verathon, Bothell, WA) (https://verathon.com; accessed November 5, 2017)
C-MAC® (www.karlstorz.com/us/en/anesthesiology-and-emergency-medicine.htm; accessed November 5, 2017) (Karl Storz Endoscopy – America, Inc., El Segundo, CA) (www.karlstorz.com/us/en/human-medicine.htm; accessed November 5, 2017)
McGrath® MAC EDL (www.medtronic.com/covidien/en-us/products/intubation/mcgrath-mac-enhanced-direct-laryngoscope.html; accessed November 5, 2017) (Medtronic, Dublin, Ireland) (www.medtronic.com/covidien/en-us/products.html; accessed November 5, 2017)
Airtraq® (www.airtraq.com/products/airtraq-avant-routine-intubations/; accessed November 5, 2017) (Airtraq LLC, Fenton, MO) (www.airtraq.com; accessed November 5, 2017)
King Vision® Videolaryngoscope (www.ambuusa.com/usa/products/anesthesia/product/king_vision_video_laryngoscope-prod18730.aspx; accessed November 5, 2017) (Ambu, Columbia, MD) (www.ambuusa.com/usa/home.aspx; accessed November 5, 2017)
Truview Video Laryngoscope™ (www.truphatek.com/video.php%3fID=1; accessed November 5, 2017) (Teleflex, Morrisville, NC) (www.truphatek.com; accessed November 5, 2017)
Pentax AWS-S200® (www.dremed.com/pentax-airway-scope-aws-video-laryngoscope/id/2111; accessed November 5, 2017) (Pentax Medical USA, Montvale, NJ) (www.pentaxmedical.com/pentax/service/usa; accessed November 5, 2017)

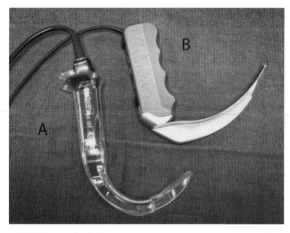

Figure 10.11 GlideScope® and C-MAC® Videolaryngoscopes. Note hyperangulated blade of the GlideScope (A). The C-MAC (B) has a blade similar in design to the conventional Macintosh blade.

required for the C-MAC. The hyperangulated blade of the GlideScope, however, may be better for some patients with limited neck mobility. Because the video feed is from the tip of the laryngoscope blade, a styleted tracheal tube is usually required to conform to the angulation of the blade for successful tracheal intubation with the GlideScope. Techniques for stylet manipulation should also be taught.

Some anesthesiologists have proposed that videolaryngoscopy should be the new standard for tracheal intubation.[58,59] Whether videolaryngoscopy becomes routine for tracheal intubation, all anesthesia providers should be thoroughly familiar with at least two different types of videolaryngoscopes.

The influence of videolaryngoscopy on tracheal intubation of patients with normal and difficult airways has been significant. The anesthesiology resident should become very proficient with both the C-MAC and GlideScope.

Flexible Fiberoptic Airway Endoscopy

Flexible fiberoptic airway endoscopy is a skill that every anesthesiology resident should master during training. The fiberoptic endoscope (bronchoscope or laryngoscope) is valuable as a tracheal intubation assist device for patients with different types of airway anomalies and is an excellent diagnostic tool for evaluation of airway problems.

Control and navigation of the flexible endoscope are the critical skills that must be mastered. Initial instruction with the basics of fiberoptic control can be done with nonanatomic models (bench models) that require a variety of manipulation skills.[60] Such models are inexpensive to construct and allow the trainee unlimited practice (Figure 10.12).

The novice endoscopist often grasps the fiberscope 25 to 30 cm from the tip of the scope (Figure 10.13A). This grip position allows the fiberscope too much freedom of movement and diminishes effective control. Holding the fiberscope closer to the tip, near the patient's mouth, permits better scope control (Figure 10.13B).

A

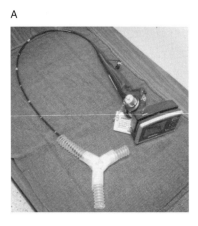

B

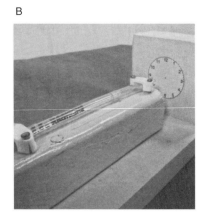

Figure 10.12 Task trainers for teaching navigation of the flexible fiberscope. (A) Simple tracheobronchial model that can be made in minutes in the operating room area. (B) More elaborate task trainer that requires finer control skills than the task trainer in 8A. The fiberscope is inserted into the tube and the trainee is asked to center each number on the circle.

A

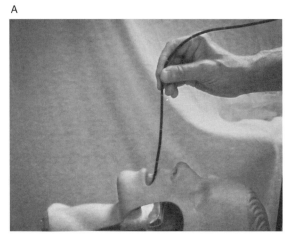

B

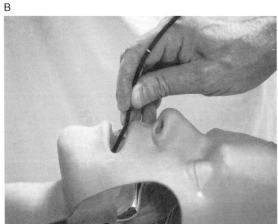

Figure 10.13 Grip position for the flexible fiberscope. (A) Incorrect position high on the fiberscope. This grip position allows the fiberscope tip too much freedom of movement. (B) Correct hand position near the patient's mouth. This grip permits better control of the fiberscope.

It is important that the resident be closely supervised during this phase to ensure that trainee learns correct fiberscope control technique. Once the trainees can demonstrate mastery of fiberscope control, they can advance to orotracheal intubation of anesthetized patients with normal airways (Figure 10.14).[61]

The anesthetized, paralyzed patient with a normal airway represents the ideal opportunity for the first orotracheal fiberoptic intubations for a resident (Table 10.11).

Most residents can become competent with orotracheal fiberoptic-assisted tracheal intubation after intubating ten anesthetized patients with normal airways.[62] Residents who perform 35 fiberoptic tracheal intubations in a six to eight week period should become proficient (Figure 10.15).

Insertion of an intubating oral airway (Ovassapian, Williams, Berman) prior to fiberoptic endoscopy can be helpful to the trainee during the initial intubations[63] (Figure 10.16).

These airways direct the fiberscope into the midline of the pharynx and open the airway to improve visualization of the glottis. After the trainee develops good fiberscope control skills, the airway may not be needed. Another assist maneuver that increases the success rate for fiberoptic intubation is the insufflation of oxygen (4–6 L/min) through the working channel (Figure 10.17).

The cool, dry oxygen will keep the lens or charge-coupled device (CCD) from fogging and the flow of oxygen through the channel will blow pharyngeal secretions away from the lens/CCD. In addition, the insufflation of oxygen may permit a longer interval of apnea before the development of hypoxemia.

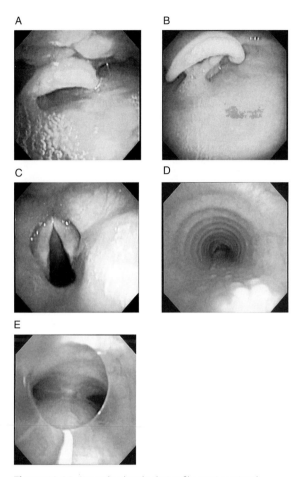

Figure 10.14 Airway landmarks during fiberoptic-assisted tracheal intubation of an anesthetized patient. (A) Before jaw thrust. Epiglottis is against the posterior pharyngeal wall; (B) The glottic inlet is now visible after jaw thrust; (C) At the level of the vocal cords; (D) The trachea; (E) Tracheal tube is above the carina.

It is not recommended that trainees begin clinical fiberoptic training with awake patients. Sedation and topical airway anesthesia for awake intubation are different skills and it is best to teach these skill sets independent of each other.

The introduction of CCD-based video fiberscopes has greatly improved the efficiency of teaching fiberoptic tracheal intubation.[64] These fiberscopes produce wide-angle, high-resolution images displayed on video monitors. Instructors can provide more effective teaching when they can see the same image as the trainee. Navigation skills are quickly taught with a task trainer and a videobronchoscope (Figure 10.18).

In addition to its use in tracheal intubation, the flexible fiberscope is an excellent diagnostic tool if the status of the airway is unknown. Preoperative

Table 10.11 Instruction program for fiberoptic-assisted tracheal intubation

Task Trainer Part I	Small group, four residents: one faculty
	Demonstration of fiberscope parts and control mechanisms
	Instruction of fiberscope navigation technique with bench model
	Residents use bench model with faculty direction
Task Trainer Part II	Resident intubates anatomic model with a videobronchoscope under faculty direction
Ten Patient Intubations with Videobronchoscope	Lean patients with normal upper airway anatomy
	General anesthesia with muscle relaxation
	Positive pressure ventilation (PPV) with face mask with 100 percent O_2
	2.5 minutes of endoscopy time (SpO_2 monitored)
	Faculty provides jaw thrust
	May use an intubating oral airway (Ovassapian airway)
	If unsuccessful after 2.5 minutes, PPV
	Another 2.5 minutes of endoscopy time

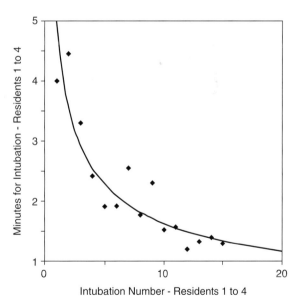

Figure 10.15 A resident's learning curve for fiberoptic tracheal intubation (Figure percent from C. Johnson, J. T. Roberts. Clinical competence in the performance of fiberoptic laryngoscopy and endotracheal intubation: A study of resident instruction. *J Clin Anesth* 1989; 1: 344–9).

fiberoptic examination of the upper airway can provide information that is useful for the development of a plan for airway management (Figure 10.19).[65]

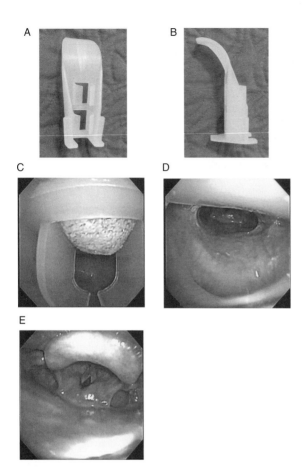

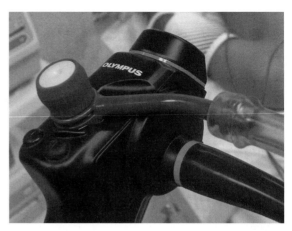

Figure 10.17 Connecting oxygen to fiberscope. Oxygen tube from the auxiliary flow meter on the anesthesia machine attached to the working channel of the fiberscope (4–6 L/min). The oxygen flow keeps secretions off the lens/CCD and prevents fogging. It may provide apneic oxygenation for the patient.

Figure 10.16 Ovassapian intubating airway. (A) Ovassapian airway from above. Notice slot for passage of tracheal tube; (B) Ovassapian airway, side view; (C) Ovassapian airway inserted; (D) Ovassapian airway keeps the fiberscope centered; (E) Fiberscope view of glottis through Ovassapian airway.

Subglottic (Invasive) Airway

Subglottic airways are techniques, which invasively enter the trachea, intended to provide emergent rescue from "cannot intubate, cannot ventilate" (CICV) situations. These procedures are rare, high stress, and high stakes. The decision to insert an invasive airway is often made only after numerous nonsurgical attempts have failed and devastating morbidity is imminent. As more effective supraglottic and video devices have been developed, the need for subglottic techniques has diminished, but situations still exist in which an invasive subglottic airway is lifesaving.[66]

Anesthesiologists should receive comprehensive instruction in invasive airway techniques. The invasive nature of these procedures poses an educational challenge because it is not feasible to electively gain experience on human subjects. Experience must be obtained with simulators, animal models, or cadavers.[67] Fresh or well-preserved cadavers provide an excellent model for invasive airway management. Logistic, ethical, and cost concerns, however, present obstacles that can be difficult to overcome to develop a cadaver program that permits all trainees to have an adequate number of attempts.[68] The most readily available method for anesthesia training programs is in the simulation laboratory with task trainers and simulators. Isolated tracheas of pigs have also been successfully used to teach both cricothyrotomy and tracheostomy.[69,70] The emergency subglottic techniques require identification of the cricothyroid membrane as the first step in the sequence. The ability to identify the cricothyroid membrane is not always easy and the trainee must receive proper instruction.[71,72] It is good practice for residents to identify the cricothyroid membrane in every patient during the preoperative airway assessment.

In clinical practice, the best resource for a patient who may require a subglottic, invasive airway is a surgeon experienced with airway surgery. If the anesthesiologist anticipates the potential need for an invasive airway technique, the immediate availability of a surgeon with these skills is sound practice.

Jet Ventilation

Transtracheal jet ventilation (TTJV) can provide effective ventilation for the CICV scenario. After

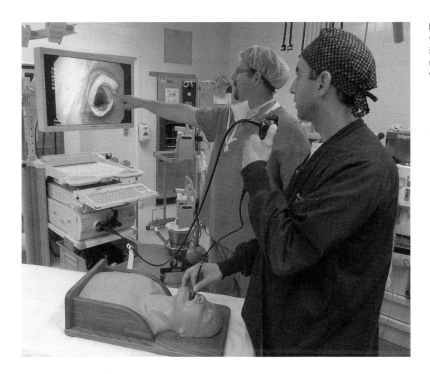

Figure 10.18 Instruction in use of videobronchoscope. An instructor instructs a trainee on fiberscope navigation with a mannequin and a videobronchoscope.

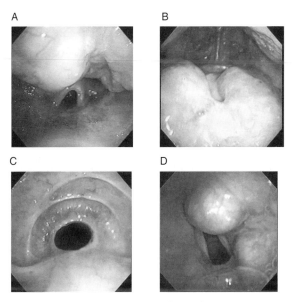

Figure 10.19 Airway pathology. The flexible fiberscope as a diagnostic device. (A) Lingual tonsil hyperplasia frequently complicates direct laryngoscopy; (B) Posterior pharyngeal tumor producing significant airway obstruction; (C) Unsuspected tracheal web; (D) Laryngeal cyst encountered during routine intubation.

insertion of a 14-, 16-, or 18-gauge catheter through the cricothyroid membrane, a high-pressure oxygen source (50 psi) can provide an oxygen flow of 500 ml/sec. The components of a TTJV system include a transtracheal catheter (14, 16, or 18 gauge), a jet oxygen injector, and noncompliant tubing that connects the catheter and the injector.[73] Skills required for TTJV are insertion of the catheter over a needle device through the cricothyroid membrane and confirmation of the catheter in the airway by aspiration of air through the catheter (Figure 10.20).

The process of transtracheal catheter placement uses equipment and skills that most anesthesiologists are comfortable with and is conceptually appealing. Furthermore, by using the transtracheal approach for airway topicalization, one can gain comfort and experience advancing a needle through the cricothyroid membrane into the trachea. Because the same procedure is required for a needle-based Seldinger cricothyrotomy technique, the transtracheal catheter can be used for conversion to a cricothyrotomy.[74] Failures of the TTJV device (42 percent) and complications associated with barotrauma (32 percent) are frequently reported with TTJV and the place of TTJV in emergency airway management has been called into question.[75] The 2015 Difficult Airway Society (DAS, United Kingdom) guidelines for management of unanticipated difficult intubation in adults recommends open surgical cricothyrotomy as the invasive airway technique of choice in the can't intubate, can't oxygenate (CICO) situation.[76] The failures

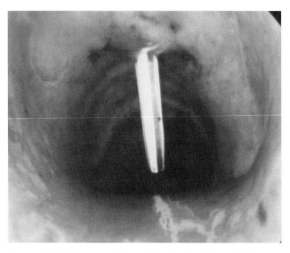

Figure 10.20 Fiberscopic view of transtracheal jet ventilation catheter. The catheter has been inserted through the cricothyroid membrane.

of TTJV, however, may simply be the result of inadequate training. The anesthesiologist is very familiar with needle or catheter insertion into the cricothyroid membrane and better training may favor TTJV for the anesthesiologist.

Cricothyrotomy

Conventional cricothyrotomy is performed by making an incision in the neck that extends through the cricothyroid membrane and allows passage of a tube of adequate diameter to permit positive pressure ventilation. Successful insertion of a subglottic device requires considerable practice and inexperienced physicians typically perform poorly with subglottic techniques.[77] Performance can be dramatically improved and better adherence to the ASA difficult airway guidelines obtained with in-depth training and frequent practice.[78,79]

Tracheostomy techniques using the Seldinger technique with exchange of a dilator and cannula over a wire are appealing and tend to perform well in simulations; however, the failure rate in clinical practice is significant and scalpel-based approaches have a higher success rate and take less time to perform. During a one-year period in the United Kingdom, emergency surgical tracheostomies and cricothyrotomies were all successful, whereas TTJV and cannula-based cricothyrotomy techniques had a 65 percent failure rate.[80] The cricothyrotomies, however, were performed by surgeons and not anesthesiologists.

Difficult Airway Management

Awake Intubation

The patient with the risk of failed ventilation after induction of anesthesia will require tracheal intubation when awake. A thorough discussion of the reason for the awake intubation must be done with the patient beforehand. The patient's safety must be emphasized during that discussion. The instructor must convey to the trainee the proper way to discuss awake tracheal intubation with the patient. Trainees who perform awake intubations must be competent with the intubation device.

Patient comfort during intubation is paramount to successful awake tracheal intubation. The patient may be sedated, but must remain cooperative during the procedure. Sedation increases patient comfort, but is no substitute for good topical anesthesia. Sedation can be achieved with small doses of benzodiazepines, fentanyl, or dexmedetomidine or a combination of the drugs.

Many methods for airway anesthesia have been described.[81] For most patients, topical anesthesia by direct application of local anesthetic to the airway mucosa will produce satisfactory anesthesia for the procedure, making nerve blocks unnecessary. Patients with head and neck tumors can have distorted anatomy that complicates performance of nerve blocks for upper airway anesthesia. Irrespective of the technique chosen to establish anesthesia of the airway, emphasis must be placed on repeated testing of the patient for lack of sensation and ablation of upper airway reflexes prior to instrumentation of the airway.

It must be stressed to the trainee that the technique for awake intubation is conscious sedation with airway anesthesia. Administration of more sedatives to compensate for inadequate airway anesthesia can result in a lost airway and a potential disaster.[82]

Advanced Planning for Difficult Airway Management

Preparation for management of the patient with a difficult airway should occur at three levels: individual, departmental, and institutional. Prediction of the difficult airway is not always easy and preparation for such events is critical to success. The individual must be responsible for developing and maintaining the necessary skills for airway management. Although basic instruction occurs during training, random experiential learning during residency is insufficient for the resident to become proficient with many techniques. Instruction can be enhanced with online programs with video and hands-on workshops. Practice of infrequently used airway management techniques in the simulation laboratory will help maintain skills. Once the patient is unconscious and airway management becomes complicated, rapid response and restoration of adequate ventilation become imperative. All anesthesia providers must know where additional equipment is stored and personnel must be able to transport the equipment to the point of care.

Difficult Airway Team

Part of the responsibility of the education process is not just to train the resident how to manage the difficult airway, but also to help them establish ways to respond to the difficult airway when they leave the protected environment of the educational program in which they are training. Not all anesthesia providers are equally skilled with management of the difficult airway. Those anesthesiologists with exceptional airway management skills can be organized into a difficult airway team. The members of this team should be summoned as soon as difficulty occurs. Practice drills will help engrain proper response techniques and minimize the time required for movement of personnel and equipment.

Compared to airway management in the operating room, airway management outside of the operating room has a significantly higher incidence of complications.[83,84] A multidisciplinary plan for management of the patient with a difficult airway who presents outside of the operating room (e.g., emergency department, intensive care unit, ward) helps reduce adverse outcomes. These multidisciplinary teams form the basis for education and ensure that expertise is present during difficult airway management, assure that airway equipment is standardized throughout the hospital, and improves awareness of difficult airways. The team approach has been shown to reduce complications of airway management in the operating room and throughout the hospital.[85-87] Identification of patients having known difficult airways with special identification bracelets is also helpful.[88] In addition, some form of "tag" on patients in the intensive care unit who experienced a difficult intubation will serve to alert personnel to contact the difficult airway team in the event of an inadvertent extubation or to make certain that a backup plan is in place at the time of planned extubation.

Simulation Laboratory

The simulation laboratory is a valuable resource for development of a comprehensive airway management instructional program. There are two levels of education that can be provided to anesthesiology residents. The first phase focuses on the use of different devices with ample time provided for instruction until the resident can properly use the different devices and techniques. The second phase is advanced airway management based on the ASA Guidelines for Management of the Patient with a Difficult Airway and is aimed at helping the resident develop and apply sound decision-making skills when confronted with airway management difficulties. This program encompasses the four typical clinical scenarios that an anesthesiologist will encounter (Table 10.4).

At the Medical University of South Carolina, residents in their first year of clinical anesthesia training receive eight hours of intensive airway training in one day (two four-hour sessions). One faculty member can instruct four residents during this program. The course is standardized and residents are objectively evaluated and debriefed at the conclusion of the workshop. During the second and third years of residency, a four-hour refresher workshop is conducted. The simulations are conducted in real time and help the resident develop integrative organizational and performance skills. Residents who have completed these workshops demonstrate logical approaches to management of both anticipated and unanticipated difficult airways that occur during clinical practice.

While simulation training is ideal, the cost of opening a simulation laboratory in terms of money, time, and personnel is significant. At the present time, the availability of commercial, "off the shelf" difficult airway management simulators, scenarios, and curricula is limited. Laerdal (Wappingers Falls, NY; www.laerdal.com/us/; accessed November 5, 2017) markets the SimMan® (www.laerdal.com/us/doc/86/SimMan; accessed November 5, 2017) and CAE Healthcare (Sarasota, FL; https://caehealthcare.com; accessed November 5, 2017) markets the CAE HPS Human Patient Simulator (https://caehealthcare.com/patient-simulation/hps; accessed November 5, 2017). The buyer must be sure that the simulator has the necessary parts and software required for airway management instruction.

Complications of Airway Management

All anesthesia trainees must develop a profound respect for the dangers of airway mismanagement. They must learn to give careful thought in preparation for airway management of both normal and abnormal airways. Because preoperative assessment methods are not perfect, seemingly normal airways can be difficult.

Failure to Ventilate and Intubate

The outcome from a failure to ventilate and oxygenate for even a short time can result in permanent neurologic injury or death. The trainee must always strive to maintain or improve ventilation and oxygenation. An airway management technique that sacrifices ventilation in an attempt to perform intubation will result in a poor outcome if intubation fails and ventilation cannot be reestablished.

Esophageal Intubation

Every experienced anesthesiologist has inadvertently intubated the esophagus. Early recognition of esophageal intubation and correct tracheal tube placement minimizes the risk of a significant adverse outcome. A capnograph or chemical carbon dioxide indicator should be monitored for every tracheal intubation.

Airway Injury

Minor airway injury is extremely common and occurs in more than 50 percent of patients. Most of the injuries are mild to moderate and consist of abrasions to the tongue, lip, or pharyngeal mucosa.[89] Although the injuries may be minor, patients may experience considerable discomfort and dissatisfaction with their anesthesiologist's care. Every effort should be made to avoid any injury to airway structures.

More serious injuries from airway management include vocal cord paralysis, arytenoid dislocation, pharyngoesophageal perforation, tracheal laceration, and death. Pharyngoesophageal perforation is difficult to diagnose and mortality exceeds 20 percent.[90,91]

Conclusion

Management of patients with difficult airways is a dynamic practice and is influenced by the patient's anatomic and physiologic abnormalities, the effect of anesthetic drugs on the airway, the type of the airway device, and the experience and clinical judgment of

Table 10.12 Airway management skills for acquisition during anesthesiology residency

Skill	Performance Level
Bag-Mask Ventilation	Expert
Pharyngeal Airways	
Supraglottic Airways (SGA)	Expert
Intubation via SGA	
Intubating LMA	
Direct Laryngoscopy	Expert
Introducers	
Stylets	
Airway Exchange Catheters	
Videolaryngoscopy	Expert
Two Types	
e.g., C-MAC and GlideScope	
Fiberoptic-Assisted Intubation	Proficient
One-Lung Ventilation/Double Lumen Tubes	Proficient
Transtracheal Jet Ventilation*	Competent
Cricothyrotomy*	Competent
Airway Crisis Management	Proficient

* Competency evaluated in simulation and/or animal laboratory

the anesthesiologist. Successful management depends on the availability of an appropriate device and the ability of the anesthesiologist to use the device.

An honest, objective evaluation of the current state of airway management education for anesthesiology residents in the United States would conclude that considerable improvement is necessary. Anesthesiology residents must sequentially learn how to use the device, when to use the device, and when to use an alternative device when the initial device fails. The airway management curriculum should be standardized for all anesthesiology residents and must contain several skill sets (Table 10.12).

The concept that airway management techniques continue to evolve must also be instilled in residents to prepare them for lifelong learning. Practicing anesthesiologists must continually study airway management, learn new techniques, and periodically practice infrequently used techniques throughout their career.[92] Educators must carefully evaluate new techniques and devices and determine when a new device may supplant an older device in the airway management scheme.

It is the responsibility of airway educators to prepare future generations of anesthesiologists to provide high-quality airway management to their patients.[93] Simulator laboratories will continue to play a vital role in the airway education mission. It is anticipated that simulators will increase in fidelity and will enhance the educational experience.

Anesthesiologists must take the lead in airway education for other healthcare providers. Educational programs can be developed in collaboration with other specialty groups to improve airway management by paramedics, medical students, emergency medicine physicians, and critical care physicians.

References

1. R. A. Caplan, K. L. Posner, R. J. Ward, F. W. Cheney. Adverse respiratory events in anesthesia: A closed claims analysis. *Anesthesiology* 1990; 72: 828–33.

2. American Society of Anesthesiologists Task Force on Management of the Difficult Airway. Practice guidelines for management of the difficult airway. A report by American Society of Anesthesiologists Task Force on Management of the Difficult Airway. *Anesthesiology* 1993; 78: 597–602.

3. American Society of Anesthesiologists Task Force on Management of the Difficult Airway. Practice guidelines for management of the difficult airway: An updated report by the American Society of Anesthesiologists Task Force on Management of the Difficult Airway. *Anesthesiology* 2003; 98: 1269–77.

4. J. L. Apfelbaum, C. A. Hagberg, R. A. Caplan et al. Practice guidelines for management of the difficult airway: An updated report by the American Society of Anesthesiologists Task Force on Management of the Difficult Airway. *Anesthesiology* 2013; 118: 251–70.

5. J. Metzner, K. L. Posner, M. S. Lam, K. B. Domino. Closed claims' analysis. *Best Pract Res Clin Anaesthesiol* 2011; 25: 263–76.

6. J. N. Koppel, A. P. Reed. Formal instruction in difficult airway management: A survey of anesthesiology residency programs. *Anesthesiology* 1995; 83: 1343–6.

7. C. A. Hagberg, J. Greger, J. E. Chelly, H. E. Saad-Eddin. Instruction of airway management skills during anesthesiology residency training. *J Clin Anesth* 2003; 15: 149–53.

8. L. M. Pott, G. I. Randel, T. Straker, K. D. Becker, R. M. Cooper. A survey of airway training among U.S. and Canadian anesthesiology residency programs. *J Clin Anesth* 2011; 23: 15–26.

9. P. A. Baker, J. Feinleib, E. P. O'Sullivan. Is it time for airway management education to be mandatory? *Br J Anaesth* 2016; 117: i13–16.

10. Accreditation Council for Graduate Medical Education. ACGME Program Requirements for Graduate Medical Education in Anesthesiology. 2017. www.acgme.org (accessed January 3, 2017).

11. R. M. Cooper. Strengths and limitations of airway techniques. *Anesthesiol Clin* 2015; 33: 241–55.

12. C. L. Carraccio, B. J. Benson, L. J. Nixon, P. L. Derstine. From the educational bench to the clinical bedside: Translating the Dreyfus developmental model to the learning of clinical skills. *Acad Med* 2008; 83: 761–7.

13. S. E. Dreyfus. The five-stage model of adult skill acquisition. *Bull Sci Tech Soc* 2004; 24: 177–81.

14. J. P. Kassirer. Teaching clinical reasoning: Case-based and coached. *Acad Med* 2010; 85: 1118–24.

15. M. Wheeler, A. G. Roth, R. M. Dsida et al. Teaching residents pediatric fiberoptic intubation of the trachea. *Anesthesiology* 2004; 101: 842–6.

16. J. A. Cook, C. R. Ramsay, P. Fayers. Using the literature to quantify the learning curve: a case study. *Int J Technol Assess Health Care* 2007; 23: 255–60.

17. E. Crosby, A. Lane. Innovations in anesthesia education: The development and implementation of a resident rotation for advanced airway management. *Can J Anaesth* 2009; 56: 939–59.

18. W. C. McGahie, B. Issenberg, E. R. Cohen et al. Does simulation-based education with deliberate practice yield better results than traditional clinical education? A meta-analytic comparative review of the evidence. *Acad Med* 2011; 86: 706–11.

19. J. Garcia, A. Coste, W. Tavares, N. Nuno, K. Lachapelle. Assessment of competency during orotracheal intubation in medical simulation. *Br J Anaesth* 2015; 115: 302–7.

20. J. J. Schaefer 3rd. Simulators and difficult airway management skills. *Paediatr Anaesth* 2004; 14: 28–37.

21. R. S. Isaacs, J. M Sykes. Anatomy and physiology of the upper airway. *Anesthesiol Clin North America* 2002; 20: 733–45.

22. K. P. Strohl, J. P. Butler, A. Malhotra. Mechanical properties of the upper airway. *Compr Physiol* 2012; 2: 1853–72.

23. G. B. Drummond. Controlling the airway: Skill and science. *Anesthesiology* 2002; 97: 771–3.

24. D. R. Hillman, P. R. Platt, P. R Eastwood. Anesthesia, sleep and upper airway collapsibility. *Anesthesiol Clin* 2010; 28: 443–55.

25. P. R. Nandi, C. H. Charlesworth, S. J. Taylor et al. Effect of general anaesthesia on the pharynx. *Br J Anaesth* 1991; 66: 157–62.

26. I. Tanoubi, P. Drolet, F. Donati. Optimizing preoxygenation in adults. *Can J Anaesth* 2009; 56: 449–66.

27. G. Bouroche, J. L. Bourgain. Preoxygenation and general anesthesia: A review. *Minerva Anesthesiol* 2015; 81: 910–20.

28. T. Shiga, Z. Wajima, T. Inoue, A. Sakamoto. Predicting difficult intubation in apparently normal patients: A meta analysis of bedside screening test performance. *Anesthesiology* 2005; 103: 429–37.

29. P. Baker. Assessment before airway management. *Anesthesiol Clin* 2015; 33: 257–78.

30. O. Langeron, E. Masso, C. Huraux et al. Prediction of difficult mask ventilation. *Anesthesiology* 2000; 92: 1229–36.

31. S. Kheterpal, R. Han, K. K. Tremper et al. Incidence and predictors of difficult and impossible mask ventilation. *Anesthesiology* 2006; 105: 885–91.

32. S. H. Kim, J. E. Kim, Y. H. Kim et al. An assessment of orophrayngeal airway position using a fibreoptic bronchoscope. *Anaesthesia* 2014; 69: 53–7.

33. A. M. Joffe, S. Hetzel, E. C. Liew. A two-handed jaw-thrust technique is superior to the one-handed "EC clamp" technique for mask ventilation in the apneic unconscious person. *Anesthesiology* 2010: 113: 873–9.

34. M. R. Hernandez, P. A. Klock Jr., A. Ovassapian. Evolution of the extraglottic airway: A review of its history, applications, and practical tips for success. *Anesth Analg* 2012; 114: 349–68.

35. J. R. Brimacombe. Placement phase. In J. R. Brimacombe, ed. *Laryngeal Mask Anesthesia: Principles and Practice*, 2nd edn. Philadelphia: Saunders, 2005; 191–240.

36. M. Lopez-Gil, J. Brimacombe, J. Cebrian, J. Arranz. Laryngeal mask airway in pediatric practice: A prospective study of skill acquisition by anesthesia residents. *Anesthesiology* 1996; 84: 807–11.

37. J. Brimacombe. Analysis of 1,500 laryngeal mask uses by one anaesthetist in adults undergoing routine anaesthesia. *Anaesthesia* 1996; 51: 76–80.

38. L. C. Berkow, J. M. Schwartz, K. Kan et al. Use of the laryngeal mask airway-Aintree intubating catheter-fiberoptic bronchoscope technique for difficult intubation. *J Clin Anesth* 2011; 23: 534–9.

39. N. S. Gerstein, D. A. Braude, O. Hung et al. The Fastrach intubating laryngeal mask airway: An overview and update. *Can J Anaesth* 2010; 57: 588–601.

40. D. G. Ostermayer, M. Gausche-Hill. Supraglottic airways: The history and current state of prehospital airway adjuncts. *Prehosp Emerg Care* 2014; 18: 106–15.

41. P. F. Fouche, P. M. Simpson, J. Bendall et al. Airways in out-of-hospital cardiac arrest: Systematic review and meta-analysis. *Prehosp Emerg Care* 2014; 18: 244–56.

42. F. Adnet, S. X. Racine, S. W. Borron et al. A survey of tracheal intubation difficulty in the operating room: A prospective observational study. *Acta Anaesthesiol Scand* 2001; 45: 327–32.

43. T. Heidegger, H. J. Gerig, B. Ulrich, G. Kreienbuhl. Validation of a simple algorithm for tracheal intubation: Daily practice is the key to success in emergencies-an analysis of 13,248 intubation. *Anesth Analg* 2001; 92: 517–22.

44. J. T. Mulcaster, J. Mills, O. R. Hung et al. Laryngoscopic intubation: Learning and performance. *Anesthesiology* 2003; 98: 23–7.

45. M. L. Buis, I. M. Maissan, S. E. Hoeks et al. Defining the learning curve for endotracheal intubation using direct laryngoscopy: A systematic review. *Resuscitation* 2016; 99: 63–71.

46. J. E. Zamora, B. J. Weber, A. R. Langley, A. G. Day. Laryngoscope manipulation by experienced *versus* novice laryngoscopists. *Can J Anaesth* 2014; 61: 1075–83.

47. S. Grape, P. Schoettker. The role of tracheal tube introducers and stylets in current airway management. *J Clin Monit Comput* 2017; 31: 531–7.

48. B. A. Marson, E. Anderson, A. R. Wilkes, I. Hodzovic. Bougie-related airway trauma: Dangers of the hold-up sign. *Anaesthesia* 2014; 69: 219–23.

49. R. M. Cooper, J. A. Pacey, M. J. Bishop, S. A McCluskey. Early clinical experience with a new videolaryngoscope (GlideScope®) in 728 patients. *Can J Anaesth* 2005; 52: 191–8.

50. Y. C. Su, C. C. Chen, Y. K. Lee et al. Comparison of video laryngoscopy with direct laryngoscopy for tracheal intubation: A meta-analysis of randomised trials. *Eur J Anaesthesiol* 2011; 28: 788–95.

51. J. McElwain, M. A. Malik, B. H. Harte et al. Comparison of C-MAC videolaryngoscope with the Macintosh, GlideScope, and Airtraq laryngoscopes in easy and difficult laryngoscopy scenarios in manikins. *Anaesthesia* 2010; 65: 483–9.

52. M. F. Aziz, A. M. Brambrink, D. W. Healy et al. Success of intubation rescue techniques after failed direct laryngoscopy in adults: A retrospective analysis from the multicenter perioperative outcomes group. *Anesthesiology* 2016; 125: 656–6.

53. K. J. Howard-Quijano, Y. M. Huang, R. Matevosian et al. Video-assisted instruction improves the success rate for tracheal intubation by novices. *Br J Anaesth* 2008; 101: 568–72.

54. F. Herbstreit, P. Fassbender, H. Haberi et al. Learning endotracheal intubation using a novel videolaryngoscope improves intubation skills of medical students. *Anesth Analg* 2011; 113: 586–90.

55. B. M. Pieters, N. E. Wilbers, M. Huijzer et al. Comparison of seven videolaryngoscopes with the Macintosh laryngoscope in manikins by experienced and novice personnel. *Anaesthesia* 2016; 71: 556–64.

56. B. Hossfeld, K. Frey, V. Doerges et al. Improvement in glottic visualization by using the C-MAC PM video laryngoscope as a first-line device for out-of-hospital emergency tracheal intubation: An observational study. *Eur J Anaesthesiol* 2015; 32: 425–31.

57. J. C. Sakles, J. Mosier, S. Chiu et al. A comparison of the C-MAC video laryngoscope to the Macintosh direct laryngoscope for intubation in the emergency department. *Ann Emerg Med* 2012; 60: 739–48.

58. J. B. Paolini, F. Donati, P. Drolet. Review article: Video-laryngoscopy: Another tool for difficult intubation or a new paradigm in airway management? *Can J Anesth* 2013; 60: 184–91.

59. C. Zaouter, J. Calderon, T. M. Hemmerling. Videolaryngoscopy as a new standard of care. *Br J Anaesth* 2015; 114: 181–3.

60. V. N. Nalik, E. D. Matsumoto, P. L. Houston et al. Fiberoptic orotracheal intubation on anesthetized patients: Do manipulation skills learned on a simple model transfer to the operating room? *Anesthesiology* 2001; 95: 343–8.

61. J. T. Roberts. Preparing to use the flexible fiber-optic laryngoscope. *J Clin Anesth* 1991; 3: 64–75.

62. C. Johnson, J. T. Roberts. Clinical competence in the performance of fiberoptic laryngoscopy and endotracheal intubation: A study of resident instruction. *J Clin Anesth* 1989; 1: 344–9.

63. K. B. Greenland, M. G. Irwin. The Williams intubator, the Ovassapian airway and the Berman airway as upper airway conduits for fibreoptic bronchoscopy in patients with difficult airways. *Curr Opin Anaesthesiol* 2004; 17: 505–10.

64. J. E. Smith, A. P. Jackson, J. Hurdley, P. J. Clifton. Learning curves for fibreoptic nasotracheal intubation when using the endoscopic video camera. *Anaesthesia* 1997; 52: 101–6.

65. W. Rosenblatt, A. I. Ianus, W. Sukhupragarn et al. Preoperative endoscopic airway examination (PEAE) provides superior airway information and may reduce the use of unnecessary awake intubation. *Anesth Analg* 2011; 112: 602–7.

66. L. C. Berkow, R. S. Greenberg, K. H. Kan et al. Need for emergency surgical airway reduced by a comprehensive difficult airway program. *Anesth Analg* 2009; 109: 1860–9.

67. G. Monreal, K. R. Moranm, M. A. Gerhardt. The in vivo skills laboratory in anesthesiology residency training. *J Educ Periop Med* 2014; 16: E075.

68. A. L. Makowski. The ethics of using the recently deceased to instruct residents in cricothyrotomy. *Ann Emerg Med* 2015; 66: 403–8.

69. H. A. McLure, D. P. Dob, M. M. Mannan, N. Soni. A laboratory comparison of two techniques of emergency percutaneous tracheostomy. *Anaesthesia* 1997; 52: 1199–201.

70. Q. Gardiner, P. S. White, D. Carson et al. Technique training: Endoscopic percutaneous tracheostomy. *Br J Anaesth* 1998; 81: 401–3.

71. A. Lamb, J. Zhang, O. Hung et al. Accuracy of identifying the cricothyroid membrane by anesthesia trainees and staff in a Canadian institution. *Can J Anaesth* 2015; 62: 495–503.

72. K. N. Hiller, R. J. Karni, C. Cai et al. Comparing success rates of anesthesia providers versus trauma surgeons in the use of palpation to identify the cricothyroid membrane in female subjects: A prospective observational study. *Can J Anaesth* 2016; 63: 807–17.

73. J. L. Benumof, M. S. Scheller. The importance of transtracheal jet ventilation in the management of the difficult airway. *Anesthesiology* 1989; 71: 769–78.

74. E. Boccio, R. Gujral, M. Cassara et al. Combining transtracheal catheter oxygenation and needle-based Seldinger cricothyrotomy into a single sequential procedure. *Am J Emerg Med* 2015; 33: 708–12.

75. L. V. Duggan, B. Ballantyne Scott, J. A. Law et al. Transtracheal jet ventilation in the "can't intubate can't oxygenate" emergency: A systematic review. *Br J Anaesth* 2016; 117(S1): i28–38.

76. C. Frerk, V. S. Mitchell, A. F. McNarry et al. Difficult Airway Society 2015 guidelines for management of unanticipated difficult intubation in adults. *Br J Anaesth* 2015; 115: 827–48.

77. P. Eisenburger, K. Laczika, M. List et al. Comparison of conventional surgical versus Seldinger technique emergency cricothyrotomy performed by inexperienced clinicians. *Anesthesiology* 2000; 92: 687–90.

78. N. Schaumann, V. Lorenz, P. Schellongowski et al. Evaluation of Seldinger technique emergency cricothyroidotomy versus standard surgical cricothyroidotomy in 200 cadavers. *Anesthesiology* 2005; 102: 7–11

79. K. E. You-Ten, M. D. Bould, Z. Friedman et al. Cricothyrotomy training increases adherence to the ASA difficult airway algorithm in a simulated crisis: A randomized controlled trial. *Can J Anaesth* 2015; 62: 485–94.

80. T. M. Cook, N. Woodall, C. Frerk. Fourth National Audit Project. Major complications of airway management in the UK: Results of the Fourth National

Audit Project of the Royal College of Anaesthetists and the Difficult Airway Society. Part 1: Anesthesia. *Br J Anaesth* 2011; 106: 617–31.

81. A. P. Reed. Preparation of the patient for awake flexible fiberoptic bronchoscopy. *Chest* 1992; 101: 244–53.

82. K. D. Johnston, M. R. Rai. Conscious sedation for awake fiberoptic intubation: A review of the literature. *Can J Anaesth* 2013; 60: 584–99.

83. S. Heinrich, T. Birkholz, A. Irouschek et al. Incidences and predictors of difficult laryngoscopy in adult patients undergoing general anesthesia: A single-center analysis of 102,305 cases. *J Anesth* 2013; 27: 815–21.

84. J. F. Heuer, T. A. Barwing, J. Barwing et al. Incidence of difficult intubation in intensive care patients: Analysis of contributing factors. *Anaesth Intensive Care* 2012; 40: 120–7.

85. J. L. Parmet, P. Colonna-Romano, J. C. Horrow et al. The laryngeal mask airway reliably provides rescue ventilation in cases of unanticipated difficult tracheal intubation along with difficult mask ventilation. *Anesth Analg* 1998; 87: 661–5.

86. L. J. Mark, K. R. Herzer, R. Cover et al. Difficult airway response team: A novel quality improvement program for managing hospital-wide airway emergencies. *Anesth Analg* 2015; 121: 127–39.

87. S. M. Nykiel-Bailey, J. D. McAllister, C. R. Schrock et al. Difficult airway consultation service for children: Steps to implement and preliminary results. *Paediatr Anaesth* 2015; 25: 363–71.

88. J. Feinleib, L. Foley, L. Mark. What we all should know about our patient's airway: Difficult airway communications, database registries and reporting systems registries. *Anesthiol Clin* 2015; 33: 397–413.

89. J. Mourao, J. Moreira, J. Barbosa et al. Soft tissue injuries after direct laryngoscopy. *J Clin Anesth* 2015; 27: 668–71.

90. K. B. Domino, K. L. Posner, R. A. Caplan, F. W. Cheney. Airway injury during anesthesia. *Anesthesiology* 1999; 91: 1703–1.

91. P. C. Pacheco-Lopez, L. C. Berkow, A. T. Hillel, L. M. Akst. Complications of airway management. *Respir Care* 2014; 59: 1006–19.

92. S. F. Dierdorf. Airway expert or expert in airway management? *Curr Opin Anaesthesiol* 2003; 16: 321–2.

93. K. R. Stringer, S. Bajenov, S. M. Yentis. Training in airway management. *Anaesthesia* 2002; 57: 967–83.

94. H. Soleimanpour, C. Gholipouri, J. P. Panahi et al. Role of anesthesiology curriculum in improving bag-mask ventilation and intubation success rates of emergency medicine residents: A prospective descriptive study. *BMC Emerg Med* 2011; 11: 8–13.

95. S. Mohr, M. A. Weigand, S. Hofer et al. Developing the skill of laryngeal mask airway insertion: Prospective single center study. *Anaesthetist* 2013; 62: 447–52.

96. K. Goldmann, D. Z. Ferson. Education and training in airway management. *Best Pract Res Clin Anaesthesiol* 2005; 19: 717–32.

97. A. Timmermann, S. G. Russo, T. A. Crozier et al. Novices ventilate and intubate quicker and safer via intubating laryngeal mask than by conventional bag-mask ventilation and laryngoscopy. *Anesthesiology* 2007; 107: 570–6.

98. M. Bernhard, S. Mohr, M. A. Weigand et al. Developing the skill of endotracheal intubation: Implication for emergency medicine. *Acta Anaesthesiol Scand* 2012; 56: 164–71.

99. M. J. Silverberg, N. Li, S. O. Acquah, P. D. Kory. Comparison of video laryngoscopy versus direct laryngoscopy during urgent endotracheal intubation: A randomized controlled trial. *Crit Care Med* 2015; 43: 636–41.

100. R. Komatsu, Y. Kasuya, H. Yogo et al. Learning curves for bag-and-mask ventilation and orotracheal intubation: An application of the cumulative sum method. *Anesthesiology* 2010; 112: 1525–31.

101. J. G. Hardman, J. S Wills. The development of hypoxaemia during apnea in children: A computational modeling investigation. *Br J Anaesth* 2006; 97: 564–70.

102. F. R. Altermatt, H. R. Munoz, A. E. Delfino, L. I. CortinezI. Pre-oxygenation in the obese patient: Effects of position on tolerance to apnea. *Br J Anaesth* 2005; 95: 706–9.

103. S. H. McClelland, D. G. Bogod, J. G. Hardman. Apnoea in pregnancy: An investigation using physiological modeling. *Anaesthesia* 2008; 63: 264–9.

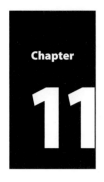

Chapter

11

Teaching and Learning Regional Anesthesia

Glenn Woodworth, Ryan Ivie, and Robert Maniker

Introduction

Historically, community practice anesthesiologists have emphasized basic regional anesthesia skills, mostly centered around neuraxial anesthesia. Peripheral nerve blocks were most often performed by those with specialized skills or interest in regional anesthesia, while the majority of anesthesiologists tended to avoid them. The advent of peripheral nerve stimulation and more recently of ultrasound-guided techniques have led to the perception that peripheral nerve blocks are now more easily performed. This has fueled a tremendous growth in the number of individuals performing nerve blocks and created an expectation that nerve blocks should be in the skill set of all anesthesiologists.[1]

The following discussion is divided into (1) specific concepts and techniques for teaching and learning regional anesthesia and (2) the opportunities and challenges for teaching and learning regional anesthesia in residency and fellowship training as well as for the continuing education of the lifelong learner.

Techniques for Teaching and Learning Regional Anesthesia

Regional anesthesia is understandably viewed as one potential component of an overall perioperative anesthetic and pain management plan; for many, however, the term is synonymous with the procedures used to address acute postoperative pain. This can lead both the educator and the learner to oversimplify the learning tasks at hand. A great deal of knowledge and judgment comes into play in deciding if a regional anesthesia procedure is appropriate for a particular patient, that is, evaluating the risks and benefits of general versus regional anesthesia, choosing the appropriate type of procedure, and recognizing and managing complications. We will not delve into this controversy other than noting its relevance to any discussion of regional

anesthesia education – *competency in regional anesthesia is much more than the technical ability to perform a set of procedures*. We will assume for the moment that the medical knowledge required for regional anesthesia can be learned in the same manner as other medical knowledge required for competency in anesthesia. Here we will focus on competency in the procedural aspect of regional anesthesia, which many find challenging.[2]

Learning Procedural Skills

The most widely accepted theory on the acquisition of procedural skills and expert performance involves the role of deliberate practice.[3] In general, the quality of performance of a skill gradually improves over time if the individual engages in practice activity that is designed to improve performance. Deliberate practice entails performance of a well-defined task, paired with immediate feedback.[4,5] The task (or a similar task) is performed repeatedly to provide opportunities for continued improvement. The key is that deliberate efforts are made to improve performance with each trial. It is important to note that the teacher or coach need not always be present. Solitary practice with intermittent instruction can be highly effective, as long as the practice sessions are directed at improving specific aspects of skill performance. (See Chapter 3 for a more detailed discussion of deliberate practice.) Ericsson et al. are widely quoted for their data from multiple domains demonstrating that true expertise is attained only after approximately 10,000 hours of deliberate practice.[3]

Deliberate practice often involves breaking a skill down into component elements and receiving feedback on the performance of each specific element. If a learner is performing a regional anesthesia skill without the guidance of an expert, feedback is typically limited to observation of success or failure (e.g., did the block work or not) and resultant complications (e.g., did a wet tap occur when attempting to place a lumbar epidural block). Regional anesthesia procedures are not innately amenable to practice and repetition-based improvement without structured feedback. This has implications for practicing physicians who may attend a weekend course to learn a new skill. When they return to their practice and begin to perform the skill, it is important that they continue to receive feedback from an expert to improve competency in the skill.

The preceding discussion provides a segue into some of the evidence for procedural skill acquisition in regional anesthesia. It is unlikely (and unnecessary) that any anesthesia trainee would practice performing epidurals for 10,000 hours. Expert performance is merely one point on a learning curve and performance of a skill at an "acceptable" level does not require the level of expertise exhibited by a master (e.g., an Olympic athlete). Even Ericsson et al., whose widely misinterpreted results are assumed to indicate that 10,000 hours of deliberate practice will result in true expertise, suggest that an acceptable standard of performance can be attained with 50 hours of deliberate practice in some skills.[3]

Medical procedure research has not focused as much on the number of hours spent practicing, but rather on the number of procedures performed to achieve competence.[6] Plotting procedure success against numbers of procedures performed is frequently used to produce a learning curve and to estimate the number of procedures necessary to achieve a desired level of performance. This research has demonstrated that the number of procedures necessary to achieve a 90 percent success rate varied by procedure (57 attempts for intubation vs. more than 90 for epidurals). It is important to note that individual attainment of acceptable performance varied considerably.

What implication does this have for learning regional anesthesia? Table 11.1 presents a list of regional anesthesia procedures that is by no means comprehensive. It is presented to highlight the challenge of learning regional anesthesia as it can encompass a large variety of procedures. It would not be possible during residency training for each resident to perform 50 to 100 of each regional anesthesia procedure.

It would seem logical that acceptable performance in one regional anesthesia procedure would translate into acceptable or near acceptable performance

Table 11.1 Partial listing of regional anesthesia and acute pain procedures to demonstrate the potential breadth of procedural skills to be mastered

Neuraxial	Epidural (lumbar)
	Epidural (thoracic)
	Spinal
	Combined spinal/epidural
	Caudal
Upper extremity	Superficial cervical plexus
	Interscalene
	Supraclavicular
	Infraclavicular
	Axillary
	Distal upper extremity peripheral nerve
Lower extremity	Ankle block
	Popliteal sciatic
	Transgluteal sciatic
	Infragluteal sciatic
	Anterior sciatic
	Proximal femoral
	Adductor canal
	Peripheral saphenous
	Obturator
	Lateral femoral cutaneous
	Pudendal
Head and neck	Mandibular
	Retrobulbar
	Occipital
	Trigeminal (Gasserian) ganglion
Airway blocks	Transtracheal
	Glossopharyngeal
	Superior laryngeal
Truncal blocks	Intercostal
	Paravertebral
	Lumbar plexus
	Transversus abdominis plane
	Rectus sheath
	Ilioinguinal/Iliohypogastric nerve
	Pecs I
	Pecs II
	Serratus plane

with a "similar" procedure and, thus, a smaller number of procedures of the second type would need to be performed to achieve acceptable competence. Unfortunately, this hypothesis has not been investigated, and it is unknown if an ultrasound-guided femoral nerve block is sufficiently similar to an ultrasound-guided popliteal sciatic nerve block to produce skills transfer and, if so, to what degree. In addition, some regional anesthesia procedures are substantially different from others (e.g., a femoral nerve block compared to a lumbar plexus block).

Component Skills

Because of the large number of procedures and the continual introduction of new techniques, training in regional anesthesia should focus on teaching some currently available procedures, while also providing learners with the tools to efficiently acquire proficiency in new procedures. Two approaches may be beneficial. The first is segmentation, wherein the complex task of performing regional anesthesia procedures is broken down into the basic components that comprise each procedure:

- Understanding of anatomy (and anatomical variants) and sonoanatomy of the relevant area;
- Equipment use (ultrasound machine, procedure trays, nerve stimulator, etc.);
- Ultrasound transducer handling to obtain and optimize an image;
- Needle guidance skills (how to plan a needle approach, skill in needle insertion/guidance under ultrasound);
- Nerve localization techniques;
- Procedure set up, patient positioning, and ergonomics;
- Sterile technique;
- Procedure flow;
- Communication;
- Assessment of patient outcomes; and
- Catheter-based techniques.

Many of these skills can be taught individually. Some (e.g., operation of the ultrasound machine) are transferrable across several procedures, while others (e.g., sonoanatomy of the relevant area) are more procedure specific. Once component skills are mastered and learners approach new procedure types, training should focus on the aspects unique to the new procedure. For example, when a student has learned the

component skill of equipment use for performing an ultrasound-guided nerve block, he or she can be expected to understand how to operate the ultrasound machine, manipulate the transducer, troubleshoot poor image quality, and so forth. When learning a new ultrasound-guided nerve block, the learning focus can be directed to the unique anatomy for the new procedure, and block-specific factors such as indications, contraindications, assessment of the block, and complications.

A second approach is to teach the process used to learn a procedure (metacognition).[7] Instructors can stress the importance of gaining a deep understanding of the anatomy of any region amenable to nerve block, including identification of the vascular and muscular anatomy, common anatomical variants, important anatomical relationships that can be used to confirm the identity of structures, sonoanatomy, surrounding structures that can result in complications, and ergonomic factors. Instructors should also stress the importance of carefully evaluating the literature on new procedures before adopting them. Repeating this process with each procedure can imbue the student with the appropriate mind-set when learning a new procedure.

Role of Simulation

Historically, acquisition of procedural skills is accomplished with personalized instruction using an apprenticeship model. Such procedural training is largely unstructured and can lead to wide variation in trainee performance and procedure knowledge. Simulation has gained popularity in medical education and is particularly suited to teaching procedural skills. Simulation provides an environment that supports deliberate practice and feedback, where learners can practice without subjecting patients to risk.[8,9] Such training has been successfully applied to teaching regional anesthesia skills.[10,11] The American Society of Regional Anesthesia and Pain Medicine and the European Society of Regional Anesthesia and Pain Therapy have issued joint recommendations on curricula and training for ultrasound-guided regional anesthesia, one of which calls for the use of simulators.[12]

Simulation in regional anesthesia can be easily introduced with lower fidelity (and less expensive) task trainers to teach component skills (e.g., needle guidance under ultrasound) or with standardized patients to teach sonoanatomy. Anecdotal experience suggests that the use of simulation early in regional anesthesia training has vastly improved resident performance. In addition, trainees are far more comfortable approaching patients after having achieved some competence during simulation. There may be significant benefit for regional anesthesia curricula to begin with extensive training on ultrasound probe handling and needle guidance under ultrasound. Based on the preceding principles, such skills training would be most effective if conducted with a deliberate practice model that provides sufficient repetition to facilitate improvement of skills as well as extensive, formalized feedback.

It is important to note that in most cases it is not necessary to use task trainers or gel phantoms to teach anatomy or sonoanatomy. Unfortunately, the anatomy of most available nerve block simulators remains highly artificial and of poor quality.[13] Instead, task trainers can be useful in teaching procedure setup, ergonomics, flow, and needle-guidance skills. Standardized patients can then be used to teach relevant anatomy and sonoanatomy. High-fidelity trainers incorporating detailed anatomy and haptic feedback have been developed, but are expensive and therefore remain somewhat impractical.

Two areas of simulation in regional anesthesia deserve special mention. The first is teaching the management of local anesthetic systemic toxicity (LAST). Treatment of this complication requires crisis resource-management skills, knowledge of how recommended guidelines for LAST differ from advanced cardiac life-support guidelines, and appropriate use of decision support tools. Simulation has been shown to be effective in teaching the management of LAST.[14] Although high-fidelity simulation can be useful, medium-fidelity simulation in-situ (in a clinical area where blocks are performed) can be helpful in teaching the learner how to access local resources (e.g., code carts, lipid emulsion, bag-valve-mask) in their working environment.

The second unique application for simulation is thoracic epidural placement. Unfortunately, this procedure is associated with a high failure rate (estimated between 20 and 30 percent), which has been attributed to inadequate training.[15] When performing a thoracic epidural, the operator has very little feedback as to the actual location of the needle tip within the tissues. Work is in progress to develop a mixed-media simulator that tracks the location of the needle tip using a high-fidelity task trainer in real time. This type of simulation technology holds tremendous promise for procedural skills training.

Cognitive Pretraining and Blended Learning

Simulation training can be considered a type of pretraining (prior to performance on patients); however, pretraining can take place even before beginning a simulator course. Almost all educational courses for procedural skills training are resource intensive. This limits their availability and the amount of trainee exposure time. In addition, the mentorship model discussed in the preceding text can provide highly variable educational experiences for trainees. Strategies to address these two concerns promote the use of blended learning. Blended learning combines online educational materials with in-person and/or in-classroom training (see Chapter 15).[16–18] Some of the online materials serve as standardized pretraining and should be completed prior to beginning classroom instruction on the topic/procedure. This can help provide a level of background information for the learners and will help them to maximize the in-classroom experience (Figure 11.1).

Using blended learning, instructors do not have to spend as much time on the didactic material, but instead can focus on the procedurals skills component. In addition, the information provides background knowledge upon which the learners can scaffold new knowledge during the in-person session. This approach is equally important for a lifelong learner attending a skills training session as it is for a resident on a regional anesthesia rotation.

Competency Assessment

Any discussion of procedural skills training must also include a discussion of competency assessment. Medical education has gradually shifted toward a competency-based model with defined sets of specific learning outcomes. An important cornerstone of competency-based education is the demonstration of competency.[19] In 2014, the Accreditation Council for Graduate Medical Education (ACGME), in conjunction with the American Board of Anesthesiology (ABA) and the Anesthesiology Review Committee, published a set of competency milestones that include milestones for technical skills in regional anesthesia (Figure 11.2).[20]

At the current time, these milestones are general statements and in many cases are not very specific. Furthermore, the milestones do not define how achievement of competency will be assessed. This might seem like an esoteric discussion; however, it is

Curriculum Components

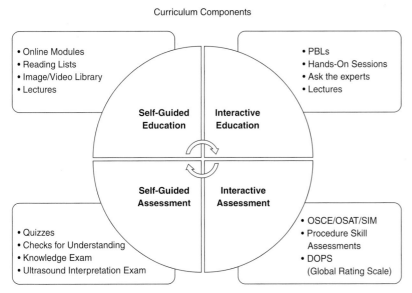

Self-Guided Education
- Online Modules
- Reading Lists
- Image/Video Library
- Lectures

Interactive Education
- PBLs
- Hands-On Sessions
- Ask the experts
- Lectures

Self-Guided Assessment
- Quizzes
- Checks for Understanding
- Knowledge Exam
- Ultrasound Interpretation Exam

Interactive Assessment
- OSCE/OSAT/SIM
- Procedure Skill Assessments
- DOPS (Global Rating Scale)

Figure 11.1 A blended learning model for regional anesthesia training that is a combination of self-guided learning and assessment, and faculty driven educational experiences and assessment.

Has not Achieved Level 1	Level 1	Level 2	Level 3	Level 4	Level 5
	Demonstrates sterile technique Administers infiltrative local anesthetics for procedures under direct supervision Identifies physiologic changes associated with local anesthesia administration and seeks help appropriately	Applies appropriate monitors and prepares resuscitative equipment prior to performing regional anesthesia procedures Performs spinal and epidural anesthesia under direct supervision Recognizes problems or complications associated with regional anesthesia, and manages them with direct supervision	Performs peripheral nerve blocks and regional anesthesia under direct supervision, including both upper and lower extremity blocks and thoracic epidurals Uses ultrasound or nerve stimulator guided techniques appropriately Performs common pediatric regional anesthetics (e.g., caudal blockade) with direct supervision Recognizes problems or complications associated with regional anesthesia and manages them with indirect supervision	Performs spinal, epidural, and peripheral nerve blocks with conditional independence Supervises junior residents in performing regional anesthetics and other health care providers on issues related to regional anesthesia Manages problems or complications associated with regional anesthesia with conditional independence	Independently performs peripheral and neuraxial regional anesthesia techniques Independently manages problems or complications associated with regional anesthesia

Figure 11.2 Patient Care 10: Technical skills: Regional anesthesia. (From the ABA / ACGME "The Anesthesiology Milestone Project.")

possible, if not likely, that in the near future physicians will need to demonstrate competency in a wide variety of procedures they intend to perform in practice. Many institutions today require credentialing for a variety of procedures (e.g., pulmonary artery catheter placement, use of fluoroscopy). It is not unreasonable to expect that at some time in the future an anesthesiologist would be asked to demonstrate competency in placement of an ultrasound-guided nerve block prior to being credentialed to do the procedure in a particular hospital. On the surface, it sounds reasonable to require a demonstration of competency in a given procedure before allowing the practitioner to perform it independently on patients. How granular credentialing will become remains to be seen. It is possible that each provider will maintain a set of procedural skills "badges" documenting that a certain level of competency has been achieved and maintained. These badges could be earned in residency, fellowship, or later.

Because demonstration of procedural skills competency has potentially far-reaching implications for restricting practice, it will be important for the specialty to develop validated competency assessment tools that can be used in high-stakes examinations. (The assessments will be high stakes because they may be required to pass board certification or to be credentialed in a hospital.)[21] Several researchers have looked at validating various tools for the assessment of competency for regional anesthesia procedural skills.[22,23] Validation studies are needed to assure that assessment tools are measuring what they intend to measure and can distinguish between different levels of competency. Passing scores (or "cut scores") will also need to be determined. While most of these assessment tools have focused on the direct observation of an individual performing the actual skill, some have addressed the assessment of component skills.[24]

Anesthesia Residency Training in Regional Anesthesia

In this section, we will briefly address some of the special considerations for residency training in regional anesthesia. In the past ten years, the majority of anesthesia training programs have been providing specific rotations (of varying length) for regional anesthesia training. In part, this was to assure that trainees could meet the minimum number of regional anesthesia procedures required by the ACGME. There are essentially three sources to guide residency programs on developing curricula:

- The ABA-defined content outline;[1]
- The ACGME program requirements;[2] and
- The ACGME Anesthesiology Milestones.[3]

It is the responsibility of individual programs to design curricula for their residents. Although this allows programs considerable flexibility, it also means that residents graduating from different programs can have widely varying experiences and training in regional anesthesia. Smith et al. published a suggested regional anesthesia curriculum for residents that details specific learning objectives, educational experiences, and resources.[25] In our program we have two four-week-long rotations dedicated to regional anesthesia. Our approach has been to utilize a blended curriculum format in which learners access online tools (quizzes, e-learning modules, reading, lecture slide set archive, etc.) to conduct self-guided learning.[18] The online system, the Anesthesia Education Toolbox[18] (www.anesthesiatoolbox.com; accessed November 5, 2017), includes a "curriculum" that residents can use as a study guide to direct their learning to key topics and resources recommended by a national committee of regional anesthesia experts. This online learning should be complemented by mentored clinical care conducted while the resident is on the regional anesthesia rotation. In addition to providing learner feedback during real-time patient encounters, faculty can conduct specific educational sessions (lectures, skills training sessions with simulators or standardized patients, problem-based learning discussions, etc.). Materials are organized into self-guided and interactive education and assessment tools (Figure 11.1). This blended learning approach helps guide self-directed learning activities, provide some quality control over educational experiences delivered by faculty, and assists the faculty in conducting high-quality educational experiences.

One unique challenge in a training environment that requires performance of high-stakes procedures is deciding when to provide autonomy. This is where the concept of entrustability and entrustable professional activities (EPAs) can be useful. In this context, entrustability is a spectrum of graduated independence that a supervisor provides to a trainee in performing a task, while EPAs are individual tasks that are amenable to the entrustability decision. For example, one EPA may be performance of an interscalene block for a patient undergoing shoulder surgery. Throughout training, the supervising physicians must decide how independent the trainee can be in performing this procedure, and it will range from constant direct supervision, likely while the trainee has minimal experience, to indirect or conditional independence, likely near the

---

[1] www.theaba.org/PDFs/ADVANCED-Exam/Basic-and-Advanced-ContentOutline (accessed November 5, 2017).
[2] www.acgme.org/Portals/0/PFAssets/ProgramRequirements/CPRs_2017-07-01.pdf (accessed November 5, 2017).
[3] www.acgme.org/Portals/0/PDFs/Milestones/AnesthesiologyMilestones.pdf (accessed November 5, 2017).

end of training. The concept of entrustability can be a very practical and convenient way to assess competency. A certain competency threshold is reached when multiple supervising physicians have determined (based on personal observations, test and assessment scores, etc.) that a particular resident can be entrusted to perform a task or procedure with a greater level of independence. This threshold will likely be achieved at different times for (1) different individual trainees and (2) various procedures. For example, the average trainee would be expected to achieve a certain level of entrustability in performing a femoral nerve block before a paravertebral block. Once an entire list of EPAs is defined and mapped, including specific assessment tools to assist supervisors in determining entrustability for each one, EPAs have the potential to be used as a framework for documenting competency in regional anesthesiology.[26]

Lifelong Learners and Regional Anesthesia

The lifelong learner presents special challenges. How do practicing physicians acquire and maintain new skills and knowledge? The most common methods for acquiring or maintaining knowledge are reading (which would require a dedicated physician to keep up with the evolving literature) or attending meetings. Unfortunately, most practicing physicians find it hard to devote adequate time to these endeavors. Social media tools may hold some promise in bridging this gap. Physicians may be able to access social media platforms that will allow them to customize news streams and engage in asynchronous online discussions with their colleagues and experts around the world (see Chapter 16).[27] Ultimately, this could be a more efficient mechanism of asking questions, accessing expert opinion, and staying abreast of current developments.

Learning a new procedural skill is an entirely different story. For this, many will attend specific workshops, which are usually no more than a day or two in duration. The main question with this type of training is whether this brief experience is sufficient to learn a new skill and begin performing it on patients. Few community practices have the capability of providing experts to mentor and provide directed feedback as a physician begins performing a newly acquired procedural skill. Many universities have tried to address this by offering extensive blended learning opportunities

to participants in a hands-on skills training workshops. This helps the learners maximize their limited time during the actual hands-on sessions. In addition, they have a resource to which they refer after the "course" has finished. Unfortunately, this may still be insufficient training for some to begin performing the new procedure on patients without expert guidance. This scenario has played out over the last ten years as the use of ultrasound-guided regional anesthesia has gained widespread popularity, presenting a unique learning challenge to practicing physicians.

The challenge to our specialty is to develop cost-effective and efficient mechanisms for lifelong learners to acquire new procedural skills. Submission of video recordings or telemedicine-type encounters may hold some promise, but there are many hurdles (practical and medico-legal) to implementation, and this will likely not be widely available for quite some time. Access to high-fidelity simulators with haptic feedback (and possibly automated expert guidance) may also be important tools for the future if they can be made economically viable. Another solution may be providing dedicated expert "trainers" in large anesthesia groups. Despite the opportunity for quality improvement, making this economically feasible will also be a challenge.

Summary

In summary, learning regional anesthesia involves far more than just repeated performance of procedures. Fortunately, the nonprocedural skills aspect may be the easiest to teach and learn for both residents and lifelong learners. Intensive procedural skills training can be easily provided in residency programs. We advocate a blended learning approach to curricula and the use of directed feedback. Simulation can also be an important tool for teaching many aspects of procedural skills. Competency assessment is in its infancy, but it is likely to play an ever-greater role in resident and fellow training and in the credentialing of practicing physicians. Lifelong learners present a special challenge when attempting to acquire new procedural skills.

References

1. B. Tsui. Ultrasound-guidance and nerve stimulation: Implications for the future practice of regional anesthesia. *Can J Anaesth* 2007; 54: 165–70.

2. B. D. Sites, B. C. Spence, J. D. Gallagher et al. Characterizing novice behavior associated with

learning ultrasound-guided peripheral regional anesthesia. *Reg Anesth Pain Med* 2007; 32: 107–15.

3. K. A. Ericsson. Deliberate practice and the acquisition and maintenance of expert performance in medicine and related domains. *Acad Med* 2004; 79: S70–81.

4. K. A. Ericsson. Deliberate practice and acquisition of expert performance: A general overview. *Acad Emerg Med* 2008; 15: 988–94.

5. K. A. Ericsson, K. Nandagopal, R. W. Roring. Toward a science of exceptional achievement: Attaining superior performance through deliberate practice. *Ann N Y Acad Sci* 2009; 1172: 199–217.

6. C. Konrad, G. Schupfer, M. Wietlisbach, H. Gerber. Learning manual skills in anesthesiology: Is there a recommended number of cases for anesthetic procedures? *Anesth Analg* 1998; 86: 635–9.

7. C. Y. Colbert, L. Graham, C. West et al. Teaching metacognitive skills: Helping your physician trainees in the quest to "know what they don't know." *Am J Med* 2015; 128: 318–24.

8. W. C. McGaghie, S. B. Issenberg, E. R. Cohen et al. Does simulation-based medical education with deliberate practice yield better results than traditional clinical education? A meta-analytic comparative review of the evidence. *Acad Med* 2011; 86: 706–11.

9. W. C. McGaghie, S. B. Issenberg, J. H. Barsuk, D. B. Wayne. A critical review of simulation-based mastery learning with translational outcomes. *Med Educ* 2014; 48: 375–85.

10. A. D. Udani, T. E. Kim, S. K. Howard, E. R. Mariano. Simulation in teaching regional anesthesia: Current perspectives. *Local Reg Anesth* 2015; 8: 33–43.

11. A. U. Niazi, N. Haldipur, A. G. Prasad, V. W. Chan. Ultrasound-guided regional anesthesia performance in the early learning period: Effect of simulation training. *Reg Anesth Pain Med* 2012; 37: 51–4.

12. B. D. Sites, V. W. Chan, J. M. Neal et al. The American Society of Regional Anesthesia and Pain Medicine and the European Society of Regional Anaesthesia and Pain Therapy joint committee recommendations for education and training in ultrasound-guided regional anesthesia. *Reg Anesth Pain Med* 2010; 35: S74–80.

13. G. Hocking, S. Hebard, C. H. Mitchell. A review of the benefits and pitfalls of phantoms in ultrasound-guided regional anesthesia. *Reg Anesth Pain Med* 2011; 36: 162–70.

14. J. M. Neal, R. L. Hsiung, M. F. Mulroy et al. ASRA checklist improves trainee performance during a simulated episode of local anesthetic systemic toxicity. *Reg Anesth Pain Med* 2012; 37: 8–15.

15. D. H. Tran, T. C. Van Zundert, J. Aliste et al. Primary failure of thoracic epidural analgesia in training centers: The invisible elephant? *Reg Anesth Pain Med* 2016; 41: 309–13.

16. D. A. Cook, A. J. Levinson, S. Garside et al. Internet-based learning in the health professions: A meta-analysis. *JAMA* 2008; 300: 1181–96.

17. Q. Liu, W. Peng, F. Zhang et al. The effectiveness of blended learning in health professions: Systematic review and meta-analysis. *J Med Internet Res* 2016; 18: e2.

18. G. Woodworth, A. M. Juve, C. E. Swide, R. Maniker. An innovative approach to avoid reinventing the wheel: The anesthesia education toolbox. *J Grad Med Educ* 2015; 7: 270–1.

19. J. R. Frank, R. Mungroo, Y. Ahmad et al. Toward a definition of competency-based education in medicine: A systematic review of published definitions. *Med Teach* 2010; 32: 631–7.

20. S. A. Schartel, C. Kuhn, D. J. Culley et al. Development of the anesthesiology educational milestones. *J Grad Med Educ* 2014; 6: 12–14.

21. E. Ben-Menachem, T. Ezri, A. Ziv et al. Objective structured clinical examination-based assessment of regional anesthesia skills: The Israeli National Board Examination in Anesthesiology experience. *Anesth Analg* 2011; 112: 242–5.

22. A. Chuan, P. L. Graham, D. M. Wong et al. Design and validation of the Regional Anaesthesia Procedural Skills Assessment Tool. *Anaesthesia* 2015; 70: 1401–11.

23. M. J. Watson, D. M. Wong, R. Kluger et al. Psychometric evaluation of a direct observation of procedural skills assessment tool for ultrasound-guided regional anaesthesia. *Anaesthesia* 2014; 69: 604–12.

24. G. E. Woodworth, P. A. Carney, J. M. Cohen et al. Development and validation of an assessment of regional anesthesia ultrasound interpretation skills. *Reg Anesth Pain Med* 2015; 40: 306–14.

25. H. M. Smith, S. L. Kopp, A. K. Jacob et al. Designing and implementing a comprehensive learner-centered regional anesthesia curriculum. *Reg Anesth Pain Med* 2009; 34: 88–94.

26. O. Ten Cate. Nuts and bolts of entrustable professional activities. *J Grad Med Educ* 2013 Mar; 5(1): 157–8.

27. C. C. Cheston, T. E. Flickinger, M. S. Chisolm. Social media use in medical education: A systematic review. *Acad Med* 2013; 88: 893–901.

Teaching Transesophageal Echocardiography

John D. Mitchell and Robina Matyal

Transesophageal echocardiography (TEE) has become an essential tool in the repertoire of the anesthesiologist. In the operating room (OR), TEE was initially utilized primarily for patients undergoing cardiac surgery. Over time, it has steadily gained acceptance in other roles as well. TEE has proven valuable in noncardiac surgery and rescue applications such as cardiac arrest and hemodynamic instability. The American Board of Anesthesiology (ABA) and the Accreditation Council on Graduate Medical Education (ACGME) have acknowledged TEE as an example element of essential milestone progression of technical skills in anesthesiology (Figure 12.1).

Further, the ABA has begun incorporating identification and assessment of TEE images into examinations, including the written exams and the Objective Structured Clinical Exam (OSCE).[1] A recent call to action by the Society of Cardiovascular Anesthesiologists endorses a need for comprehensive education in perioperative ultrasound including TEE.[8] Thus, it is clear that TEE teaching should be integrated into anesthesiology residency. The goal of this chapter is to explore existing approaches and best practices for the teaching of this complex skill set.

Elements of Echocardiography

To effectively teach TEE, it is important to enhance learning of each element involved in this skill set, including knowledge, dexterity, and workflow (Figure 12.2).

Without experience in all these areas, trainees will be unable to successfully obtain and interpret images. Therefore, a program of training must address each of these in the context of the procedure. To ensure a successful educational experience, appropriate didactic methodologies must be applied to each of these elements. A comprehensive curriculum can then be assembled that leverages appropriate resources and addresses learner needs (Figure 12.3).

Knowledge

There is a substantial amount of knowledge that is required to successfully obtain, optimize, and interpret TEE images. Foundational knowledge related to principles of ultrasound physics, probe positioning and orientation, artifacts, and image optimization form the bedrock for solid imaging techniques. Proper image interpretation also requires understanding of normal and abnormal anatomy as well as sonoanatomy. Diagnosis and management are higher levels of application of knowledge that can be integrated later. Teaching this information benefits from multimodal approaches to enhance efficiency of delivery, facilitate retention, and address the needs of learners with differing learning preferences or styles. Standard textbooks and lectures are helpful but do not adequately address the needs of learners in this highly visual pursuit; supplemental approaches include online modules (described in the following text) and electronic books that allow for large volumes of video content to be integrated into the learning process. Table 12.1 and Figure 12.1 demonstrate some of the teaching approaches recommended to enhance knowledge acquisition.

Assessments of knowledge are most commonly undertaken with written examinations. The National Board of Echocardiography (NBE) offers well-designed examinations for Basic and Advanced Perioperative TEE (Basic PTeEXAM and Advanced PTeEXAM, respectively). While expensive on a per-learner basis, they have been rigorously designed and form the basis for a certification process for these skill sets.

Other examinations have been designed for the purposes of verification of competency to begin training in the clinical environment or to verify that concepts taught in courses have been adequately learned.[3] Some of these examinations, published as part of research protocols, have shown reasonable ability to

Has not Achieved Level 1	Level 1	Level 2	Level 3	Level 4	Level 5
	Demonstrates the correct use of standard monitoring devices, including blood pressure (BP) cuff, electrocardiogram (ECG), pulse oximeter, and temperature monitors Interprets data from standard monitoring devices, including recognition of artifacts	Performs pre-anesthetic equipment and machine checks Inserts arterial and central venous catheters with direct supervision Demonstrates use of ultrasound for placement of invasive catheters Interprets data from arterial and central venous catheters Recognizes and appropriately troubleshoots malfunctions of standard ASA monitoring equipment and anesthesia machines	Inserts arterial catheters with conditional independence and central venous catheters with indirect supervision Performs advanced monitoring techniques for assessing cardiac function (e.g., pulmonary artery catheterization, transesophageal echocardiography) with direct supervision Applies data from advanced monitoring devices (e.g., electroencephalogram [EEG], motor evoked potentials [MEPs], somatosensory evoked potentials [SSEPs], fetal monitors) with indirect supervision Recognizes and appropriately troubleshoots malfunctions of advanced monitoring equipment	Obtains vascular access in complex or difficult situations with conditional independence Performs advanced monitoring techniques for assessing cardiac function (e.g., pulmonary artery catheterization, transesophageal echocardiography) with indirect supervision Supervises other members of the health care team in the placement and interpretation of monitoring techniques Recognizes equipment malfunctions and troubleshoots appropriately	Independently selects and uses basic and advanced monitoring techniques

Figure 12.1 Patient Care 9: Technical skills: Use and interpretation of monitoring and equipment. Note reference to TEE in Level 3 and Level 4.

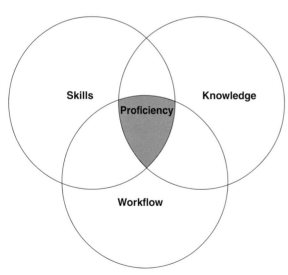

Figure 12.2 Elements of proficiency. Knowledge, skills, and workflow must all be learned to become a proficient echocardiographer (adapted from L. Yeh, M. Montealegre-Gallegos, F. Mahmood, P. E. Hess, M. Shnider, J. D. Mitchell et al. Assessment of perioperative ultrasound workflow understanding: A consensus. *J Cardiothorac Vasc Anesth* 2016; 31: 197–202).[2]

Table 12.1 Suggested educational program elements

Number	Element
1	Structured curriculum based on goals and objectives
2	Learning environment that is optimal and adequately resourced
3	Information and skills repeated to ensure retention
4	Graduated complexity and progression from normal to abnormal
5	Flexible adaptable learning environment/ curriculum
6	Incorporation of multiple learning strategies
7	Timely and objective feedback provided to participants
8	Performance and compliance measures designed and incorporated

Source: Adapted from J. D. Mitchell, F. Mahmood, R. Bose, P. E. Hess, V. Wong, R. Matyal. Novel, multimodal approach for basic transesophageal echocardiographic teaching. *J Cardiothorac Vasc Anesth* 2014 Jun; 28(3): 800–9.[3]

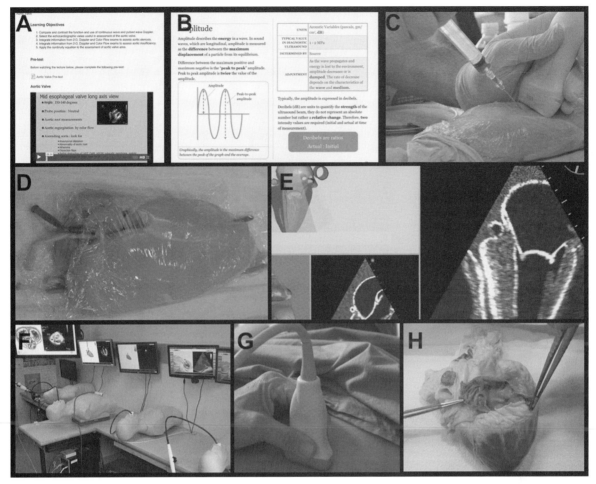

Figure 12.3 Beth Israel Deaconess Medical Center perioperative ultrasound course elements. The elements of the course include (A) online learning modules; (B) iBooks; (C) hands-on with phantom models; (D) hands-on with tissue models; (E) simulator work for Transthoracic Echocardiography (TTE), Transesophageal Echocardiography (TEE), Focused Assessment with Sonography for Trauma (FAST), and Focused Assessed Transthoracic Echo (FATE) examinations; (F) simulator acquired metrics for hand motion analysis; (G) live model workshops for TTE, regional, vascular access, and abdominal ultrasound; and (H) heart dissection workshops (adapted from J. D. Mitchell, M. Montealegre-Gallegos, F. Mahmood, K. Owais, V. Wong, B. Ferla et al. Multimodal perioperative ultrasound course for interns allows for enhanced acquisition and retention of skills and knowledge. *AA Case Rep* 2015 Oct; 5(7): 119–23).[4]

detect gaps in knowledge but none are fully validated. One struggle is to determine the appropriate length of an examination to ensure participation while retaining ability to discriminate adequacy of understanding. Other approaches to verifying knowledge acquisition include oral examinations, and OSCEs, but these approaches are under development.

Dexterity/Image Acquisition

Manual skills and dexterity are required to handle the probe and obtain adequate images. Traditionally, these are observed directly or inferred based on the number of exams a trainee completed. More recently, motion metrics have been developed and tested as a possible approach to assess proficiency.[7] These motion metrics can track probe motion in the x, y, and z coordinates (roll, pitch, and yaw) and generate three-dimensional plots that can be tracked over time. Patterns of probe manipulation change over time from novice to experienced echocardiographer. Ongoing research seeks to compare trainee performance to that of experts as well as establish the number of exams needed to be ready to acquire images without assistance.

Manual skills for TEE have traditionally been taught and practiced in the ORs on anesthetized patients. This approach allows for learners to practice under direct

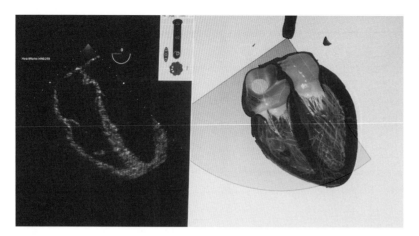

Figure 12.4 TEE simulator. A side-by-side view from a HeartWorks simulator showing the TEE image juxtaposed to a cutaway of the heart. Note that the TEE image is illustrated on the cutaway of the heart by the "fan" from the ultrasound probe (image for HeartWorks simulator).

observation and guidance but results in a small but incremental increase in risk to the patient compared to an exam conducted by the mentor. Echo simulators have allowed for this process to be undertaken without patient involvement, resulting in elimination of risks and time constraints for learners. Simulation also allows for several additional differences from conventional training. Split-screen settings available on most simulators allow the learner to simultaneously see the anatomic location of the probe and the resulting ultrasound image, potentially enhancing understanding of imaging planes (Figure 12.4).

Some simulators can also be programmed in a testing mode to identify an ideal target-imaging plane. The student can then be asked to obtain the desired image. The degree of difference from the ideal image can be calculated and feedback provided to the leaner quantitatively instead of just qualitatively.

Workflow

Workflow is the least well studied and most difficult to assess of the elements of TEE competency. Workflow encompasses elements of machine setup, equipment selection, patient management, data acquisition, image storage, and report generation. While these are essential elements necessary for appropriate conduct of TEE, instruction in workflow has been traditionally accomplished through direct mentorship and apprenticeship and has not been formally studied. Recently, efforts have been made to define and prioritize elements of ultrasound and echocardiographic workflow. A national expert consensus was developed and is being used to develop a curriculum and metrics to teach and evaluate the essential elements of workflow.

Checklists and OSCEs appear to be feasible ways to assess this area, but further work needs to be done to validate these approaches.

Didactic Modalities

Aside from apprenticeship models, the most common teaching approaches described for TEE are lecture and textbook based. While texts are valuable resources, they often are unable to convey the highly visual content necessary to fully understand concepts in echocardiography. Many have adapted by offering companion materials either on DVDs or websites to address this issue. An example of a textbook with an accompanying DVD is *Practical Perioperative Transesophageal Echocardiography with Critical Care Echocardiography*, second edition, by Davide Sidebotham, Alan F. Merry, Malcom E. Legget, and Mark L. Edwards. This excellent basic text comes with an extensive supplemental library of images and cases. Another extensive resource with a supplemental DVD included is *Transesophageal Echocardiography Multimedia Manual*, second edition, by Andre Y. Denalt, Pierre Couture, Annette Vegas, Jean Buitheieu, and Jean-Claude Tardif.

Another adaptation of the traditional textbook to accommodate this highly visual discipline is the e-book. Several ultrasound texts exist in e-book format with significant quantities of embedded video and questions allowing for a more interactive learning experience. Some are versions of hard-copy textbooks published in one or more electronic formats (e.g., Adobe's Portable Document Format – pdf; International Digital Publishing Forum's electronic publishing format – epub; or Mobipocket Reader's format – MOBI). Other e-books may be published solely in an electronic format. One limitation of most e-book formats is that answers to questions cannot be stored and tabulated for later review.

Numerous websites exist that offer resources for TEE teaching. Perhaps the best known is the virtual TEE website hosted by Toronto General Hospital Department of Anesthesia[1]. This interactive web resource allows the user to view and manipulate cut planes of an anatomic heart model at the same time as viewing the corresponding echo images. The site also contains descriptions of how to obtain the view and anatomic labels that can be shown to facilitate learning. Other popular sites include a basic course in TEE available from Open Anesthesia (www.openanesthesia.org/basic-course-in-tee/). Learning management systems (LMS) take web-based learning modules and add the ability to ask questions, grade tests, and send curriculum and assignments, making them versatile teaching tools for learners separated in space and time. The Anesthesia Toolbox Project[2] offers a variety of interactive learning modules in echocardiography to more than 40 member departments aimed at teaching TEE and transthoracic echocardiography (TTE) skills as part of cardiac and intensive care unit curricula. Other individual departments also host and share content related to TEE teaching and will be discussed further in the following section.

Whether textbooks, e-books, or websites, the number of resources available for teaching echocardiography is expanding so rapidly and the content is being updated so frequently that a list that would be exhaustive at the time this chapter was written would be out of date by the time this book is published.

Comprehensive Curricula

Most cardiothoracic anesthesia fellowships have developed curricula based on mentored examinations, readings, and lectures. These curricula typically run through the course of a year and are tailored to meet the sophisticated requirements of the NBE Advanced PTeEXAM. Fellowships traditionally rely heavily on an apprenticeship model with intraoperative examinations making up the majority of the learning experience. By virtue of time limits and more limited goals of residency-based echo training, a more focused curriculum is required for most anesthesiology core training programs. Several curricula have been proposed and incorporated for residents; while not exhaustive, the profiles that follow represent several different approaches to ensuring a comprehensive education in TEE and perioperative ultrasound.

University of North Carolina

The Department of Anesthesiology at the University of North Carolina published the first randomized controlled trial of perioperative ultrasound training demonstrating the benefits of a simulator-based training program.[5] Training in TEE occurs biweekly for residents and incorporates simulation and case presentations to supplement teaching based in the OR. Easy, round-the-clock access to a TEE simulator allows residents to engage in self-directed learning as well as faculty-led hands-on TEE skills training. All clinical anesthesia residents experience at least four weeks of TEE rotation to supplement their experiences during CA-2 and CA-3 cardiac rotations. Additionally, CA-3 residents can spend elective time on intraoperative TEE or with cardiology, in their echo lab, to learn TTE. Residents are encouraged to take NBE's Basic PTeEXAM because most residents easily achieve the minimum required number of hands-on cases as well as cases reviewed. They also incorporate OSCE exams to assess echo learning. Residents in this department also cross-train with cardiology fellows and cardiothoracic surgeons in an effort to facilitate multidisciplinary collaboration and use of ultrasound to improve patient care.

University of California – Irvine

The Department of Anesthesiology and Perioperative Care at University of California – Irvine has developed a comprehensive perioperative ultrasound course that involves echocardiography as well as scanning of abdomen, eye, trachea, and multiple other organs. Training involves classroom work, simulation, and hands-on management of patients. They have demonstrated an impact of their educational efforts in the patient care arena.

University of Utah

The Department of Anesthesiology at the University of Utah has a comprehensive training program in

---

1 https://pie.med.utoronto.ca/TEE/ (accessed November 5, 2017).

2 www.anesthesiatoolbox.com (accessed November 5, 2017).

perioperative ultrasound for its residents and fellows. It runs the echocardiography service (TEE, TTE, and stress echocardiography) at the affiliated Veterans' Administration Hospital and thus conducts close to 1,000 exams per year. This provides a source of content as well as live exams to learners. The curriculum also incorporates simulator-based training. The department also offers free online introductory lectures, interesting cases, and question banks, and the option to pay for continuing medical education (CME) credit that will be discussed further in that section.[3] Graduates of this program routinely take and pass the NBE Advanced PTeEXAM.

University of Kentucky

The Department of Anesthesiology at the University of Kentucky has a long-standing and highly successful TEE training program for its residents. The program incorporates in-OR experiences, case conferences, weekly echo simulator experiences, and online learning. A hallmark of this program is the extensive library of clips that learners are required to review to gain a comprehensive understanding of different abnormalities and conditions. The echo simulator used for didactics is also available to the residents at all times for review and independent skills practice. The program is longitudinal and begins with initial simulations in first Clinical Anesthesia (CA-1) year, but increases in complexity as learners enter cardiac anesthesia rotations and echo electives as senior residents. The coursework includes a dedicated five-day rotation in each the first two cardiothoracic anesthesia rotations (occurring in in the first or second CA year) year as well as two weeks during their cardiac rotation in the third CA year. In addition, monthly "Echo Rounds" are incorporated as part of the weekly General Competencies Conference (aka "Grand Rounds"). The spaced approach allows for initial orientation and later application of knowledge at a higher level once a clinical context is better appreciated. This group has been tracking their outcomes over multiple years. They have created significant opportunities for reading echocardiograms with experts (average of more than 42 studies per resident) that are increasing over time. They also have demonstrated significant

improvements in exam scores following the first TEE experience (mean scores increased from 40.2 before the course to 87.5 after the course) (personal correspondence). Residents are encouraged to take the NBE Basic PTeEXAM; there has been a 100 percent pass rate for those who have opted to take the exam. Other ultrasound skills including transthoracic ultrasound are also taught; the Sonosim and HeartWorks simulators are used in part for this training. The group is working on developing an OSCE examination to test learner knowledge as well.

Beth Israel Deaconess Medical Center

The Department of Anesthesia, Critical Care and Pain Medicine at Beth Israel Deaconess Medical Center has developed and incorporated an extensive approach to teaching perioperative ultrasound, including hand motion metrics for evaluation of dexterity, written exams for knowledge assessment, and OSCE-type exams to assess workflow. The curriculum began as eight sessions throughout a month, but has evolved over time into a longitudinal course that spans the entire training program. Starting with a three-week immersive course in the first postgraduate year (see Table 12.2), it is buttressed with a refresher boot camp at the start of the CA-1 year.

The curriculum includes workshops, as well as live model and simulator sessions, which run every six to eight weeks throughout training to ensure constant exposure to the full range of perioperative ultrasound skill (Table 12.3).

Course didactics are managed through an online LMS and supported with a collection of specially designed e-books that permit a highly visual, interactive experience to prime learners prior to live learning sessions.

Live sessions incorporate focused questions, review, and problem-based discussions to augment simulator-based drills and diagnosis of unknown lesions. Residents apply their skills clinically during their CA-1 and CA-2 cardiac rotations as well as senior electives in cardiac anesthesia and TEE. They also apply TTE during intensive care unit and vascular anesthesia rotations and the use ultrasound guidance during regional, pain, and obstetric anesthesia rotations. Testing for knowledge is done through the online LMS. Technical skills are assessed by analysis of probe motion data. Workflow is assessed through the OSCE exam. A proficiency index is under

---

[3] http://medicine.utah.edu/anesthesiology/echo/ (accessed November 6, 2017).

Table 12.2 Beth Israel Deaconess Medical Center intern course curriculum

Day	Topic	Daily Activities
1	Basic physics	• Orientation • Pretest • Lecture: Ultrasound physics (Part 1) • Lecture: Ultrasound-guided vascular access • Workshop: Vascular access (chicken and balloon model and Blue Phantom [Sarasota, FL]) • Interactive questions with faculty
2	Physics, Regional anesthesia	• Shadowing/self-study • Lecture: Ultrasound physics (Part 2) and Doppler • Interactive questions with faculty • Lecture: Ultrasound machine overview and imaging basics with live models • Workshop: Knobology; tissue phantom and vascular access • Lecture: Upper extremity regional anesthesia
3	Regional anesthesia	• Workshop: Upper extremity regional anatomy with live models • Lecture: Lower extremity regional anesthesia • Lecture: Local anesthetics • Lecture: Trunk blocks • Case studies: Vascular access and regional anesthesia
4	Cardiac anatomy	• Shadowing/self-study • Workshop: Lower extremity, upper extremity, and trunk blocks with live models • Lecture: Probe position and manipulation and basic TEE imaging planes • Hands-on practice with haptic TEE simulators • Workshop: Heart dissection with homemade models
5	TEE	• Shadowing/self-study • Review: Basic imaging planes and probe position • Hands-on practice with haptic TEE simulators • Lecture: Left ventricular function and regional wall motion abnormalities • Hands-on practice with haptic TEE simulators
6	TEE	• Shadowing/self-study • Lecture: Right ventricular function • Hands-on practice with haptic TEE simulators • Lecture: Aortic valve • Case studies: TEE • Hands-on practice with haptic TEE simulators
7	TEE	• Shadowing/self-study • Lecture: Mitral valve • Hands-on practice with haptic TEE simulators • Lecture: Point-of-care TEE • Case studies: TEE • Hands-on practice with haptic TEE simulators
8	TTE	• Lecture: TTE imaging planes and probe positions • Hands-on practice with haptic TTE simulators • Lecture: Pericardial effusion and tamponade • Hands-on practice with haptic TTE simulators
9	TTE	• Shadowing/self-study • Review: Basic TTE imaging planes • Hands-on practice with haptic TTE simulators • Lecture: Artifacts and anatomic pitfalls (TEE and TTE) • Workshop: TTE and regional anesthesia with live models

(continued)

Table 12.2 (*continued*)

Day	Topic	Daily Activities
10	TTE	• Shadowing/self-study • Workshop: Hemodynamics • Hands-on practice with haptic TTE simulators • Hands-on practice with haptic TEE and TTE simulators (with hemodynamics and pathologies) • Case studies: TEE and TTE
11	FAST[a]/RUSH[b]	• Shadowing/self-study • Lecture: FAST, extended FAST, and RUSH exams • Interactive case studies TEE, TTE, FAST, and RUSH • Workshop: TTE, FAST, and lung ultrasound with live models
12	Summary	• Shadowing/self-study • Lecture: Lung ultrasound and BLUE[c] protocol • Mixed simulation: TEE, TTE, FAST, and Rush
13	Final	• TEE, TTE, FAST, and RUSH exams refresher with mixed simulation • Posttest • Final skills testing

[a] FAST: Focused Assessment with Sonography for Trauma.
[b] RUSH: Rapid Ultrasound for Shock and Hypotension.
[c] BLUE: Bedside Lung Ultrasound in Emergency.

Table 12.3 Beth Israel Deaconess Medical Center perioperative ultrasound course elements

Teaching Goal	Tools	Description	Metrics
Knowledge	Live teaching	• Live lectures • Shadowing in the OR	• Online pre- and posttest
	Apple iBooks (Apple, Cupertino, CA)	• Self-study • 3 electronic books with interactive videos, questions, and figures • Topics: physics, regional anesthesia, and TTE	
	Online modules	• Self-study • Online modules with videos, questions, and interactive practice exercises • Topics: TTE and TEE	
Skills	High-fidelity simulators	• Hands-on practice of manual TTE, TEE, and RUSH and FAST exam skills on HeartWorks (Inventive Medical Ltd., London, UK) and VIMEDIX (CAE Healthcare, Montreal, Canada) haptic simulators	• Probe motion data provided by haptic simulator software
	Live workshops	• Manual skills practice on: ◦ Live human models ◦ Task models, including Blue Phantom, beef, and chicken models ◦ Porcine hearts • Topics: regional anesthesia, vascular access, lung ultrasound, FAST exam, and TTE	• Scoring of the quality of images acquired on live human models and need for assistance
Workflow	Interactive workstations	• Workflow workshop sessions • Supervised hands-on practice in OR	• OSCE exam

development to assess overall adequacy of training. Residents are encouraged to take the NBE basic echo exam and become basic TEE certified. To date, all residents who have chosen to take the exam have passed, including several CA-1 residents.

Continuing Medical Education Courses and Preceptorship Experiences for Graduates

Learning must continue over time, both for those who have acquired TEE skills in training and for those who wish to develop them later in their careers.

For those who have completed training, there are several different CME courses and preceptorships available to learn TEE skills. Live courses and workshops are easily accessible, but their episodic nature is better suited to maintenance of knowledge and hands-on workshops are usually limited.

Online Learning

The Society for Cardiovascular Anesthesiologists (SCA)[4] offers an extensive online course collection including a series of courses and case scenarios that allows learners to fulfill the CME and case requirements to become certified by the NBE in basic echocardiography provided they pass the NBE PTeEXAM. The SCA also offers more advanced teaching programs in collaboration with iTeachU.[5] While comprehensive and thoughtfully designed, the courses run from $50 for some individual topics to $2,300 for more complete curricula. The Division of Perioperative Echocardiography in the Department of Anesthesiology at the University of Utah[6] offers a similar menu of online courses and case scenarios as well as live seminars and courses.

Preceptorships

Preceptorships of three to five days duration can allow learners to receive small group instruction customized to their personal needs and integrate OR-based teaching with simulation and classroom didactics. Preceptorships are offered at several institutions including the Department of Anesthesiology at Duke University and Beth Israel Deaconess Medical Center but require significant tuition and time away from work to participate. Therefore, some programs, including the University of Utah and Beth Israel Deaconess Medical Center also offer on-site training to departments in perioperative ultrasound skills as an option. While more costly than other options, the convenience and customization of learning objectives are attractive for some departments or groups with specific goals such as mastering 3D echo, adding transthoracic approaches for experienced TEE providers, or learning how to use new equipment. When adding new equipment, manufacturers also may provide complimentary workshops to help familiarize staff with features and workflow.

Conclusion

TEE represents a complex interplay of knowledge, skills, and workflow. Traditional apprenticeship models have been successful, but require substantial time commitments and significant numbers of patients for adequate exposure to achieve the full depth and breadth of conditions and skills required of the learner. Simulation represents an important advance in teaching of TEE by allowing for progression from normal to abnormal anatomy, unlimited practice without risk of harm to patients, and analysis of hand motion to track progression of learners. When applied in the context of a curriculum that builds knowledge and workflow skills in parallel, learning can be achieved quickly and successfully. While further work needs to be done to develop assessment metrics, existing programs have converged on similar methodologies that incorporate the best of simulation, online, and OR-based learning.

References

1. American Board of Anesthesiology. Applied Examination: Objective Structured Examination. www.theaba.org/PDFs/APPLIED-Exam/APPLIED-OSCE-ContentOutline (accessed November 17, 2017).

2. L. Yeh, M. Montealegre-Gallegos, F. Mahmood et al. Assessment of perioperative ultrasound workflow understanding: A consensus. *J Cardiothorac Vasc Anesth* 2016; 31: 197–202.

3. J. D. Mitchell, F. Mahmood, R. Bose, P. E. Hess, V. Wong, R. Matyal. Novel, multimodal approach for basic transesophageal echocardiographic teaching. *J Cardiothorac Vasc Anesth* 2014 Jun; 28(3): 800–9.

[4] http://scahq.org/default.aspx (accessed November 6, 2017).
[5] www.iteachu.com/catalogue/sca/ (accessed November 6, 2017).
[6] http://medicine.utah.edu/anesthesiology/echo/ (accessed November 6, 2017).

4. J. D. Mitchell, M. Montealegre-Gallegos, F. Mahmood, K. Owais, V. Wong, B. Ferla et al. Multimodal perioperative ultrasound course for interns allows for enhanced acquisition and retention of skills and knowledge. *A & A Case Reports* 2015 Oct; 5(7): 119–23.

5. F. Mahmood, R. Matyal, N. Skubas et al. Perioperative ultrasound training in anesthesiology: A call to action. *Anesth Analg* 2016; 122: 1794–804.

6. J. D. Mitchell, M. Montealegre-Gallegos, F. Mahmood et al. Multimodal perioperative ultrasound course for interns allows for enhanced acquisition and retention of skills and knowledge. *AA Case Rep* 2015; 5: 119–23.

7. R. Matyal, J. D. Mitchell, P. E. Hess et al. Simulator-based transesophageal echocardiographic training with motion analysis: a curriculum-based approach. *Anesthesiology* 2014; 121: 389–99.

8. N. A. Ferrero, A. V. Bortsov, H. Arora et al. Simulator training enhances resident performance in transesophageal echocardiography. *Anesthesiology* 2014; 120: 149–59.

Chapter 13

Teaching Point-of-Care Ultrasound (POCUS) to the Perioperative Physician

Davinder Ramsingh and Jason Gatling

Introduction

Early ultrasound devices were large, and often confined to imaging laboratories (cardiology, radiology, and obstetrics). With recent advances in ultrasound technology, these devices have become smaller, more portable, less expensive, and usable at the patient's bedside.[1,2] Point-of-care ultrasound (POCUS) refers to the use of portable ultrasonography at the patient's bedside for diagnostic and therapeutic purposes.[3] Kendall et al. described seven characteristics of emergency ultrasounds (Box 13.1).[3]

It is important to note that the American Medical Association passed a resolution (#802) stating that all medical specialties have the right to use ultrasound in accordance with specialty-specific practice standards.[4] Within the hospital, POCUS has proved to serve a vital role in the rapid assessment of the patient's cardiac, pulmonary, hemodynamic, vascular, neurologic, ocular, and gastrointestinal status.[5] As is often the case with new technologies in medicine, the clinical value of POCUS gained acceptance before guidelines could be established. The critical care and emergency medicine specialties have led the development in this area, with the first policy statement regarding its utility having been published in 2001.[6–9]

While these specialties continue to demonstrate clinical utility with this new patient-assessment tool, they are also continuing to develop guidelines on scope of practice, credentialing, training, and proficiency evaluation. In addition, several societies in emergency medicine and critical care have developed educational programs to establish a standard level of proficiency for POCUS.[5,10,11] In fact, both emergency medicine and critical care medicine list POCUS training as a key index procedure in which current trainees must demonstrate proficiency.[5,10,11]

For the perioperative environment, until approximately 2010 the utility of POCUS had primarily focused on central venous access and regional anesthesia. While use of ultrasound has resulted in significant improvement in patient care in critical care and emergency medicine,[12–15] the full potential of POCUS for the perioperative setting is still being explored. The ability of POCUS to assist with various perioperative issues including airway evaluation, determination of gastric volume, assessment of pulmonary pathology, diagnosis of free intra-abdominal fluid, and assessment of cardiovascular function is just beginning to be investigated.[16–20] Recent potential POCUS topics that are relevant to the perioperative environment have been published (Table 13.1) along with a call to action for anesthesiologists to develop a systematic approach of integrating POCUS as done by other acute care specialties.[5]

The validity of POCUS in the perioperative setting is further supported by the increase in ultrasound-related content for the American Board of Anesthesiology (ABA) certification examinations, including the use of ultrasound in cardiac and hemodynamic assessment.[21] This change highlights the growing awareness amongst anesthesiologists in 2017 of the utility of POCUS. In conjunction with

> **Box 13.1** Characteristics of emergency ultrasound (as described by Kendall et al.)[3]
>
> An emergency ultrasound should
>
> 1. Have a well-defined purpose linked to improving patient outcomes;
> 2. Be focused and goal directed;
> 3. Have findings that are easily recognizable;
> 4. Involve a technique that is easily learned;
> 5. Be easily performed;
> 6. Have a direct effect on clinical decisions; and
> 7. Be able to be performed at the bedside.

Table 13.1 Current and potential uses for perioperative ultrasound

Target	Estimation, Evaluation, or Procedural Guidance
Vessels	Guide central and peripheral venous access, guide arterial access, detect aortic dissection, evaluate carotid artery
Regional anesthesia	Guide peripheral nerve blocks, neuraxial blocks (spinal, epidural), and trunk blocks (paravertebral, transversus abdominal, rectus sheath blocks)
Lung	Detect pneumothorax, pulmonary edema, pleural effusion, pneumonia; evaluate dyspnea
Abdomen	Evaluate for bleeding (Focused Assessment with Sonography in Trauma: FAST); determine gastric volume
Heart	Evaluate cardiac function (contractility, valvular function, volume status), detect pericardial effusion, diagnose tamponade
Eye	Detect elevated intracranial pressure (optic nerve sheath diameter), retinal detachment, vitreous hemorrhage, lens dislocation, retrobulbar hematoma, foreign body
Airway	Predict difficult laryngoscopy (soft tissue in anterior neck), assess vocal cord function, guide cricothyroid membrane puncture/cricothyrotomy, determine subglottic airway diameter/predict tracheal tube size, detect position of laryngeal mask airway, confirm tracheal intubation, guide tracheostomy, detect tracheal tube position, determine position of double lumen tracheal tube, assess cervical spine, suggest cause of extubation failure in intensive care unit
Procedures	Determine need for urinary catheter, guide thoracentesis and pericardiocentesis, detect pacing capture, guide bladder aspiration, detect joint effusions, guide abscess drainage

recognition of the significance of POCUS, however, lies the dilemma of training perioperative providers for this new skill set.

One method of training and integrating perioperative POCUS into the curriculum of an anesthesiology residency has been demonstrated. In 2011, a novel "whole body" comprehensive perioperative POCUS examination and training program was developed.[22] This examination, abbreviated FORESIGHT (Focused periOperative Risk Evaluation Sonography Involving Gastro-abdominal, Hemodynamic, and Transthoracic ultrasound, Figure 13.1), was implemented to assess its impact on residency education and perioperative care.

The curriculum was structured and had defined education and certification targets.[22] This study demonstrated the interest amongst anesthesiology residents in the topic of POCUS and highlighted clinical utility after appropriate training.

In addition to preparing residents to be able to use a technology with rapidly expanding, recognized indications, it is also important to educate them on subject matter that will appear on examinations. The ABA recognizes the importance of ultrasound by including the subject in the content outline[21] for both parts of the Part 1 Examination (previously known as the "written boards"). Ultrasound images are examples of video

questions on the In-Training Examination (ITE)[1]. It should be anticipated that POCUS will be included in the new Objective Structured Clinical Examination (OSCE) portion of the ABA Applied Exam (previously known as "oral boards").

As anesthesiology continues to embrace POCUS, the specialty will face challenges similar to the other acute care specialties regarding defining a scope of practice, education, and certification. This chapter focuses specifically on the development of an educational framework for perioperative POCUS training in an anesthesiology residency training program. The concepts discussed are what were used in the design of the FORESIGHT curriculum. Components of this chapter include:

- A review of the qualities of a good clinical educator with reference to the differences of the adult learner;
- A presentation of an effective educational strategy for perioperative POCUS training;
- Highlights of a validated instrument to assess the impact of POCUS training; and
- Examples from the FORESIGHT curriculum.

---

[1] www.theaba.org/TRAINING-PROGRAMS/In-training-Exam/Video-Questions (accessed November 18, 2017).

F.O.R.E.S.I.G.H.T. Comprehensive Perioperative Ultrasound Examination

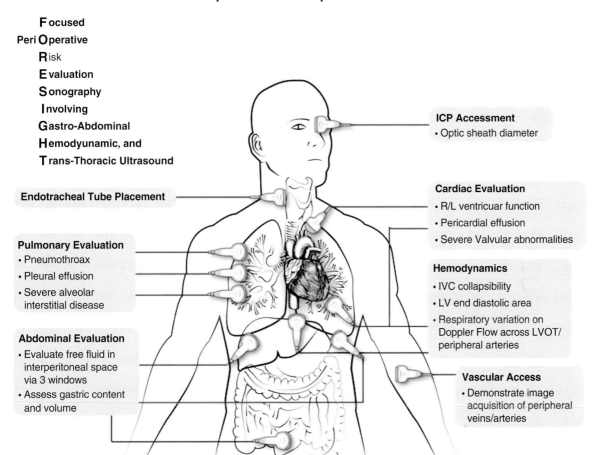

Focused
Peri **O**perative
Risk
Evaluation
Sonography
Involving
Gastro-Abdominal
Hemodyunamic, and
Trans-Thoracic Ultrasound

ICP Accessment
• Optic sheath diameter

Endotracheal Tube Placement

Cardiac Evaluation
• R/L ventricuar function
• Pericardial effusion
• Severe Valvular abnormalities

Pulmonary Evaluation
• Pneumothroax
• Pleural effusion
• Severe alveolar
  interstitial disease

Hemodynamics
• IVC collapsibility
• LV end diastolic area
• Respiratory variation on
  Doppler Flow across LVOT/
  peripheral arteries

Abdominal Evaluation
• Evaluate free fluid in
  interperitoneal space
  via 3 windows
• Assess gastric content
  and volume

Vascular Access
• Demonstrate image
  acquisition of peripheral
  veins/arteries

Figure 13.1 FORESIGHT examination.

The Good Clinical Educator and the Adult Learner

It is important to emphasize that very few studies have evaluated systems to teach attending physicians how to be good educators; rather it is assumed that "if you understand your discipline you should be able to teach it." A review article on what makes a good clinical teacher in medicine identified five common themes, of which medical expertise was only one component.[23] The remaining four noncognitive elements included (1) development of a positive relationship, (2) emotional activation, (3) generativity, and (4) self-awareness.[23] An explanation of each noncognitive skill set and how it is important in perioperative POCUS education is provided as follows.

1. **Development of a positive relationship:**
   A good clinical educator must develop a positive relationship with the student such that the student feels engaged in the process. This "positive relationship" has been defined as one in which communication is bidirectional and in which the student is given immediate feedback.[23] Because POCUS can be viewed as a new physical examination tool for all levels of medical providers, the educator must be aware that there will be opportunities in which both the student and teacher are learning simultaneously. The environment to stimulate this bidirectional learning should be encouraged.

2. **Emotional activation**: A good clinical educator must exhibit a sincere connection with the

student such that they share in the educator's enthusiasm to teach. The teacher must be engaging to stimulate the learner to want to learn this information and acquire this skill. The teacher should also suggest ways in which this skill, which is currently not a mandated clinical competency, may have clinical relevance.

3. **Generativity:** A good clinical educator must be able to gauge the student's abilities and provide a stepwise assumption of responsibility. Because POCUS education covers topics that vary greatly in required level of training and practice (e.g., bladder scan vs. evaluation for aortic stenosis), a graduated system for POCUS education is probably appropriate for most residents. This system should start with the basic topics and allow the student to advance after established metrics have been achieved.

4. **Self-awareness:** A good clinical educator must be sensitive to feedback from the students and be willing to dynamically alter teaching style based on the characteristics of the learner(s). For POCUS education, this directly relates to prior ultrasound education/knowledge. A wide spectrum of experience with ultrasound may exist in a specific group of learners (e.g., some residents may have no experience, some may have experience with ultrasound through use of transesophageal echocardiography [TEE] during a cardiac anesthesia rotation, and some may have extensive TEE experience gained through an elective in addition to the routine experience attained through cardiac anesthesia rotations). The teacher should be aware of the varying levels of experience and must be able to adjust teaching strategy to match the audience.

Adult Learner

Along with these traits a good clinical teacher must be aware of the characteristics of the "adult learner." The term *andragogy* is used to describe the methods and practices used to teach adults. When compared with the strategy used to educate children, termed *pedagogy*, there are stark differences. Pedagogy is the traditional one-way communication pathway from teacher to student. In this environment the teacher is viewed as the only disseminator of information and all students are dependent solely on that individual's

teaching style and fund of knowledge. In addition, teachers have control of the curriculum and determine performance using their established evaluation system. These points are in distinct contrast to the andragogy method of education. This method focuses on self-directed and/or cooperative learning between the adult students and teacher. The students in this model have much more control over their learning experience and two-way education is encouraged. Lastly, the evaluation strategies under the andragogy method are focused on evaluating utility of the education process on the learner's career activities. Embracing these concepts of the adult learner is key for medical education; it has been suggested that graduate medical education is doing a disservice to trainees by providing pedagogy-style learning strategies.[24,25] Multiple chapters in this book address various components of education for adult learners. Examples include Chapter 3, Chapters 14–18, and Chapter 20.

Thus, to implement any new educational strategy/curriculum in medical education, one needs to understand the key factors of a good educator as well as the characteristics of the adult learner. For the development of a perioperative POCUS educational curriculum, the team that developed the FORESIGHT curriculum utilized the preceding concepts.

Designing a POCUS Educational Strategy

Acquisition of an ultrasound image requires selecting the correct probe and the ability to place it appropriately on the patient and then manipulate it correctly. Interpretation of an ultrasound image requires knowledge of appropriately obtained images in normal and pathologic conditions. There is evidence that use of a model/simulation task trainer is more effective than conventional didactic lectures in teaching POCUS.[11] Models are useful for teaching probe selection, positioning, and manipulation but presumably limit ultrasound findings to normal anatomy and physiology. Multiple types of ultrasound task trainers are available. Currently marketed simulation devices offer the ability to

- Connect a dummy probe to a laptop with the option to run multiple modules with normal and abnormal conditions to practice manipulation of a probe and interpretation of resulting images;

- Demonstrate predetermined pathology by placing "stickers" containing pathologic images on a model when a dummy probe is connected to a laptop;
- Use "stickers" to integrate ultrasound with a human patient simulator mannequin; or
- Practice with any device on a dedicated ultrasound simulation task trainer.

(Chapter 17 provides more details on available ultrasound task trainers.) Vendors also offer extensive libraries of training modules that include everything from basic instruction on ultrasound to complex techniques including calculation of left ventricular outflow tract (LVOT) diameter and velocity time integral (VTI). Simulators offer an opportunity to present pathologic conditions but may limit realistic practice in correct positioning and manipulation of the probe – skills that are important to novice learners. Currently available devices that permit the learner to position and manipulate the probe on a mannequin generally have limited capacity to display pathologic findings.

With the understanding of how the adult medical trainee learns, one needs to develop an appropriate educational curriculum that incorporates these principles. One group developed an educational curriculum through a process of consultation (using a survey of anesthesiology residency program directors in the United States and consulting with POCUS experts in the areas of emergency medicine and critical care medicine) and reference to the Accreditation Council for Graduate Medical Education (ACGME) core competencies. This task force ultimately formulated clinical objectives for the total body perioperative ultrasound exam (FORESIGHT) with the main areas of the curriculum being assessment of the (1) heart, (2) lungs, (3) hemodynamic status, (4) abdomen, (5) airway, (6) blood vessels for advanced vascular access, and (7) intracranial pressure (Figure 13.1).[22]

Cardiac Ultrasound

The focus on cardiac ultrasound was chosen because of the incidence of cardiac events in the perioperative setting and due to the potential impact of these events on patient outcome. In addition, transthoracic examination of the cardiopulmonary system using bedside POCUS technology has proven to be a reliable tool when compared to formal echocardiography[26] and can be taught to noncardiologists.[27,28] Recently,

guidelines have been published for POC cardiac ultrasound by noncardiologists for the intensive care unit (ICU) setting.[28]. Considering the similarity between the ICU and the operating room (OR), the curriculum incorporated similar guidelines.

Pulmonary Ultrasound

The high prevalence of events involving the lung and the pleura during the perioperative period, as well as the potential impact of these events on patient outcome, resulted in the inclusion of pulmonary ultrasonography in the curriculum. Ultrasonography has been shown to be more accurate than auscultation or chest radiography for the detection of pleural effusion, consolidation, and alveolar interstitial syndrome in the critical care setting.[29,30] POCUS has also proven to be a valuable tool for the detection of pneumothorax.[31,32] Consequently, assessment of pneumothorax, evaluation of air-space disease, and evaluation of pleural effusion were included in the curriculum.

Hemodynamic Monitoring

POCUS incorporates several modalities that allow determining the ventricular filling pressures and fluid responsiveness, which are frequent concerns in the perioperative setting. Specifically, the collapsibility of the inferior vena cava (IVC)[33] as well as decreased left ventricular end diastolic area have been shown to be accurate measurements of reduced filling pressures[34–36] and were incorporated in the curriculum together with dynamic predictors of fluid responsiveness using ultrasound.[37,38]

Abdominal Ultrasound

Focused assessment with sonography for trauma (FAST)[39] is the most-studied example of focused clinical ultrasound in trauma care[34] and was incorporated in the curriculum. Interpretation of this exam should allow determination of the etiology of hemodynamic instability if it is secondary to injury of the pericardial and/or peritoneal space resulting in free fluid. POCUS performed by anesthesiologists at the bedside has been used to assess gastric content and volume[18,19] and a recent grading system based exclusively on qualitative sonographic assessment of the gastric antrum has shown strong correlation with gastric volume.[19] Given the critical importance of gastric content as it relates to the risk of aspiration, this topic was included in the curriculum.

Airway Ultrasound

Unrecognized malposition of the tracheal tube (TT) can lead to severe complications.[9,40] The use of POCUS for adjunct confirmation of tracheal versus esophageal intubation has been demonstrated[41] and a recent study showed successful ability of POCUS to verify correct TT position in the trachea.[42] For these reasons, this technique was added to the curriculum.

Vascular Access

The use of ultrasound to aid with vascular access has advanced beyond widespread use for central venous access.[43] Specifically, ultrasound has proven to reliably aid in the placement of difficult peripheral intravenous catheters[44–45] and intra-arterial catheters.[46,47] The utility of this skill set is obvious for perioperative medicine as these are procedures that are performed every day, and therefore they were included in the curriculum.

Intracranial Pressure Assessment

POCUS has been shown to provide rapid detection of elevated intracranial pressures (ICP) based on the assessment of optic nerve sheath diameter (ONSD).[48] The relationship between the ONSD and ICP has been well established. Because of the potential impact of increased ICP on patients' outcome in the perioperative setting it was decided to add this assessment to the curriculum.

Once the topics were identified the next step was development of the best strategy for teaching these topics. The task force involved in the FORESIGHT curriculum implemented an educational strategy based on the use of models and simulation task trainers.[22] This approach was based on prior research on teaching POCUS that demonstrated this teaching strategy is more effective for the adult medical learner than traditional didactics.[25] The task force developed two different educational strategies for POCUS education. One strategy involved a weekly 20-minute focused lecture on one of the objectives of the FORESIGHT exam that is immediately followed by a 25-minute human model practice period. Another strategy was a 2.5-hour monthly session, with approximately 60 minutes of lecture followed by 1 to 1.5 hours of model/

simulation practice.[22] In both strategies, the curriculum focuses on the adult learner by providing at least half of the allocated time to hands-on training with direct peer-to-peer feedback.[22,25] In addition, topics were designed to address key issues for the trainees' everyday clinical practice. The FORESIGHT curriculum was structured to start in August during its initial inaugural year of implementation and then be repeated every year (Table 13.2).

The curriculum is designed to repeat approximately every six months such that the course would cycle six times during each anesthesiology resident's training. This is intentional by the FORESIGHT task force to ensure uniform and adequate exposure to the curriculum for all anesthesiology residents.

Regarding evaluating improvement in understanding as one progresses through training, the FORESIGHT task force monitored for continued improvement in scores (see "Educational Curriculum Impact Assessment") throughout training. Because the vast majority of POCUS topics are new to perioperative physician trainees, the FORESIGHT task force sought to focus on designing a curriculum with built-in repetition to allow residents multiple opportunities to learn the topics.

In addition to determining what topics should be presented, it is also important to decide on the order in which topics are taught to optimize the trainees' learning. The FORESIGHT task force arranged the sequence of the determined curriculum topics such that the overview of POCUS and physics and knobology were the first topics. These were followed by

Table 13.2 FORESIGHT curriculum timeline

Month	Subject
1st	Prelecture tests/volume status
2nd	Cardiac
3rd	Pulmonary
4th	Vascular access
5th	Additional topics
6h	Volume status
7th	Cardiac
8th	Pulmonary
9th	Vascular access
10th	Additional topics
11th	Written and model examinations

POCUS topics with gradually increasing degrees of difficulty. The order determined by the FORESIGHT team is:

1. Ultrasound physics;
2. Assessment of volume status/mechanisms of hypotension;
3. Cardiac;
4. Pulmonary;
5. Vascular access; and
6. Additional advanced topics.

Finally, the FORESIGHT task force realized that while the curriculum was designed for resident education, the training of supervising faculty is also crucial. To encourage faculty training, the task force held small group training sessions for faculty only. Sessions were offered weekly as an alternative to the hour-long Grand Rounds lecture. The sessions were similar in structure to the resident lectures (a brief didactic presentation followed by use of ultrasound on models or simulation task trainers). By separating the lecture series for faculty from the program for residents, it allowed the attending physicians to learn the topics with their peers without pressure to prioritize the trainees' education.

Educational Curriculum Impact Assessment

Once a curriculum has been determined it is important to identify the tool that can be used to evaluate its impact. Kirkpatrick's educational model is well recognized as a method to evaluate the effectiveness of a new educational intervention. The model evaluates outcomes based on four criteria:

1. The participants' affective responses to training content (reaction and satisfaction);
2. The impact of the training on improving knowledge (learning and performance on a test);
3. The application of the new information (behavior and execution of the intervention); and
4. Use of the new training to improve patient care (clinical impact on the organization).[49]

While, ideally, any new educational intervention should attain level 4 in Kirkpatrick's instrument, this is not easily achievable due to the fact that it can be challenging to demonstrate a direct relationship between the educational intervention and an improvement in the quality of clinical care. The benefit of perioperative POCUS has been demonstrated at each Kirkpatrick level.[16–20,22,50]

The group involved with the FORESIGHT exam evaluated participating trainees using the Kirkpatrick model at different intervals. Resident satisfaction surveys (Kirkpatrick level 1) and content examinations (Kirkpatrick level 2) were performed at the end of each six-month course completion. Model practicums were performed every year for all residents to evaluate the trainees' ability to perform the ultrasound exams (Kirkpatrick level 3). Specific categories of evaluation were image quality, anatomy identification, and acquisition time. After one year of training and completion of at least ten complete FORESIGHT exams, the clinical impact assessment was assessed through a survey of the primary anesthesiology team after the POCUS studies (Kirkpatrick level 4). Importantly, this study required all documented exams to be performed under the supervision of an attending anesthesiologist who was department certified after completing 50 FORESIGHT exams.[22] It is important to state that currently there is no certification process for perioperative POCUS and the departmental requirement of 50 FORESIGHT exams is based on the limited evidence suggesting that POCUS topics can be trained after 10 to 50 examinations.[51] Similarly, while the definition of *improvement* in POCUS education is highly subjective, literature supports a 20 percent increase in score to represent improvement.[22–52]

Highlights of a Perioperative POCUS Curriculum

This section highlights key concepts of a perioperative POCUS curriculum and provides examples on how these topics can be effectively taught by utilization of the preceding concepts. The key topics include:

1. Basic ultrasound physics and knobology;
2. Preload and fluid responsiveness;
3. Assessment of cardiac status and mechanisms of shock;
4. Assessment of pulmonary and airway status;
5. Vascular access; and
6. Additional topics.

Ultrasound Physics and Probe Selection

The topic of ultrasound physics is often viewed as challenging for the trainee to grasp. To encourage learning

Transducer type	Linear	Curvilinear	Phased array
	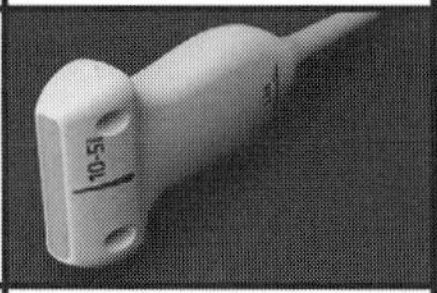	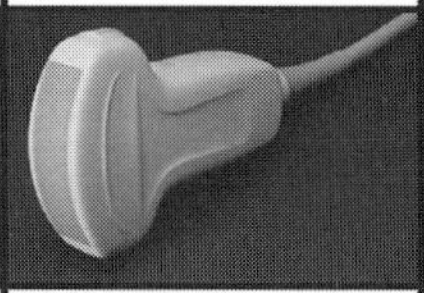	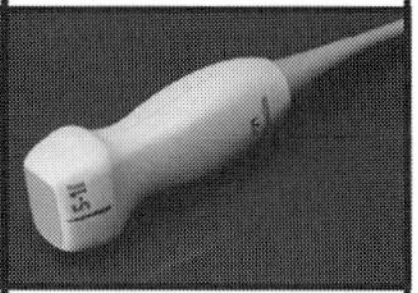
Frequency range	5–10 MHz	2–5 MHz	1–5 MHz
Imaging depth	9 cm	30 cm	35 cm
Footprint	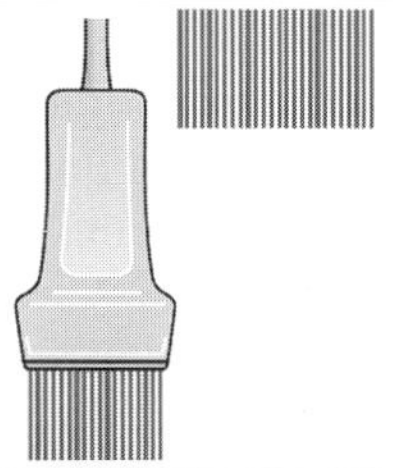	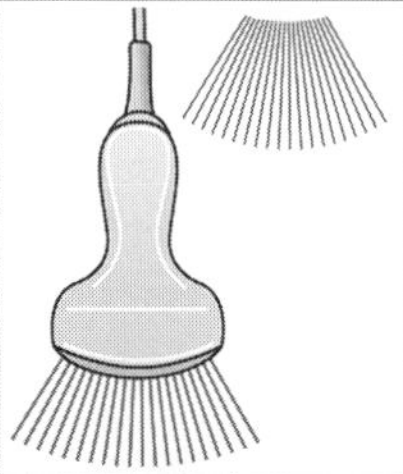	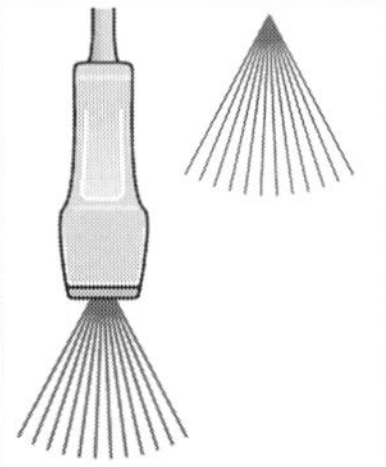
Image	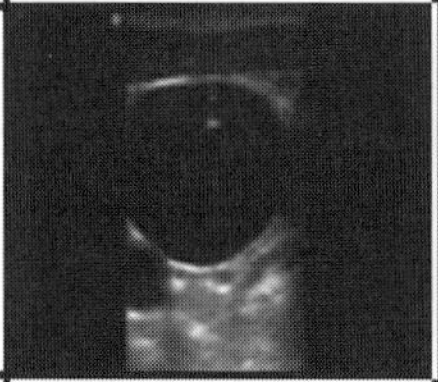	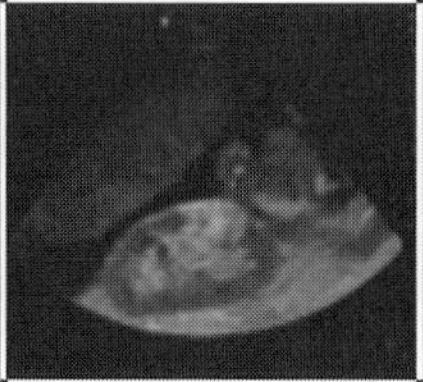	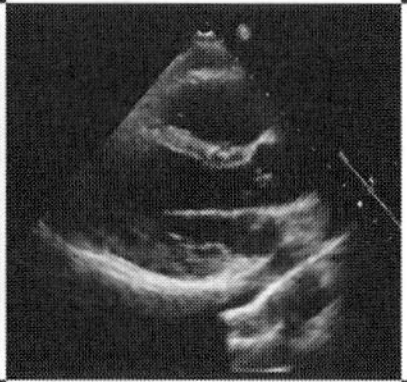
Applications	Arteries/veins Procedures Pleura Skin/soft tissues Musculoskeletal Testicles/hernia Eyes Breast	Gallbladder Liver Kidney Bladder Abdominal aorta Abdominal free fluid Uterus/ovaries	Heart Inferior vena cava Lungs Pleura Abdomen

Figure 13.2 Common ultrasound probe types (modified from Figure 3.5 of N. J. Soni, R. Arntfield, P. Kory, eds. *Point of Care Ultrasound*. Philadelphia: Saunders, 2015).

on this topic one must understand the learners' prior knowledge (highly variable across medical trainees) and place a strong emphasis on clinical relevance. For example, demonstration of how alterations to settings of the ultrasound device impact image quality followed by an explanation of the physics of ultrasound can be useful. This approach can be used to address knobology, probe type, and the acoustic windows used for image acquisition (Figure 13.2).

For example, the attached video file (Video 13.1) demonstrates how the ultrasound image can be altered by the use of different ultrasound probes that have their distinct qualities (e.g., high vs. low frequency). Finally, a demonstration of how one should maneuver the ultrasound probe and the terminology to define these movements are crucial as this is the mechanism by which one can learn how to improve their insonation skills (Figure 13.3 and Video 13.2).

Preload and Fluid Responsiveness

Fluid management is of key importance in perioperative care. The education of how POCUS can be useful in this area relies on establishing a connection between POCUS and the current methods used to assess preload and volume responsiveness in the perioperative period. For example, in certain circumstances (e.g., positive pressure ventilation with relatively large tidal volumes and in the absence of spontaneous ventilation) pulse pressure variation (PPV) derived from an arterial line has been demonstrated to predict volume responsiveness.[53] To validate use of ultrasound preload assessment one can compare how ultrasound techniques (Doppler ultrasound of major structures with pulsatile flow) have demonstrated a high degree of correlation with PPV.[37,38,54]

Ultrasound techniques (measurement of IVC diameter) have also been demonstrated to correlate with the clinically used parameter of central venous pressure.[33] The diameter of the IVC and its percent collapsibility from a maximal negative inspiratory

breath has been shown to correlate with right atrial pressures. To obtain IVC measurements one places a low-frequency probe in the subxiphoid position in the sagittal plane (Figure 13.4). It is important to note that due to the changes in intrathoracic pressures a spontaneous inspiratory breath will cause a decrease in IVC diameter while a mechanical inspiratory breath will cause an increase in IVC diameter. Specific guidelines for IVC measurements and their corresponding atrial pressures have been identified.[55,56]

Another modality that helps determine cardiovascular filling pressures involves the direct measurement of left ventricular end-diastolic area (LVEDA) from a parasternal short axis view. Several studies have shown the utility of LVEDA in helping predict preload status in ventilated patients.[35–37] Key reference values from these studies suggest that reduced filling pressures may be present when the LVEDA is less than 8 cm^2.

Similar to central venous pressure, measurement of the IVC diameter or LVEDA are "static" measurements of volume status; individual response is variable and patients may not respond to fluid boluses as expected.[57,58] In addition, impaired tissue oxygenation from decreased cardiac output may not be identified by these static parameters.[59] Thus, while these assessments may be more reliable than less invasive markers of hypovolemia such as urine output, they may not always predict fluid responsiveness.

In comparison, dynamic flow parameters may be used to predict the fluid responsiveness of a patient; fluid responsiveness is generally defined as an increase in stroke volume by 10 percent following a fluid bolus (steep portion of the Frank-Starling curve). Dynamic

Transducer Movements

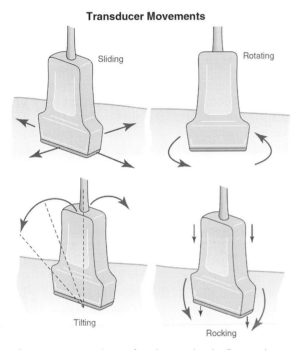

Figure 13.3 Manipulation of an ultrasound probe. From each transducer position the target structure is focused by three major movements: (1) Tilt, which is scanning in the left–right direction (used to position structures in the middle of the screen); (2) Angle, which is scanning in the anterior–inferior direction; (3) Rotation (clockwise–counterclockwise) (modified from Figure 4.4 of N. J. Soni, R. Arntfield, P. Kory, eds. *Point of Care Ultrasound.* Philadelphia: Saunders, 2015).

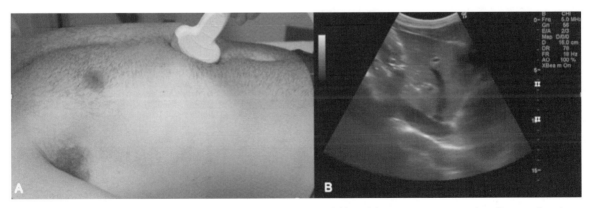

Figure 13.4 Measurement of IVC diameter. Picture of probe position on model for IVC diameter measurements (curvilinear or phased-array probe should be used) (A) and ultrasound image (B) (modified from D. Ramsingh, *Perioperative Point of Care Ultrasound Educational Manual,* epublished, available at www.foresightultrasound.com/ebook [accessed November 18, 2017]).

flow parameters require not simply recording a static measurement, but also involve comparing these measurements through several cardiac cycles. This makes it possible to monitor the hemodynamic effects of controlled intrathoracic pressure changes occurring during mechanical ventilation. Briefly, this cardiopulmonary interaction is based on controlled cyclic inspiration and expiration during mechanical ventilation, which induces a regular change in intrathoracic pressure. This cyclic change stresses the filling condition of the heart to a degree that is correlated with intravascular volume of the patient. An example of a dynamic parameter that can be used to guide fluid management during controlled ventilation is evaluating the change in IVC diameter (dIVC) utilizing POCUS. Using a threshold of 18 percent change, dIVC had a 90 percent sensitivity and a 90 percent specificity in differentiating those who responded to a fluid bolus from those who did not.[33] More intricate methods of using POCUS to determine volume status include the use of Doppler ultrasonography to measure the area under the flow curve, VTI, for structures that transmit the pulsatile systemic blood flow. For example, once the apical four-chamber cardiac view is obtained, assessment of the respiratory variation during positive pressure mechanical ventilation of the VTI across the LVOT has been shown to indicate fluid responsiveness (Figure 13.5).[37,38]

Accurate interpretation of this parameter relies on controlled mechanical ventilation with a uniform positive inspiratory pressure. In this situation, a greater amount of respiratory variation of the VTI correlates with greater "preload dependence" or a greater increase in cardiac output from a fluid bolus. Across the multitude of studies measuring dynamic indices of fluid responsiveness, it is almost universally agreed that a 15 to 20 percent variation in VTI indicates that the patient will be "fluid responsive." Feissel et al. found that a respiratory variation of the maximal flow velocity across the aorta of greater than 12 percent or the VTI of greater than 20 percent was a predictor of fluid responsiveness (Video 13.3).[60] The same concepts are the basis for similar measurements performed across the brachial and other peripheral arteries.[38, 39, 55]

Teaching POCUS Assessment of Preload and Fluid Responsiveness

Probe position is critical in measuring IVC diameter; even if the probe is appropriately aligned with the long axis of the vena cava, failure to have the probe centered on the long axis will result in a spuriously low value for the IVC diameter (the so-called cylinder effect). Accordingly, probe positioning needs to be taught on patients. In addition to acquiring the image, residents need to know how to perform ultrasound

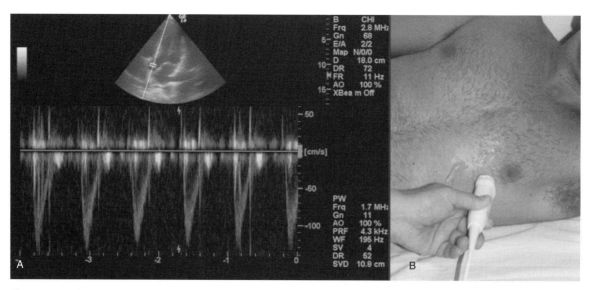

Figure 13.5 Velocity time integral: (A) image of the VTI waveform from the LVOT and (B) picture of probe (phased array) position (6th rib space inferolateral to nipple with indicator at 3 o'clock position) (modified from D. Ramsingh, *Perioperative Point of Care Ultrasound Educational Manual*, epublished, available at www.foresightultrasound.com/ebook [accessed November 18, 2017]).

measurements. This can be taught using a library of ultrasound images on which to practice before using the technique at the bedside. Because placement of the probe is critical and because simulation devices are generally not able to reproduce the ventilation-associated changes in the IVC, teaching this technique requires practice on patients. (Although use of a video clip from a library would allow the resident to practice measuring the IVC, the use of video clips does not ensure that the probe is positioned appropriately.)

Assessment of Cardiac Status and Mechanisms of Shock

The concept of ultrasound to help management of a patient in shock and for gross cardiac evaluation has been used for years by other medical specialties (emergency medicine and critical care). To support training of this section to all providers in perioperative care one should highlight how the perioperative setting has the same patient demographics as the emergency room and ICUs. The emphasis being that the primary assessment tool should not change because of the patient's location, especially if there is significant evidence to support the superiority of a specific technique (e.g., ultrasound). Therefore, when it comes to teaching this section, one should highlight the utility it has demonstrated in these other patient care settings. For example, a study performed in the ICU demonstrated that when a POCUS examination was performed on primarily medical patients upon admission to the ICU, the admitting diagnosis was modified 25 percent of the time.[61] Thus, connecting the perioperative provider to the literature on the utility POCUS in assessing the mechanism of shock by other specialists is an important method to gain the learners' interest. Finally, highlighting a validated perioperative point of care cardiac examination is also important. The "FATE" (Focus Assessed Transthoracic Echocardiography; http://usabcd.org/sites/default/files/FATE_card_Prof_Erik_Sloth.pdf; accessed November 9, 2017) exam is a validated examination designed by perioperative physicians and has demonstrated significant positive patient care impact.[62,63]

FAST POCUS Exam

The FAST (Figure 13.6) exam is the most studied example of focused clinical ultrasound in trauma care.[64,65]

The purpose of bedside ultrasound in trauma is to rapidly identify free fluid (usually blood) in the peritoneal, retroperitoneal, pericardial, or pleural spaces.

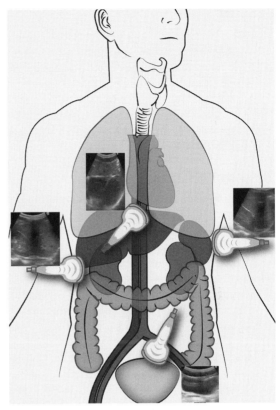

Figure 13.6 FAST (1. Right Upper Quadrant, 2. Subxiphoid, 3. Left Upper Quadrant, 4. Suprapubic) – performed with either phased array or curvilinear probes (modified from D. Ramsingh, *Perioperative Point of Care Ultrasound Educational Manual*, epublished, available at www.foresightultrasound.com/ebook [accessed November 18, 2017]).

The FAST exam has been shown to reliably detect > 200 ml in body cavities. Indications include acute blunt or penetrating torso trauma, trauma in pregnancy, pediatric trauma, and subacute torso trauma. For the perioperative physician the application of this exam allows rapid determination if hemodynamic instability is secondary to cardiac or abdominal injury resulting in free fluid.

Studies have demonstrated that 20–40 percent of patients with significant abdominal injuries may initially have a normal physical examination of the abdomen.[66,67] The FAST exam has proven to be a highly effective tool in the detection of clinically significant hemoperitoneum, hemothorax, or hemopericardium in the unstable patient.[39, 64,68–70] The value of the FAST exam is not limited to trauma patients. A patient who is hypotensive following surgery may also benefit from a FAST exam.

Training in FAST

Simulators are available to train residents to perform a FAST exam. Devices that accurately represent images that would be seen depending on the position of the probe are presumably more useful than devices that present an image only when a probe is placed over a "sticker." Again, because probe location is critical, bedside exams of patients are also an essential element of instruction.

Assessment of Cardiac Function

Transthoracic examination of the cardiopulmonary system using bedside POCUS technology has proven to be a reliable tool when compared to formal echocardiography performed in a cardiac catheterization laboratory.[71] Assessments of global left ventricular (LV) function, abdominal aorta size, and presence of pericardial effusion showed a very strong correlation (r ≥ 0.92) between POCUS and TEE examinations.[73] Similarly, correlation was also shown between right ventricular (RV) function and valvular function (excluding aortic stenosis) (r > 0.81).[72] POCUS cardiac examination has been demonstrated to correlate well with pulmonary artery catheter (PAC) data regarding cardiac function and volume status.[71] The parasternal short axis cardiac view is specifically useful to assess cardiac function. This view is performed by placing the phased array ultrasound probe at the left parasternal border at the 3rd or 4th rib space with the indicator at the 2 to 3 o'clock position (Figure 13.7).

This view has been integrated into POCUS protocols used to assess acute care patients.[39] For example, it has been demonstrated that ten one-hour tutorial sessions consisting of lectures, reviews of videotapes, and observing demonstration of image acquisition and interpretation were sufficient to train noncardiologists to perform and interpret a limited transthoracic echocardiographic (TTE) exam that focused on assessment of LV function.[27,28]

Guidelines have been published for POC cardiac ultrasound by noncardiologists for the intensive care setting [28] These guidelines suggest that the curriculum should include general knowledge (e.g., indications and contraindications for TTE and TEE, physics of ultrasound, and acquisition of standard cardiac views), assessment of the heart (e.g., evaluation of valvular and aortic disease, heart failure, tamponade), and specific problems (e.g., assessment of hypotension, calculation of cardiac output, measurement of chamber sizes, assessment of regional wall motion abnormalities, detection of thrombus). Given the strong similarity of the ICU to the OR, it would seem beneficial that the perioperative physician adopt similar guidelines.

Training in Assessment of Cardiac Function

Instruction in the use and interpretation of TEE should be an essential element of training in cardiothoracic anesthesia. POCUS TTE training should build on the elements of TEE assessment. TTE can be taught by simulation devices that present dynamic changes; these devices are preferable to simulators that present a static image (see Chapter 12 and Chapter 17). As with other elements of POCUS, there is no substitute for bedside instruction by skilled clinicians performing evaluations on real patients.

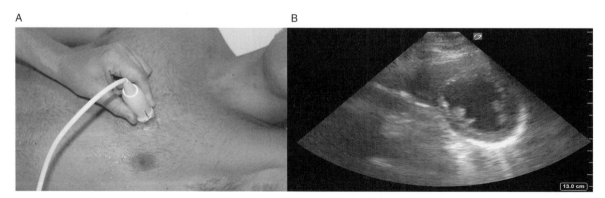

A   B

Figure 13.7 Transthoracic assessment of cardiac function. (A) Probe (phased array) position for parasternal short axis cardiac view (third rib space immediately lateral to sternum with indicator at 2 o'clock position); (B) Ultrasound image of parasternal short axis with tracing of left ventricular end diastolic area (modified from D. Ramsingh, *Perioperative Point of Care Ultrasound Educational Manual*, epublished, available at www.foresightultrasound.com/ebook [accessed November 18, 2017]).

Assessment of Pulmonary and Airway Status

As discussed in the cardiac section, a similar approach should be used to highlight the utility of pulmonary and airway ultrasound for perioperative care. Ultrasonography has been shown to be more accurate than chest auscultation or radiography for the detection of pleural effusion, consolidation, and alveolar interstitial syndrome in the critical care setting.[29,30] In addition, it has been demonstrated that even using a handheld device novice learners can detect lung pathology (e.g., "ultrasound lung comets") with essentially the same accuracy as an experienced ultrasonographer using a full-featured system.[73,74]

The Bedside Lung Ultrasound in an Emergency (BLUE) protocol, a POCUS pulmonary examination that has been demonstrated to assist evaluation of patients in respiratory failure in the intensive care setting,[75] is a four-point exam over each hemithorax with a documented accuracy in excess of 90 percent in diagnosing the cause of respiratory failure (Figure 13.8).

The presence of "lung sliding," a shimmering appearance due to the motion of the visceral and parietal pleura against one another (Video 13.4), effectively rules out the presence of a pneumothorax or a pleural effusion under the area being scanned. Repetitions of the pleural line at equally spaced intervals result in "A lines," which occur in aerated lungs in the absence of fluid or gas in the pleural space (Figure 13.9).

A lines occur because air in the lung parenchyma prevents ultrasound waves from penetrating past the pleura thereby resulting in reverberations that appear as lines identical to the pleural line at distances equal to the distance between the transducer and the pleura. A lines are not an indication of the absence of pathology in the underlying lung; they may occur with asthma, chronic obstructive pulmonary disease, pulmonary embolism, or any condition in which the lung underlying the probe is aerated and in which there is no pneumothorax, pleural effusion, or hemothorax.

B lines (Figure 13.10) may occur as a result of fluid in the septa (due to pulmonary edema, pneumonia, etc.) or chronic fibrosis.

Because a normal fissure may also produce a single B line in a scan, it is generally recommended that three B lines must be seen in a single scan to be classified as representing pathology. B lines that are symmetrical at multiple points across the anterior chest wall generally indicate the presence of pulmonary edema while the lack of symmetry is consistent with pneumonia, lung scarring, or respiratory distress syndrome.

Lung consolidation, due to pneumonia, or atelectasis, results in the ability to visualize lung parenchyma by ultrasound. Because the consolidated lung tissue resembles the liver, this is sometimes described as "hepatization" of the lung (Figure 13.11).

The utility of perioperative POCUS to identify the location of the endotracheal tube has been demonstrated (Figure 13.12).[20]

Teaching Pulmonary Assessment

Because probe location is not as critical in pulmonary assessment (it only needs to be located between the ribs) as in other modalities, simulators capable of displaying pathologic conditions are ideally suited for teaching this technique.

Vascular Access

The use of ultrasound for vascular access is now routine for placement of central venous lines. Highlighting the evidence of ultrasound to decreased risk of cannulation failure, arterial puncture, hematoma, and hemithorax is important to emphasize its importance for perioperative education.[45] In addition, ultrasound has proven to reliably aid in the placement of difficult intravenous[43,44] and intra-arterial catheters.[46,47] Use of ultrasound for peripheral venous access also has shown to significantly increase success rates.[76]

Teaching Advanced Vascular Access

Simulators are ideally suited for teaching the use of ultrasound for placement of central venous catheters in the presence of normal anatomy. (See Chapter 17 for a detailed discussion of the use of simulation in training for central venous access.) Instruction in the use of ultrasound for the placement of difficult peripheral venous or arterial catheters probably needs to be done at the bedside.

Additional Topics

The utility of perioperative POCUS is still being explored, and it is important to highlight this point when teaching this topic. Two more areas of emerging focus of POCUS assessment include assessment of gastric volume and estimation of intracranial pressure.

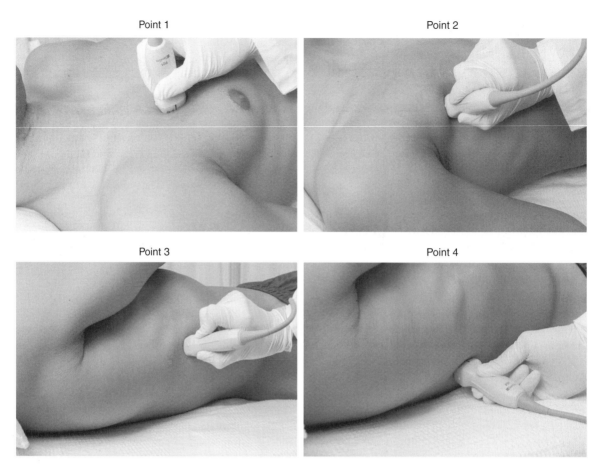

Figure 13.8 Bedside Lung Ultrasound in an Emergency Exam. Point 1 is located on the mid-clavicular line at approximately the second intercostal space. Point 2 is located on the anterior axillary line at approximately the fifth intercostal space, usually just lateral to the nipple in men. Point 3 is located along the diaphragm in mid-axillary line. Point 4 is also called the posterolateral alveolar pleural syndrome (PLAPS) point and is the most posterior point along the diaphragm. Note the probe face is pointing to the sky with patient back rotated off the bed (from Figure 8.6 of N. J. Soni, R. Arntfield, P. Kory, eds. *Point of Care Ultrasound*. Philadelphia: Saunders, 2015).

Gastric Volume Assessment

POCUS has been used for assessment of gastric contents and volume[18,19] and a recent grading system based exclusively on qualitative sonographic assessment of the gastric antrum has shown strong correlation with predicted gastric volume (Figure 13.13).[19]

Perlas et al. reported that the presence of fluid in the antrum identified by ultrasound in the supine and right lateral decubitus positions correlated with a clinically significant volume of gastric contents (180 +/- 83 ml).[18] This ability of POCUS to detect gastric volume may provide a method to assess aspiration risk.

Intracranial Pressure Estimation

POCUS has been shown to provide rapid assessment of ICP based on the assessment of ONSD. The optic nerve sheath is contiguous with the dura mater and has a trabeculated arachnoid space through which cerebrospinal fluid circulates. This relationship between ONSD and ICP has been well established.[77,78] The sensitivity of the ultrasonography in detecting elevated intracranial pressure was 96 percent and specificity was 80 percent.[79] An ONSD greater than 5.2 mm, at a point approximately 2 mm from the retina, suggests elevated ICP (Figure 13.14).

Teaching Additional Topics

Both of these techniques need to be taught at the bedside. Encouraging the learner to evaluate other possible emerging areas is another strategy to improve learning.

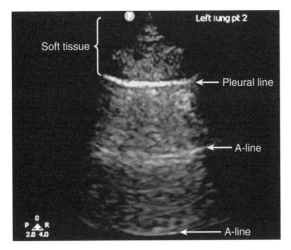

Figure 13.9 "A" line reverberation artifact. Horizontal, hyperechoic lines are seen deep to the pleural line, repeating at the same distance as the transducer is to the pleural line (from Figure 9.2 of N. J. Soni, R. Arntfield, P. Kory, eds. *Point of Care Ultrasound*. Philadelphia: Saunders, 2015).

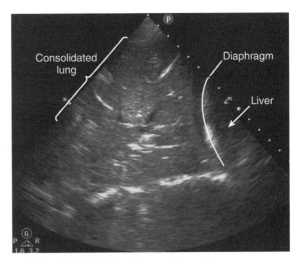

Figure 13.11 Hepatization of lung. Alveolar consolidation pattern with echogenicity similar to liver (from Figure 9.7 of N. J. Soni, R. Arntfield, P. Kory, eds. *Point of Care Ultrasound*. Philadelphia: Saunders, 2015).

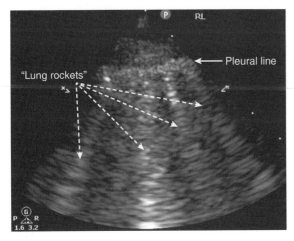

Figure 13.10 B-line pattern. Also called "lung rockets" or "comet tails." These are B lines, seen when interstitium is widened with fluid or scarring (from Figure 9.5 of N. J. Soni, R. Arntfield, P. Kory, eds. *Point of Care Ultrasound*. Philadelphia: Saunders, 2015).

Summary

The preceding review indicates that POCUS has the capability to help the perioperative physician with far more than central venous access and regional anesthesia. POCUS has become increasingly vital within critical care medicine[80] and its positive impact in the perioperative arena has been demonstrated.[4,81,82] Courses for advanced ultrasound have been taught at the Society of Critical Care Medicine, American College of Chest Physicians, and the America College of Surgeons for years. As the critical care physicians of the perioperative arena, POCUS may benefit the anesthesiologist throughout the entire perioperative period – in preoperative evaluation, management in the OR, as well as postoperative care in the recovery area. However, one needs to consider the differences of adult learner and the importance of incorporating model and simulation-based educational strategies. Several curricula have been established with this in mind.[23,81]

It is reasonable to remember that both probe placement and manipulation, as well as normal and abnormal findings, need to be taught. A variety of simulators, each with its own advantages and disadvantages, are currently available. Growth in simulators is dramatic and innovations may be expected to result in even better teaching possibilities. Devices that focus on differentiating normal from abnormal findings are useful but are probably less useful to novice learners than those that provide both educational elements. In the final analysis, however, there is little substitute for performing multiple scans on multiple patients while being supervised by someone with expertise in the field.

As POCUS becomes more readily available in the OR, the perioperative physician must be ready to use the technology effectively to help elevate their level of patient care into the twenty-first century. The

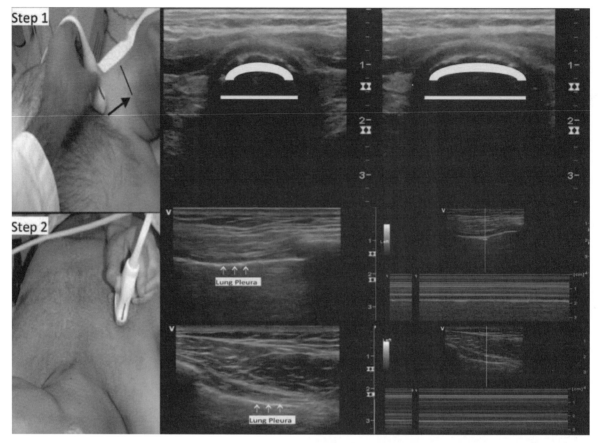

Figure 13.12 Pulmonary tree and lung expansion ultrasound study (PLUS) examination. Step 1: Tracheal dilation assessment – ultrasound probe placed transversely on the anterior neck approximately 2 cm superior to the suprasternal notch and scanned cranially to the cricothyroid membrane. The marker for endotracheal cuff is tracheal dilation with balloon inflation. The image on the left in step 1 shows a nondilated trachea, and the one on the right shows a dilated trachea secondary to balloon inflation. Absence of tracheal dilation suggests that the endotracheal cuff is not in the area examined. Step 2: Pleural sliding assessment – ultrasound placed vertically on the anterior chest at the third rib space midclavicular line bilaterally. Assessment of lung expansion evaluated by the detection of the horizontal movement of the two pleural linings with respiration. Use of M-mode facilitates pleural sliding assessment. The top image for step 2 examination shows normal pleural sliding verified with M-mode identification of pleural motion. The bottom image for step 2 examination shows absence of pleural sliding verified with no motion identified with M-mode (modified from D. Ramsingh, *Perioperative Point of Care Ultrasound Educational Manual*, epublished, available at www.foresightultrasound.com/ebook [accessed November 18, 2017]).

formulation of a structured curriculum and method of education is essential. Further development in this area is needed to establish the perioperative physician at the top of this advancing patient care modality.

References

1. J. S. Alpert, J. Mladenovic, D. B. Hellmann. Should a hand-carried ultrasound machine become standard equipment for every internist? *Am J Med* 2009; 122: 1–3.

2. C. Prinz, J. U. Voigt. Diagnostic accuracy of a hand-held ultrasound scanner in routine patients referred for echocardiography. *J Am Soc Echocardiogr* 2011; 24: 111–16.

3. J. L. Kendall, S. R. Hoffenberg, R. S. Smith. History of emergency and critical care ultrasound: The evolution of a new imaging paradigm. *Crit Care Med* 2007; 35(Suppl 5): S126–30.

4. American Medical Association. House of Delegates Policy H-230.960. Privileging for Ultrasound Imaging. https://searchpf.ama-assn.org/SearchML/searchDetails.action?uri=%2FAMADoc%2FHOD.xml-0-1591.xml (accessed April 28, 2017).

5. F. Mahmood, R. Matyal, N. Skubas et al. Perioperative ultrasound training in anesthesiology: A call to action. *Anesth Analg* 2016; 122: 1794–804.

A B

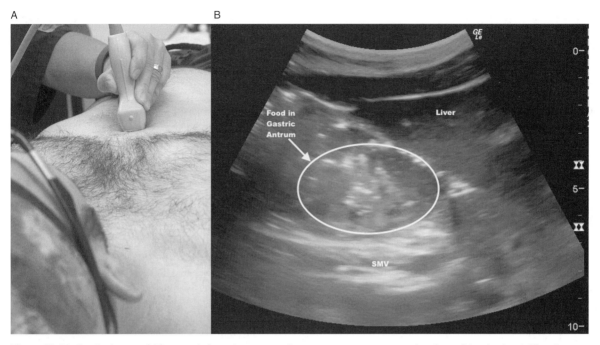

Figure 13.13 Gastric ultrasound. Ultrasound of gastric antrum and measurements to assess gastric volume; (A) probe (curved linear) position for gastric antrum acquisition; (B) ultrasound image (modified from D. Ramsingh, *Perioperative Point of Care Ultrasound Educational Manual*, epublished, available at www.foresightultrasound.com/ebook [accessed November 18, 2017]).

A B

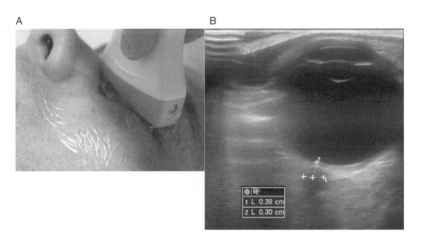

Figure 13.14 Ultrasound of optic nerve sheath diameter. (A) probe (linear) position; (B) Ultrasound image (modified from D. Ramsingh, *Perioperative Point of Care Ultrasound Educational Manual*, epublished, available at www. foresightultrasound.com/ebook [accessed November 18, 2017]).

6. E. Cardenas. Emergency medicine ultrasound policies and reimbursement guidelines. *Emerg Med Clin North Am* 2004; 22: 829–38.

7. American College of Emergency Physicians. American college of emergency physicians. ACEP ultrasound guidelines – 2001. *Ann Emerg Med* 2001; 38: 470–81.

8. A. J. Labovitz, V. E. Noble, M. Bierig et al. Focused cardiac ultrasound in the emergent setting: A consensus statement of the American Society of Echocardiography and American College of Emergency Physicians. *J Am Soc Echocardiogr* 2010; 23: 1225–30.

9. S. Price, G. Via, F. Guarracino et al. Echocardiography practice, training and accreditation in the intensive care: Document for the World Interactive Network Focused on Critical Ultrasound (WINFOCUS). *Cardiovasc Ultrasound* 2008; 6: 49.

10. American College of Emergency Physicians. Policy statement: Ultrasound guidelines: Emergency,

point-of-care, and clinical ultrasound guidelines in medicine. www.acep.org/Clinical---Practice-Management/Ultrasound/ (accessed November 18, 2017).

11. International Federation for Emergency Medicine. Point-of-care ultrasound curriculum guidelines. 2014. www.ifem.cc/wp-content/uploads/2016/07/IFEM-Point-of-Care-Ultrasound-Curriculum-Guidelines-2014.pdf (accessed November 18, 2017).

12. AHRQ issues critical analysis of patient safety practices. *Qual Lett Healthc Lead* 2001; 13: 8–12.

13. D. Hind, N. Calvert, R. McWilliams et al. Ultrasonic locating devices for central venous cannulation: Meta-analysis. *BMJ* 2003; 327: 361.

14. J. M. Neal, R. Brull, J. L. Horn et al. The Second American Society of Regional Anesthesia and Pain Medicine evidence-based medicine assessment of ultrasound-guided regional anesthesia: Executive summary. *Reg Anesth Pain Med* 2016; 41: 181–94.

15. A. G. Randolph, D. J. Cook, C. A. Gonzales, C. G. Pribble. Ultrasound guidance for placement of central venous catheters: A meta-analysis of the literature. *Crit Care Med* 1996; 24: 2053–8.

16. D. J. Canty, C. F. Royse, D. Kilpatrick et al. The impact of focused transthoracic echocardiography in the pre-operative clinic. *Anaesthesia* 2012; 67: 618–25.

17. B. Cowie. Three years' experience of focused cardiovascular ultrasound in the peri-operative period. *Anaesthesia* 2011; 66: 268–73.

18. A. Perlas, V. W. Chan, C. M. Lupu et al. Ultrasound assessment of gastric content and volume. *Anesthesiology* 2009; 111: 82–9.

19. A. Perlas, L. Davis, M. Khan et al. Gastric sonography in the fasted surgical patient: a prospective descriptive study. *Anesth Analg* 2011; 113: 93–7.

20. D. Ramsingh, E. Frank, R. Haughton et al. Auscultation versus point-of-care ultrasound to determine endotracheal versus bronchial intubation: A diagnostic accuracy study. *Anesthesiology* 2016; 124: 1012–20.

21. The American Board of Anesthesiology. Primary certification content outline. www.theaba.org/PDFs/BASIC-Exam/Basic-and-Advanced-ContentOutline (accessed November 8, 2017).

22. D. Ramsingh, J. Rinehart, Z. Kain et al. Impact assessment of perioperative point-of-care ultrasound training on anesthesiology residents. *Anesthesiology* 2015; 123: 670–82.

23. G. Sutkin, E. Wagner, I Harris, R. Schiffer. What makes a good clinical teacher in medicine? A review of the literature. *Acad Med* 2008; 83: 452–66.

24. M. S. Knowles, E. F. Holton, R. A. Swanson. *The Adult Learner: The Definitive Classic in Adult Education and Human Resource Development*, 7th edn. New York: Routledge, 2012.

25. D. Ramsingh, B. Alexander, K. Le et al. Comparison of the didactic lecture with the simulation/model approach for the teaching of a novel perioperative ultrasound curriculum to anesthesiology residents. *J Clin Anesth* 2014; 26: 443–54.

26. G. N. Andersen, B. O. Haugen, T. Graven et al. Feasibility and reliability of point-of-care pocket-sized echocardiography. *Eur J Echocardiogr* 2011; 12: 665–70.

27. A. R. Manasia, H. M. Nagaraj, R. B. Kodali et al. Feasibility and potential clinical utility of goal-directed transthoracic echocardiography performed by noncardiologist intensivists using a small hand-carried device (SonoHeart) in critically ill patients. *J Cardiothorac Vasc Anesth* 2005; 19: 155–9.

28. R. M. Mazraeshahi, J. C. Farmer, D. T. Porembka. A suggested curriculum in echocardiography for critical care physicians. *Crit Care Med* 2007; 35(Suppl 8): S431–3.

29. D. Lichtenstein, I. Goldstein, E. Mourgeon et al. Comparative diagnostic performances of auscultation, chest radiography, and lung ultrasonography in acute respiratory distress syndrome. *Anesthesiology* 2004; 100: 9–15.

30. P. Vignon, C. Chastagner, V. Berkane et al. Quantitative assessment of pleural effusion in critically ill patients by means of ultrasonography. *Crit Care Med* 2005; 33: 1757–63.

31. B. Bouhemad, M. Zhang, Q. Lu, J. J. Rouby. Clinical review: Bedside lung ultrasound in critical care practice. *Crit Care* 2007; 11: 205.

32. K. Ueda, W. Ahmed, A. F. Ross. Intraoperative pneumothorax identified with transthoracic ultrasound. *Anesthesiology* 2011; 115: 653–5.

33. C. Barbier, Y. Loubieres, C. Schmit et al. Respiratory changes in inferior vena cava diameter are helpful in predicting fluid responsiveness in ventilated septic patients. *Intensive Care Med* 2004; 30: 1740–6.

34. L. M. Gillman, C. G. Ball, N. Panebianco et al. Clinician performed resuscitative ultrasonography for the initial evaluation and resuscitation of trauma. *Scand J Trauma Resusc Emerg Med* 2009; 17: 34.

35. K. Scheuren, M. N. Wente, C. Hainer et al. Left ventricular end-diastolic area is a measure of cardiac preload in patients with early septic shock. *Eur J Anaesthesiol* 2009; 26: 759–65.

36. B. Subramaniam, D. Talmor. Echocardiography for management of hypotension in the intensive care unit. *Crit Care Med* 2007; 35(Suppl 8): S401–7.

37. O. Broch, J. Renner, M. Gruenewald et al. Variation of left ventricular outflow tract velocity and global end-diastolic volume index reliably predict fluid responsiveness in cardiac surgery patients. *J Crit Care* 2012; 27: 325 e7–e13.

38. C. Charron, V. Caille, F. Jardin, A. Vieillard-Baron. Echocardiographic measurement of fluid responsiveness. *Curr Opin Crit Care* 2006; 12: 249–54.

39. G. S. Rozycki, M. G. Ochsner, J. A. Schmidt et al. A prospective study of surgeon-performed ultrasound as the primary adjuvant modality for injured patient assessment. *J Trauma* 1995; 39: 492–8.

40. R. L. Keenan, C. P. Boyan. Cardiac arrest due to anesthesia: A study of incidence and causes. *JAMA* 1985; 253: 2373–7.

41. J. E. Utting, T. C. Gray, F. C. Shelley. Human misadventure in anaesthesia. *Can Anaesth Soc J* 1979; 26: 472–8.

42. B. Muslu, H. Sert, A. Kaya et al. Use of sonography for rapid identification of esophageal and tracheal intubations in adult patients. *J Ultrasound Med* 2011; 30: 671–6.

43. W. Brunel, D. L. Coleman, D. E. Schwartz et al. Assessment of routine chest roentgenograms and the physical examination to confirm endotracheal tube position. *Chest* 1989; 96: 1043–5.

44. T. G. Costantino, A. K. Parikh, W. A. Satz, J. P. Fojtik. Ultrasonography-guided peripheral intravenous access versus traditional approaches in patients with difficult intravenous access. *Ann Emerg Med* 2005; 46: 456–61.

45. L. E. Keyes, B. W. Frazee, E. R. Snoey et al. Ultrasound-guided brachial and basilic vein cannulation in emergency department patients with difficult intravenous access. *Ann Emerg Med* 1999; 34: 711–14.

46. S. Y. Wu, Q. Ling, L. H. Cao et al. Real-time two-dimensional ultrasound guidance for central venous cannulation: a meta-analysis. *Anesthesiology* 2013; 118: 361–75.

47. A. Ashworthand, J. E. Arrowsmith. Ultrasound-guided arterial cannulation. *Eur J Anaesthesiol* 2010; 27: 307.

48. S. Shiver, M. Blaivas, M. Lyon. A prospective comparison of ultrasound-guided and blindly placed radial arterial catheters. *Acad Emerg Med* 2006; 13: 1275–9.

49. C. Dubost, A. Le Gouez, V. Jouffroy et al. Optic nerve sheath diameter used as ultrasonographic assessment of the incidence of raised intracranial pressure in preeclampsia: A pilot study. *Anesthesiology* 2012; 116: 1066–71.

50. D. L. Kirkpatrick. Effective supervisory training and development, Part 2: In-house approaches and techniques. *Personnel* 1985 62: 52–6.

51. J. Neelankavil, K. Howard-Quijano, T. C. Hsieh et al. Transthoracic echocardiography simulation is an efficient method to train anesthesiologists in basic transthoracic echocardiography skills. *Anesth Analg* 2012; 115: 1042–51.

52. E. M. AlEassa, M. T. Ziesmann, A. W. Kirkpatrick et al. Point of care ultrasonography use and training among trauma providers across Canada. *Can J Surg* 2016; 59: 6–8.

53. J. A. Town, P. A. Bergl, A. Narang, J. F. McConville. Internal medicine residents' retention of knowledge and skills in bedside ultrasound. *J Grad Med Educ* 2016; 8: 553–7.

54. M. M. Berger, I. Gradwohl-Matis, A. Brunauer et al. Targets of perioperative fluid therapy and their effects on postoperative outcome: A systematic review and meta-analysis. *Minerva Anestesiol* 2015; 81: 794–808.

55. M. I. Monge Garcia, A. Gil Cano, J. C. Diaz Monrove. Brachial artery peak velocity variation to predict fluid responsiveness in mechanically ventilated patients. *Crit Care* 2009; 13: R142.

56. S. R. Ommen, R. A. Nishimura, D. G. Hurrell, K. W. Klarich. Assessment of right atrial pressure with 2-dimensional and Doppler echocardiography: A simultaneous catheterization and echocardiographic study. *Mayo Clin Proc* 2000; 75: 24–9.

57. M. E. Prekker, N. L. Scott, D. Hart et al. Point-of-care ultrasound to estimate central venous pressure: A comparison of three techniques. *Crit Care Med* 2013; 41: 833–41.

58. P. E. Marik, M. Baram, B. Vahid. Does central venous pressure predict fluid responsiveness? A systematic review of the literature and the tale of seven mares. *Chest* 2008; 134: 172–8.

59. S. Gelman. Venous function and central venous pressure: a physiologic story. *Anesthesiology* 2008. 108: 735–48.

60. M. D. Howell, M. Donnino, P. Clardy et al. Occult hypoperfusion and mortality in patients with suspected infection. *Intensive Care Med* 2007; 33: 1892–9.

61. M. Feissel, F. Michard, I. Mangin et al. Respiratory changes in aortic blood velocity as an indicator of fluid responsiveness in ventilated patients with septic shock. *Chest* 2001; 119: 867–73.

62. E. Manno, M. Navarra, L. Faccio et al. Deep impact of ultrasound in the intensive care unit: The "ICU-sound" protocol. *Anesthesiology* 2012; 117: 801–9.

63. M. B. Jensen, E. Sloth, K. M. Larsen, M. B. Schmidt. Transthoracic echocardiography for cardiopulmonary monitoring in intensive care. *Eur J Anaesthesiol* 2004; 21: 700–7.

64. M. R. Jorgensen, P. Juhl-Olsen, C. A. Frederiksen, E. Sloth. Transthoracic echocardiography in the perioperative setting. *Curr Opin Anaesthesiol* 2016; 29: 46–54.

65. A. C. Quinn, R. Sinert. What is the utility of the Focused Assessment with Sonography in Trauma (FAST) exam in penetrating torso trauma? *Injury* 2011; 42: 482–7.

66. D. Stengel, G. Rademacher, A. Ekkernkamp et al. Emergency ultrasound-based algorithms for diagnosing blunt abdominal trauma. *Cochrane Database Syst Rev* 2015; 14: CD004446.

67. A. Rodriguez, R. W. DuPriest Jr., C. H. Shatney. Recognition of intra-abdominal injury in blunt trauma victims: A prospective study comparing physical examination with peritoneal lavage. *Am Surg* 1982; 48: 457–9.

68. J. F. Perry Jr., J. E. DeMeules, H. D. Root. Diagnostic peritoneal lavage in blunt abdominal trauma. *Surg Gynecol Obstet* 1970; 131: 742–4.

69. T. M. Scalea, A. Rodriguez, W. C. Chiu et al. Focused Assessment with Sonography for Trauma (FAST): Results from an international consensus conference. *J Trauma* 1999; 46: 466–72.

70. J. S. Rose. Ultrasound in abdominal trauma. *Emerg Med Clin North Am* 2004; 22: 581–99.

71. A. W. Kirkpatrick, M. Sirois, K. B. Laupland et al. Prospective evaluation of hand-held focused abdominal sonography for trauma (FAST) in blunt abdominal trauma. *Can J Surg* 2005; 48: 453–60.

72. M. Gunst, V. Ghaemmaghami, J. Sperry et al. Accuracy of cardiac function and volume status estimates using the bedside echocardiographic assessment in trauma/critical care. *J Trauma* 2008; 65: 509–16.

73. G. N. Andersen, B. O. Haugen, T. Graven et al. Feasibility and reliability of point-of-care pocket-sized echocardiography. *Eur J Echocardiogr* 2011; 12: 665–70.

74. G. Bedetti, L. Gargani, A. Corbisiero et al. Evaluation of ultrasound lung comets by hand-held echocardiography. *Cardiovasc Ultrasound* 2006; 4: 34.

75. K. L. Eibenberger, W. I. Dock, M. E. Ammann et al. Quantification of pleural effusions: Sonography versus radiography. *Radiology* 1994; 191: 681–4.

76. D. A. Lichtenstein, G. A. Meziere. Relevance of lung ultrasound in the diagnosis of acute respiratory failure: The BLUE protocol. *Chest* 2008; 134: 117–25.

77. L. A. Stolz, U. Stolz, C. Howe et al. Ultrasound-guided peripheral venous access: A meta-analysis and systematic review. *J Vasc Access* 2015; 16: 321–6.

78. H. C. Hansen, K. Helmke. Validation of the optic nerve sheath response to changing cerebrospinal fluid pressure: Ultrasound findings during intrathecal infusion tests. *J Neurosurg* 1997; 87: 34–40.

79. V. S. Tayal, M. Neulander, H. J. Norton et al. Emergency department sonographic measurement of optic nerve sheath diameter to detect findings of increased intracranial pressure in adult head injury patients. *Ann Emerg Med* 2007; 49: 508–14.

80. M. Raffiz, J. M. Abdullah. Optic nerve sheath diameter measurement: A means of detecting raised ICP in adult traumatic and non-traumatic neurosurgical patients. *Am J Emerg Med* 2017; 35: 150–3.

81. K. Killu, V. Coba, M. Mendez et al. Model point-of-care ultrasound curriculum in an intensive care unit fellowship program and its impact on patient management. *Crit Care Res Pract* 2014; 2014: 934796

82. D. Ramsingh, J. C. Fox, W. C. Wilson. Perioperative point-of-care ultrasonography: An emerging technology to be embraced by anesthesiologists. *Anesth Analg* 2015; 120: 990–2.

83. D. Ramsingh, V. Gudzenko, R. D. Martin. Point-of-care ultrasound: Novel Technology to Routine Perioperative Assessment Tool. *Anesth Analg* 2017; 124: 709–11.

Chapter 14

How to Design Multimedia Presentations

Richard E. Mayer

Introduction: Applying the Science of Learning to Medical Education

Suppose we asked a cohort of medical students to attend a series of introductory-level classes on key medical specialties. Each class session involves a narrated slideshow, consisting of a lecture by a specialist in the field accompanied by PowerPoint slides. Does research from the science of learning provide any guidance in how best to design effective slideshows that promote deep learning – reflected in being able to apply what was taught? If we take an existing slideshow lecture and redesign the slides predicated on research-based principles, will that improve student learning on transfer tests – that is, tests that ask students to use the material in new situations?

This question was addressed in an experiment by Issa and colleagues,[1] in which third-year medical students received a slideshow lecture on shock using traditionally designed slides or redesigned slides that followed research-based principles of multimedia instruction as articulated by Mayer.[2,3] Although the groups did not differ significantly on a pretest, the group taught with the redesigned slides significantly outperformed the traditional group on a posttest involving transfer questions given one hour after the lecture, yielding an effect size of $d = 0.83$, which is considered a large effect. In a follow-up study using the same methodology but with the addition of delayed tests, Issa and colleagues[4] found that the group taught using redesigned slides significantly outscored the traditional group on an immediate transfer test (with an effect size of $d = 0.76$), a delayed transfer test given one week later (with an effect size of $d = 0.83$), and a delayed transfer test given four weeks later (with an effect size of $d = 1.17$). These experiments demonstrate that student learning can be improved greatly when traditional slides from a medical lecture are redesigned to follow research-based principles.

How Multimedia Learning Works

What Is Multimedia Learning?

Multimedia learning involves learning from words and pictures, such as in a narrated slideshow. The words can be in print or spoken form and the pictures can be static (such as diagrams, drawings, or photos) or dynamic (such as animation or video). For the past 25 years, as summarized in the *Cambridge Handbook of Multimedia Learning*,[5] researchers have been trying to understand how multimedia learning works and how to design multimedia instruction that fosters learning.

Three Principles of Multimedia Learning

Table 14.1 summarizes three key principles from cognitive science that are particularly relevant to designing multimedia instruction – dual channels, limited capacity, and active learning. The dual channels principle is that people have somewhat separate channels for processing auditory/verbal information and visual/pictorial information. The limited capacity principle is that people can actively process only a few pieces of information in each channel at any one time. The active learning principle is that deep learning – learning that supports transferring what is taught to new situations – depends on the degree to which learners engage in appropriate cognitive processing during instruction, including attending to relevant incoming information, mentally organizing the information into a coherent structure, and integrating it with relevant existing knowledge from long-term memory. Thus, the challenge for instructional designers concerns how to promote the appropriate cognitive processing needed for active learning within an information processing system that has limited capacity in each channel.

Table 14.1 Three principles from the science of learning that are relevant for multimedia learning

Principle	Definition
Dual Channels	Learners have separate channels for processing auditory/verbal information and visual/pictorial information
Limited Capacity	Learners can process only a few pieces of information in each channel at any one time
Active Processing	Deep learning occurs when learners engage in the cognitive processes of selecting, organizing, and integrating during learning

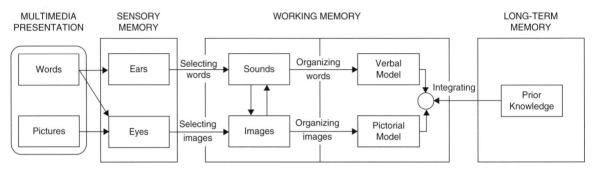

Figure 14.1 A cognitive model of multimedia learning.

The Human Information Processing System

Figure 14.1 shows a model of the human information processing system, consisting of three memory stores (i.e., sensory memory, working memory, and long-term memory), three cognitive processes (i.e., selecting, organizing, and integrating), and two channels (i.e., verbal and pictorial). When a multimedia message is presented, such as a narrated slideshow, the spoken words impinge on the ears and enter auditory sensory memory while the graphics and printed words impinge on the eyes and enter visual sensory memory. Auditory sounds and visual images are held for a fraction of a second in their sensory form. If the learner attends to parts of the incoming words and images, they are transferred to working memory as indicated by the *selecting* arrows, where they can be held as words and images but need to be rehearsed within about half a minute to stay alive in working memory. Next, the learner mentally organizes the incoming images into a pictorial model, and the incoming words into a verbal model (including printed words that are converted into the verbal channel), as indicated by the *organizing* arrows. Finally, the learner activates relevant knowledge from long-term memory and combines it with incoming information, as indicated by the *integrating* arrows.

Three Kinds of Learning Outcomes

Table 14.2 summarizes three kinds of learning outcomes. When a learner fails to engage in all three processes of selecting, organizing, and integrating, no learning occurs, resulting in poor performance on retention tests (i.e., remembering the presented information) and transfer tests (i.e., using the information to solve new problems). When the learner selects the relevant information, but does not try to make sense of it by reorganizing it and integrating it, rote learning occurs, resulting in good retention but poor transfer performance. When the learner selects, organizes, and integrates, the result is deep learning, resulting in good retention and good transfer performance. In medical education, although retention is a necessary outcome, the key focus is on transfer in order for physicians to be able to apply knowledge in new situations.

How Multimedia Instruction Works: Research-Based Principles

Three Key Goals in Multimedia Design

Table 14.3 lists three key goals in designing effective multimedia instruction – reducing extraneous

Table 14.2 Three kinds of learning outcomes

Learning Outcome	Learning Process	Retention Test	Transfer Test
No learning	None	Poor	Poor
Rote learning	Selecting	Good	Poor
Deep learning	Selecting, organizing, and integrating	Good	Good

Table 14.3 Three key goals in multimedia instruction

Goal	Definition	Example
Reduce extraneous processing	Cognitive processing that does not support the learning objective, caused by poor instructional design	Exclude irrelevant material
Manage essential processing	Cognitive processing needed to mentally represent the essential material, caused by the complexity of the essential material	Break explanation into bite-sized pieces
Foster generative processing	Cognitive processing needed to deeply understand the material, caused by the learner's motivation	Use conversational language

processing, managing essential processing, and fostering generative processing. Extraneous cognitive processing occurs when the learner wastes precious processing capacity on cognitive processing that does not support the learning objective. This can be caused by poor instructional design, such as having highly interesting but irrelevant facts and graphics in the lesson. Essential processing occurs when the learner selects the essential material and constructs a representation of it in working memory. Difficulties can arise when the essential material is so complex for the learner that it cannot all be processed at once in working memory. Generative processing occurs when the learner strives to make sense of the essential material by reorganizing it and integrating it with relevant prior knowledge from long-term memory. This depends on the learner's motivation to exert the effort needed to understand the material.

Suppose you have prepared a slideshow lesson for a class in anesthesiology, but you would like to redesign the slides based on multimedia design principles. In this section, we examine ten principles of multimedia design that have been shown in numerous research studies to produce effect sizes greater than $d = 0.4$ on transfer tests,[2] which is considered educationally significant in intervention studies. Effect size (based on Cohen's d), calculated by subtracting the mean score of the control group from the mean score of the experimental group and dividing by the pooled standard deviation, is a common metric used to summarize the effectiveness of an instructional intervention.

Principles for Reducing Extraneous Processing

Table 14.4 reviews five principles summarized by Mayer and Fiorella[5] aimed at reducing extraneous processing – coherence, signaling, redundancy, spatial contiguity, and temporal contiguity. Based on the coherence principle, your first step in building effective slides is to weed out extraneous words and graphics, such as getting rid of unneeded use of color or eye-catching background frames around each slide. Each slide should have a clear instructional goal, and material not directly relevant to that goal should be deleted. For example, Figure 14.2 shows a slide from a lesson on how a virus causes a cold; the slide has extraneous sentences in the form of seductive details – interesting but irrelevant facts – or does not have extraneous sentences. Students learn better from the version without extraneous sentences.

Second, based on the signaling principle, you can highlight the most important material on screen, such as placing an arrow to show where to look or using a heading for the slide that briefly describes the main point. For example, a lesson on how airplanes achieve lift can have slides without headings for each paragraph and illustration, or slides with headings such

Table 14.4 Five design principles for reducing extraneous processing

Principle	Definition	Effect Size (n)
Coherence	Weed out extraneous words and graphics	0.86 (23)
Signaling	Highlight key words and parts of graphics	0.41 (28)
Redundancy	Do not add onscreen text that duplicates narration	0.86 (16)
Spatial contiguity	Place printed words next to corresponding part of graphics	1.10 (22)
Temporal contiguity	Present narration at same time as corresponding graphics	1.22 (9)

n = number of comparisons

With extraneous sentences

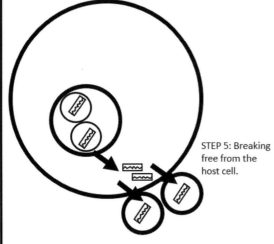

Step 5: Breaking Free from the Host Cell
The new parts are packaged into new virus within the host cell. The new viruses break free from the host cell. In some cases, they break the host cell open, destroying the host cell in the process, which is called lysis. In other cases, they punch out of he cell membrane surrounding them, which is called budding. A study conducted by researchers at Wilkes University in Wilkes-Barre, Pennsylvania, reveals that people who make love once or twice a week are more immune to colds than folks who abstain from sex. Researchers believe that the bedroom activity somehow stimulates an immune-boosting antibody called IgA.

STEP 5: Breaking free from the host cell.

Without extraneous sentences

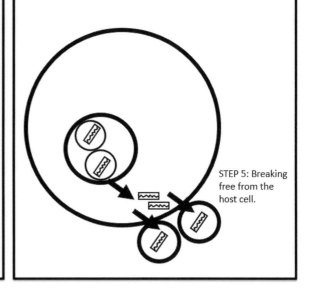

Step 5: Breaking Free from the Host Cell
The new parts are packaged into new virus within the host cell. The new viruses break free from the host cell. In some cases, they break the host cell open, destroying the host cell in the process, which is called lysis. In other cases, they punch out of he cell membrane surrounding them, which is called budding.

STEP 5: Breaking free from the host cell.

Figure 14.2 Coherence principle: Does deleting interesting but irrelevant details improve learning?

as "Wing shape: Curved upper surface is longer," "Air speed: Air moves faster across top of wing," and "Air pressure: Air pressure on top is less."

Third, if you have a slide that is full of words that you also read to the class, this creates verbal redundancy, which can cause the learner to waste processing capacity by trying to reconcile the two verbal streams.

For example, Figure 14.3 shows a frame from a narrated animation on how lightning storms develop that either does or does not have a redundant caption printed at the bottom of the screen. People learn better without the caption. Based on the redundancy principle, you should greatly reduce the number of printed words on the screen so that only one, two, or

Animation and Narration

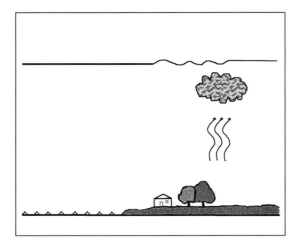

"As the air in this updraft cools, water vapor
condenses into water droplets and forms a cloud."

Animation, Narration, and On-Screen Text

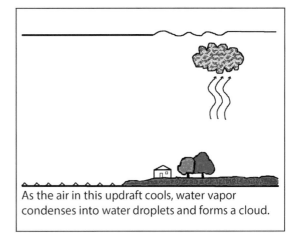

"As the air in this updraft cools, water vapor
condenses into water droplets and forms a cloud."

Figure 14.3 Redundancy principle: Which instructional method leads to better learning from a narrated animation?

Separated Presentation

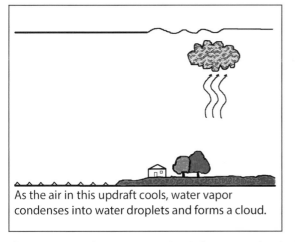

As the air in this updraft cools, water vapor
condenses into water droplets and forms a cloud.

Integrated Presentation

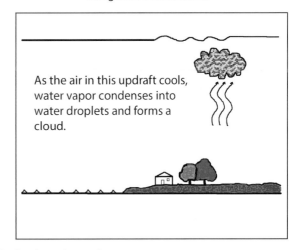

Figure 14.4 Spatial contiguity principle: Which instructional method leads to better learning?

three words summarize each point, then use your narration to explain graphics and points on the screen in more detail.

Fourth, your existing lesson may include a slide that has an illustration along with a caption below it (as shown in the left side of Figure 14.4). This creates a split attention problem in which learners must scan between the words and the corresponding part of the graphic, thereby wasting precious processing capacity. According to the spatial contiguity principle, the

solution is to place the printed words next to the part of the graphic to which they refer (as shown in the right side of Figure 14.4). Fifth, according to the temporal contiguity principle, the words you are speaking should correspond to the graphics that are on the screen, so they can help guide where the learner looks on the screen.

As you can see in Table 14.4, using techniques such as these have been shown to increase transfer test performance – with median effect sizes of 0.86 for the

Table 14.5 Three design principles for managing essential processing

Principle	Definition	Effect Size (n)
Segmenting	Break a complex screen into manageable parts	0.79 (10)
Pretraining	Provide pretraining on names and characteristics of key elements	0.75 (16)
Modality	Present main verbal message as spoken text	0.76 (61)

n = number of comparisons

Segmented: With "Continue" button

Continuous: Without "Continue" button

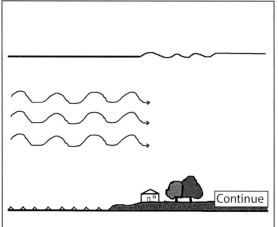
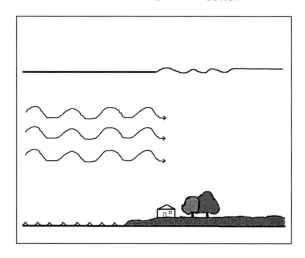

"Cool moist air moves over a warmer surface and becomes heated."

"Cool moist air moves over a warmer surface and becomes heated."

Figure 14.5 Segmenting principle: Do people learn better when a "Continue" button is added after each segment?

coherence principle, 0.41 for the signaling principle, 0.86 for the redundancy principle, 1.10 for the spatial contiguity principle, and 1.22 for the temporal contiguity principle.

Principles for Managing Essential Processing

Table 14.5 summarizes three principles examined by Mayer and Pilegard[6] aimed at managing essential processing – segmenting, pretraining, and modality. First, suppose you have a complicated diagram showing several subsystems and multiple steps in a process, with so much detail that it is likely to overload the learner's working memory. You can't weed out material because all of it is essential, but in accord with the segmenting principle, you can present it in bite-size pieces rather than filling the slide all at once. This way, the learner can digest one segment before moving on to the next one. For example, Figure 14.5 shows

a frame from a narrated animation on lightning that contains a CONTINUE button after a segment or does not. People learn better when they can control the pace of presentation by clicking on the CONTINUE button, thereby creating bite-sized segments rather than a continuous presentation.

Another approach to the problem of having to explain a complex system is to provide pretraining in the names and characteristics of the key parts in the system, in accord with the pretraining principle. For example, pretraining can be presented using printed materials, a video, or even interacting with a concrete model of each key part. Figure 14.6 shows some pretraining frames for a lesson on how a car's braking system works, in which the learner sees what a piston is and how it moves before receiving a narrated animation explaining how the whole system works as a cause-and-effect chain. Pretraining helps free up processing capacity when those terms are used later in the

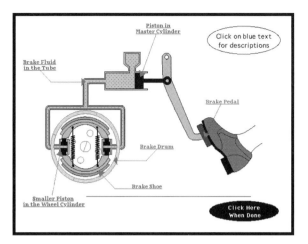 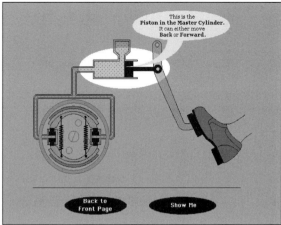

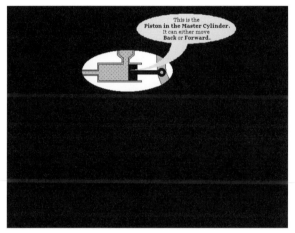

Figure 14.6 Pretraining principle: Do people learn better when they receive pretraining in the names and characteristics of key parts?

context of explaining a complex system, because the learner already knows the parts.

Finally, based on the modality principle, when you explain a complex system it is best to use the slide for presenting a graphic with a minimum of words on it, along with narration that systematically explains the graphic (as shown in the left side of Figure 14.7) rather than presenting the verbal information as onscreen text (as shown in the right side of Figure 14.7). By off-loading the printed words from the screen to spoken words, you create more capacity for processing the visual information, while not overloading the verbal channel.

As you can see in Table 14.5, using techniques such as these have been shown to increase transfer test performance – with median effect sizes of 0.79 for the segmenting principle, 0.75 for the pretraining principle, and 0.76 for the modality principle.

Principles for Fostering Generative Processing

Table 14.6 summarizes two principles articulated by Mayer[7] aimed at fostering generative processing – personalization and embodiment. To prompt learners to try harder to understand the material, it is useful to use social cues that make learners feel like they are in a conversation with the instructor. One important social cue is conversational language, such as using first- and second-person constructions (i.e., "I," "we," and "you") rather than third-person constructions, which are more formal and traditional. Another is polite wording, such as saying "Shall we press the ENTER key?" rather than "Press the ENTER key." Both conversational language and polite language are consistent with the personalization principle, and are intended to build a social partnership between the

157

Words as Narration

Words as On-Screen Text

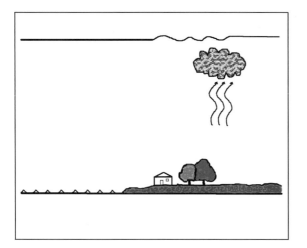

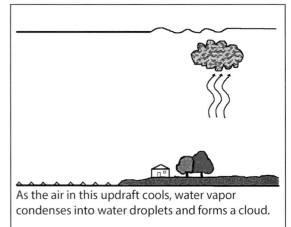

As the air in this updraft cools, water vapor condenses into water droplets and forms a cloud.

"As the air in this updraft cools, water vapor condenses into water droples and forms a cloud."

Figure 14.7 Modality principle: Which instructional method leads to better learning?

Table 14.6 Two design principles for fostering generative processing

Principle	Definition	Effect Size (n)
Personalization	Use conversational or polite wording	0.79 (17)
Embodiment	Use appropriate gestures, facial expression, eye gaze, or hand-drawing movement	0.36 (11)

n = number of comparisons

learner and the instructor, which can foster better learner motivation.

In addition to using personalized wording, you can focus on your bodily movements while instructing. According to the embodiment principle, students learn more deeply when instructors use appropriate gestures, facial expressions, and eye gazes during instruction, rather than simply stand motionless and expressionless. Similarly, recent research by Fiorella and Mayer[8] shows that students learn better when they watch instructors draw illustrations as they orally explain them (as shown in the left side of Figure 14.8 for a lesson on the Doppler effect) rather than view already drawn illustrations (as shown in the right side of Figure 14.8). Rather than being a disembodied voice, the instructor can help foster generative processing by using embodied social cues such as gesture, facial expression, eye contact, and even drawing by hand.

As you can see in Table 14.6, using techniques such as these have been shown to increase transfer test performance – with median effect sizes of 0.79 for the personalization principle and 0.36 for the embodiment principle.

Conclusion

To what extent can the principles listed in Tables 14.4, 14.5, and 14.6 be applied successfully to the design of multimedia instruction in medical education, such as anesthesiology? Most of the content used in the evidence base involves science, technology, engineering, and mathematics (STEM) fields, particularly explanations of how cause-and-effect systems work, ranging from how the human heart works to how lightning storms develop to how a car's braking system works. Most are short-term studies – with lessons less than one hour – involving immediate tests in lab environments

Narration as instructor draws by hand:

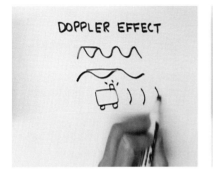

Narration of static graphics:

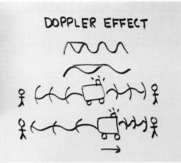

Figure 14.8 Embodiment principle: Which method leads to better learning from a lecture?

with low-knowledge learners. Therefore, it is necessary to examine how these multimedia design principles work when applied to courses in medical school, in line with the useful preliminary studies by Issa and colleagues[1,4] described in the chapter introduction. I will consider this chapter to be a success if it helps you create more effective slideshow lessons and if it fosters continued research on applying multimedia design principles to medical education.

References

1. N. Issa, M. Schuller, S. Santacaterina et al. Applying multimedia design principles enhances learning in medical education. *Med Educ* 2011; 45: 818–26.

2. R. E. Mayer. *Multimedia Learning,* 2nd edn. New York: Cambridge University Press, 2009.

3. R. E. Mayer. Applying the science of learning to medical education. *Med Educ* 2010; 44: 543–9.

4. N. Issa, R. E. Mayer, S. Schuller et al. Teaching for understanding in medical classrooms using multimedia design principles. *Med Educ* 2013, 47: 388–96.

5. R. E. Mayer, L. Fiorella. Principles for reducing extraneous processing in multimedia learning: Coherence, signaling, redundancy, spatial contiguity, and temporal contiguity principles. In R. E. Mayer, ed. *The Cambridge Handbook of Multimedia Learning,* 2nd edn. New York: Cambridge University Press, 2014; 279–315.

6. R. E. Mayer, C. Pilegard. Principles for managing essential processing in multimedia learning: Segmenting, pretraining, and modality principles. In R. E. Mayer, ed. *The Cambridge Handbook of Multimedia Learning,* 2nd edn. New York: Cambridge University Press, 2014; 316–44.

7. R. E. Mayer. Principles based on social cues in multimedia learning: Personalization, voice, image, and embodiment principles. In R. E. Mayer, ed. *The Cambridge Handbook of Multimedia Learning,* 2nd edn. New York: Cambridge University Press, 2014; 345–68.

8. L. Fiorella, R. E. Mayer. Effects of observing the instructor draw diagrams on learning from multimedia lessons. *J Educ Psychol* 2016; 108: 528–46.

Chapter 15

The Interactive Classroom

Susan M. Martinelli and Edwin A. Bowe

Introduction

The superiority of active learning over traditional teaching methods has been well established[1,2] and is, in fact, a topic evaluated by the National Research Council.[3]

Advantages to active learning include:[4]

- Increased knowledge gain;
- Increased retention of knowledge;
- Increased sense of community; and
- Increased motivation to become lifelong learners.

Educators generally accept the fact that meaningful learning, that is, construction of a mental model that can be used to solve problems, is determined by the cognitive activity of the learner during the learning session. While lecturing may be an efficient way to transfer factual information to a large group of learners who passively take notes and regurgitate factual information on an exam, meaningful learning rarely occurs in that situation.

There are a variety of ways to stimulate active learning. The methods described in this chapter have been used by one or both authors, and those experiences, in combination with a literature review, constitute the basis for the information and recommendations.

Several words of caution.

- First, as described in Chapter 2, there are multiple different learning styles. What works well for one resident may not work for someone else.
- Second, the objective of teaching should not be simply to pass factual information to residents; the objective should be to help them establish a mental model so they can use the information in combination with clinical reasoning (Chapter 3) to solve problems they have not previously encountered.
- Third, because the goal of active learning is improving application of knowledge as opposed to facilitating transfer of factual information, it is unlikely that comparing scores between

multiple-choice pretests and posttests will demonstrate a benefit of active learning techniques. It is, however, much more challenging to have any form of standardized testing effectively measure the application of knowledge.

- Fourth, it is difficult to demonstrate a statistically significant advantage of one technique over another in part because it is difficult to avoid confounding variables in learning environments. Unlike a genetically consistent strain of rats who receive an experimental drug, the learners participating in any didactic presentation have different motivations and interests. An undergraduate freshman biology class is likely to include some students who are seeking entry into medical school and will study hard to achieve a good grade in an effort to enhance their chances of admission, but it will also likely include some English or history majors who simply want to achieve a passing score to fulfill a requirement. Trying to document an effect of a teaching modality on test scores from that group of learners will be difficult. While not quite as striking in diversity, a resident who is naturally interested in cardiovascular physiology may be more likely to be attentive and try to construct a mental model from a lecture on that subject than a resident who is anticipating a fellowship in pain management. (Furthermore, if nothing else, anesthesia residents have demonstrated their proficiency at taking multiple-choice tests. They are motivated to accumulate the information necessary to pass written board exams and will likely acquire the majority of that factual information even if it's not formally presented.)
- Fifth, it is extremely difficult to get a study population large enough to demonstrate statistical significance when working in graduate medical education.

- Finally, there is a phenomenon of too much of a good thing. (In the 1700s lobsters were so plentiful that in New England they washed ashore in piles up to two feet high. The result was that they were used as an inexpensive form of protein for prisoners and slaves. Reportedly some servants had written into their contracts that they would not have to eat lobster more than twice per week.)[5] A diverse educational experience, including both the interactive modes described in this chapter and some aspects of more traditional teaching methods, should have some elements that appeal to each resident's individual learning style.

Description of Interactive Learning

Historically, didactic teaching has primarily occurred through prepared lectures with minimal interaction between teachers and learners (Figure 15.1).

This passive, teacher-centered educational method serves as a means to transfer factual knowledge without ensuring that learners have the necessary tools to apply the material. This is primarily how the generations that preceded Generation Y (i.e., Baby Boomer Generation and Generation X) were taught (Table 15.1).

Most current anesthesia faculty are members of either the Baby Boomer Generation or Generation X. Consequently, they were primarily taught through traditional lectures or the Socratic method and had minimal experience with an interactive classroom. Knowledge was primarily attained through reading textbooks and journal articles. Although technologic advances (e.g., the personal computer and Microsoft PowerPoint) became available during the education of Generation X, they played little role in learning. Now these individuals are the educators for the new generation of anesthesia residents, most of whom belong to Generation Y. Members of Generation Y achieve their learning goals by different means than the faculty whose responsibility it is to teach them. Generation Y learners do not want to listen to lectures. They do not want to be put on the spot with Socratic questioning. They desire a learner-centered educational process that incorporates discussion and teamwork, utilizes a variety of educational resources, and functions with the educator as a facilitator[6,7] (Figure 15.2).

This is a technology-native group of learners that wants to incorporate technology into their learning. As such, this generation of learners will likely benefit from an interactive classroom. An interactive classroom utilizes active learning techniques to facilitate the learner-centered education desired by Generation Y anesthesia residents.

This environment does not focus on the passive transfer of factual knowledge from teacher to student, as students no longer primarily rely on teachers to acquire basic knowledge. Instead students utilize

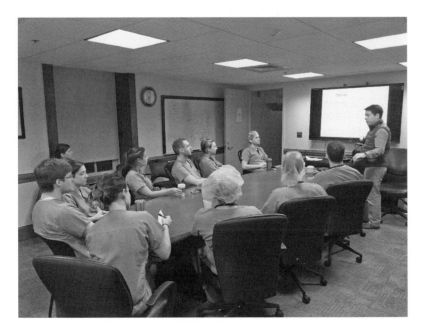

Figure 15.1 Traditional classroom. The educator is delivering a lecture to the learners, who are passive participants.

Table 15.1 Characteristics of different generations. Definitions, including years of birth, vary between sources. Characteristics are generalizations

	Baby Boomers	Gen X	Gen Y (Millennials)
Year of Birth	1945–63	1963–80	1980–95
Tech Savvy	Low; technology requires learning	Moderate; little exposure to computers in elementary school	High; have always had computers; information primarily obtained from web
Work Ethic	Hardworking	Moderate	Self-absorbed; appear lazy
Work Expectations	Work more important than family	Commitment is to self instead of organization	Want low stress with support and accolades
Adaptability	Low	High	High
Teams	Team oriented	Individualistic	Prefer to work in teams

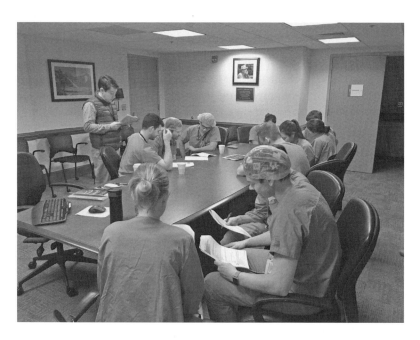

Figure 15.2 Interactive classroom. The educator is functioning as a facilitator for the learners who are actively engaged in problem solving as a group.

classroom time to clarify concepts, apply knowledge, and solve problems. There are multiple teaching methods that utilize the active learning approach, but they have many commonalities. All require student participation wherein students share in the responsibility of their education. Control of the educational environment shifts toward the learners. Students utilize higher-order thinking in the application of knowledge. Although the evidence is minimal in graduate medical education, data from other health fields suggest multiple benefits of the interactive classroom. As students work to solve problems, educators will have a better understanding of where knowledge gaps lie. By applying newfound knowledge, it is expected that

students will utilize higher-order thinking and retain more information than through rote memorization. Development of professionalism and team-based skills may be expected to occur through group work. Students' motivation to learn will likely increase.[8]

Problem-Based/Case-Based Learning

The educational concepts of problem-based learning (PBL) and case-based learning (CBL) have been some of the most utilized interactive teaching methods in medical education. Although the concepts of PBL and CBL have some subtle differences,[9] for the purposes of this discussion the two will be equated and will be referred to as PBL. While the definition of PBL varies in nuance, there are some common themes among most descriptions. PBL is a learner-centered process that begins with an authentic patient-care scenario or problem. Learners work in small groups to determine and discover what knowledge is needed to diagnose and treat the patient.

Educators take on the role of facilitator rather than the traditional teacher role. Ideally, the educator would have prior training in this new role, but frequently that isn't the case. Instead of providing solutions, the facilitator functions as a guide, asking open-ended questions and challenging the learners' thinking. If the group is heading off course, the facilitator guides it back on track, ensuring that the educational objectives are met. It is controversial whether the facilitator must be a content expert in the educational objectives of the session, but it has been suggested that this might allow the learners a more complete educational experience.[10]

There are multiple proposed benefits of PBL[10,11]:

- Working together to care for their patient fosters teamwork, communication, leadership, and problem-solving skills.
- Students will develop the lifelong learning attributes of self-directed learning.
- The interactive nature and connection of basic science with real-life scenarios may prove to be more enjoyable for learners.
- Students may develop a deeper understanding of concepts through their self-directed research.

PBLs have long been utilized in undergraduate medical education, where it was first introduced into McMaster University by Howard Barrows more than 50 years ago. Currently most medical schools are utilizing a form of PBL for at least a part of their curriculum, and some use PBL for almost the entirety of their curriculum.[10] The American Society of Anesthesiologists (ASA) has been using PBL as a method of continuing medical education at their Annual Meetings since 1991.[12]

Evidence

There have been several studies done comparing PBL programs to traditional learning techniques (primarily lecture-based learning) in undergraduate medical education, graduate medical education, and continuing medical education. (Unlike most of the other active learning techniques discussed in this chapter, research

on PBL has been the subject of many studies involving thousands of students; longitudinal studies involving undergraduate medical students in particular have had enough subjects that it should have been possible to demonstrate an advantage for PBL if one existed.)[9,13–16] None of these studies have demonstrated an educational advantage for the PBL format. Studies have found that students[9,13] and educators[9] enjoyed the PBL format more than traditional lectures.

Sakai et al. investigated the use of PBL for teaching anesthesia residents the fundamentals of research.[17] They developed a case in which the residents served as the primary investigators on a prospective randomized clinical trial. The residents went through the research process including determining the research question, finding a mentor, applying for a grant, and so forth. There were more residents from the PBL group who participated in research (and asked for help with research) than in the group that was not exposed to the PBL. (It is unclear if the group of residents not exposed to the PBL had a different educational intervention or no intervention regarding the basics of research.)[17]

Implementation

There are several factors that must be included in the development of a PBL scenario. As with all learning activities, the first step should be to decide upon the learning objectives. After there is agreement on the objectives, if PBL is determined to be an appropriate teaching method, a case scenario can be developed. Ideally, a real patient encounter will form the foundation of the scenario, but some details may need to be modified for all learning objectives to be met. The case should be written in steps so that the learners can make decisions on diagnoses and medical management. Additional information regarding the patient's condition should be provided to the learners based on the decisions they have made.

Traditionally, learners research the problem or case in their small groups or as a homework assignment allocated among team members. In the situations in which team members are assigned homework, they bring their findings to their small group at the next session meeting. This format may work better in undergraduate medical education than in graduate medical education due to time constraints. When the learners are residents, it might be helpful to guide their fund of knowledge by providing "homework" to read prior to the session. The residents can then come to class prepared to discuss the case and ideally diagnose and treat the patient. (This is the format of PBLs used for the ASA Annual Meetings.)[12]

As previously mentioned, the faculty member functions as a facilitator and not a teacher when implementing a PBL. The facilitator should keep the learners on track, ask questions, and ensure the learning objectives are met.

Korin and colleagues have suggested some specific methods to increase learner engagement in PBLs. As the learners are working through a case, the decisions they make may lead to alternative patient outcomes. One of these outcomes is ideal and the others may lead to significant complications. To complement the case description, a video clip of a standardized patient presenting his or her history may bring more realism to the scenario. Different learners may be assigned opposing views of a topic or decision to debate in class. Similarly, each group member may be assigned a role to play in the scenario (i.e., surgeon, operating room nurse, patient) to demonstrate different perspectives that have an impact on patient care. Finally, two different diagnoses with different management but similar clinical presentations can be discussed.[18]

Barriers

Because PBLs have long been utilized in medical education, this form of active learning may be easier to implement than most. Compared to other active learning techniques with which faculty members may have little or no experience, familiarity with PBLs may facilitate adoption of this modality. Most faculty, however, are not trained to facilitate these sessions and may not be comfortable or proficient in this role.

In addition, there is criticism directed at PBLs. Some learners are concerned that they will not be adequately prepared for exams as the knowledge conveyed can be fragmented, less organized, or incomplete.[9,10,15] If PBLs are implemented in the traditional format, the learning can be time consuming for the students due to the independent research component. In addition, there is criticism that teachers are not being used efficiently to transmit knowledge to their learners when they are functioning as facilitators.[10]

Conclusion

Although PBLs have been prevalent in medical education, there is a paucity of data demonstrating their

benefit over traditional learning techniques. Even so, both learners and educators enjoy this process that connects classroom learning to realistic patient encounters. Although PBL may be criticized for the scattered manner of learning, the students tend to gain depth of knowledge on the subject and build a knowledge bank linked to patient cases that may help with recall when they are presented with similar situations in the future.

Flipped Classroom

Face-to-face class time has traditionally been utilized for educators to passively transmit knowledge through lectures. In elementary and undergraduate education, learners use the time outside of class to apply this knowledge through problem solving for homework assignments. The flipped classroom (FC) is a form of blended learning (typically defined as a combination of digital/online delivery of content with face-to-face classroom time) that reverses this process. Foundational knowledge is delivered to the learner prior to class as homework, frequently in the form of a brief video. Classroom time is then utilized for active learning and problem solving (Figure 15.3).

Evidence

The FC has long been utilized in K–12 education and has more recently gained popularity in higher learning, including graduate education. Although there is some evidence supporting improved knowledge gain with FC in medical education, it is primarily limited to allied health fields and may be subject-specific. [19-21] A recent review of the medical education literature found FC to be as beneficial, but not superior to, traditional methods of education, but the studies were primarily conducted in undergraduate medical education.[22] Martinelli et al. did a large multicenter study in anesthesia graduate medical education in which FC led to a small increase in knowledge retention ($d = 0.56$, $p = 0.01$) and no significant increase (but a trend in this direction) in knowledge acquisition ($d = 0.48$, $p = 0.06$) compared to traditional lectures.[23]

It has been postulated that FC learning may lead to an improvement in higher-order cognition such as problem solving and critical thinking. This theory was tested in a first-year medical student anatomy course in which the multiple-choice exam questions were categorized according to cognition level (knowledge, application, or analysis). They found that FC students

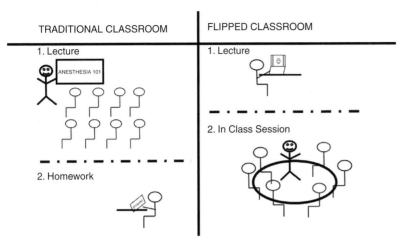

Figure 15.3 Traditional vs. flipped classroom. In a traditional classroom, the lecture is delivered passively to the learners. The learners do homework after class on their own time. For the flipped classroom, the learners receive the foundational knowledge content on their own time outside of class. They then use in-class time to problem solve and apply the newfound knowledge.

performed better on analysis questions but equal on knowledge and application questions.[24] Evidence supporting learner preference for the FC compared to traditional learning techniques is more ubiquitous throughout the literature, but again is primarily demonstrated in allied health fields.[19,25–27] Martinelli et al.'s study also demonstrated a preference for the FC by those residents that had been exposed to this learning technique.[23]

Implementation

Implementing the FC in anesthesia residency education requires few additional resources. This method can be incorporated into an entire educational program (e.g., basic board review curriculum) or can be utilized by an individual faculty member for a single assigned presentation (e.g., "lecture" on aortic stenosis). The two major components necessitating development are the presession "homework" and the in-class active learning experience.

The purpose of the presession homework is for the learner to acquire the foundational knowledge pertaining to the session. This is often provided as a brief video, but that is not a requirement. (The educator may choose to instead utilize a reading assignment, a web-based module, or anything else that conveys this material.) An assigned video may be a natural vehicle for transfer of information to this primarily Generation Y group of learners given that they tend to embrace technology and appreciate the defined time

requirement associated with video review. In addition, videos are generally easy to create.

When creating a video, it should be no longer than 15–20 minutes to maintain the attention of the learner. A traditional slide-based lecture covering the foundational concepts of the material can be created, keeping in mind the concepts described in Chapter 14. A standard voice-over software program can then be used to capture the oral delivery of the slide-based lecture. (There are currently numerous such software programs available that are fairly straightforward to use.) Although the educator may want to create a video specific to the material to be covered, a preexisting video that provides the same information may be available. (Example is shown in Video 15.1 in the supplemental online material.)

Once the educator has established the presession homework, it is necessary to communicate this information to the learners. It is important to ensure that the residents understand what their homework assignment is, that completion is required prior to the classroom session, and the time frame in which they are expected to complete it.

The second component of the FC necessitating development is the active learning in-class session. Multiple active learning techniques including, but not limited to, audience response questions, think-pair-share (TPS) questions, think-group-share questions, and CBL can be utilized. (See example in Video 15.2 in the supplemental online material.) Ideally, a variety of these techniques will be used throughout the session.

(The details of these activities are explained elsewhere in this chapter.)

It may be helpful to use a slide-based presentation as the scaffolding of this session. Each question/case can be written on a slide. The subsequent slide(s) can provide a detailed explanation that is viewed after the group had the opportunity to work through the problem. It is important to keep in mind that the educator should function as a facilitator or coach for the leaners in this environment. Instead of providing an answer, the educator may want to ask more leading questions to direct the learners toward the solution. Be mindful of the time that is allotted for the session; on occasion, discussions consume more time than anticipated. The most important material should be presented at the beginning of the session to ensure that it is covered. Ideally, the educator will have extra questions/cases available in case the group of learners progresses faster than expected.

Barriers

There are barriers to the implementation of the FC method of teaching. The faculty must embrace the concept. Many are accustomed not only to learning, but also to teaching through traditional slide-based lectures. In addition, the traditional approach provides the teacher complete control over the learning environment. With FC, the leader relinquishes control and must be adaptable because there is no way to accurately predict what issues will be raised in the session. Faculty educators probably will not have had formal training on the implementation of these newer techniques and therefore may be reluctant to step out of their comfort zone. Some may not be familiar with the technology associated with these techniques such as the voice-over software used to create the presession video. Others may be concerned that changing the format of their delivery will be too time consuming.

Conclusion

The FC has been an established teaching method in various educational settings. Evidence is suggestive of a benefit in knowledge acquisition and retention in anesthesia residents utilizing the FC compared to traditional lectures in some subject content. It has been demonstrated across multiple healthcare fields, including anesthesia graduate medical education, that learners prefer the FC to traditional lectures. Incorporating the FC into anesthesia residency education should not require many additional resources and can be done

incrementally (i.e., one lecture at a time) or as a whole (i.e., changing an entire curriculum).

Educational Games

Perhaps the biggest examples of educational games come from the military. The US Department of Defense has made extensive investments in gamification for the education of trainees. Their work showed that, compared to traditional training methods, those trained through games demonstrated substantial improvement in several areas (Box 15.1).[28,29]

Box 15.1 Demonstrated advantages of gamification for military trainees

- Increased confidence (20 percent);
- Increased procedural knowledge (14 percent);
- Increased knowledge recall (11 percent);
- Increased knowledge retention (9 percent).

There are two major commonalities for any format of an educational game: predetermined rules and a component of competition. Although simulation, virtual environments, and other types of computer games can be utilized for educational purposes, this section will focus on social and cooperative games such as board games and games mimicking TV game shows as they align more with interactive classroom learning. Perceived benefits of educational games include utilization of active learning, eliciting higher levels of thinking, perception of fun and excitement amongst learners, and employing problem-solving skills.[30] In addition, game playing provides learners with immediate feedback and can facilitate peer teaching.

Advocates for gamification in medical education theorize that engaging learners to voluntarily participate in a fun activity may lessen the likelihood of burnout associated with the long hours spent accumulating knowledge.

Evidence

There are multiple examples of the use of educational games in the medical education literature. Shiroma et al. utilized an interactive game board similar in format to Jeopardy!™ to teach third-year medical students psychopharmacology. The control group received traditional lectures. Although there was no significant difference in knowledge gain between groups, the students who played the game perceived that it was more effective.[31] O'Leary et al. also utilized a Jeopardy! style game to teach third-year medical students about ectopic pregnancy with traditional lectures for their control group. Although there was no difference in knowledge gain between groups, an attitudinal survey found that the students who played the game felt it helped with knowledge retention, it was more enjoyable, there was more substantial faculty/student interaction, and that they were more engaged in the classroom sessions.[32] Telnar et al. compared game-based learning to CBL in the continuing medical education population utilizing a game based on Snakes and Ladders™. Similar to the other studies, there was no knowledge difference between groups, but the learners preferred the game-based teaching approach.[33]

As is suggested by the aforementioned studies, there is little evidence of improved test scores when using educational games. The most recent Cochrane review compared educational games to CBL and a mode that involved video modules. The Cochrane review was unable to determine if there was knowledge benefit from game-based learning and recommended further study in this area.[34]

Implementation

The first step in developing an educational board/TV game is determining what game format to utilize.

Hollywood Squares,™ Monopoly,™ and Jeopardy! are formats that can readily be converted into medical education classroom games. An anesthesiologist at the University of North Carolina utilized a Monopoly board template to teach topics related to cardiovascular anesthesia (Figure 15.4).

Templates for the game board and related game spaces can be downloaded from Internet sites such as Pinterest. Properties and railroads can be named according to question topics such as Hemostasis Easy Street or ACLS Avenue. One may also consider working in factors unique to the institution. For example, the jail space can be renamed according to an undesirable clinical assignment such as Interventional Radiology and free parking can be renamed the "Break Room." The Chance and Community Chest cards can also be renamed to something anesthesia-specific such as You Got Paged. When a learner lands on a property, they must answer a question worth the monetary amount designated on the space (instead of having the option to purchase the property). If the question is answered correctly, the learner earns the monetary value of the property. There is no penalty for answering incorrectly. Questions of varying difficulty must be written for each topic. The monetary worth of the question is based on the difficulty level of the question asked (i.e., higher monetary values will be associated with more difficult questions). The winner is determined to be the player with the most

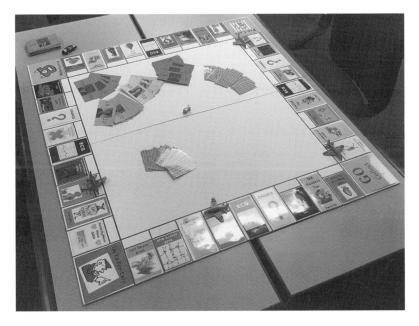

Figure 15.4 Anesthesia Monopoly game board. Developed by Dr. Lavinia Kolarczyk.

money at the end of the game. (Please see Video 15.3 for a demonstration of this game.)

Jeopardy! is another game format that can be readily adapted to medical education. The game board can be developed electronically to be interactive (in which the answers for which the contestants must provide a question appear when you click the hyperlink in the chosen square), it can be very low tech (in which the board is drawn on a dry erase board or large piece of paper and squares that have been played are erased or covered), or it can fall somewhere in between. There are electronic gameboard templates that can be downloaded from the Internet (Figure 15.5).

To be consistent with the game show format, the game board should have six categories listed horizontally across the top. Each category will have five questions of increasing monetary worth and difficulty level listed vertically under the category heading. When choosing the categories for the game, one may consider adding a fun category such as something specific to the institution or department, geographical area, sports, current events, and so forth. The other categories should be topic-specific based on the material that needs to be covered. To stay true to the nature of the TV game, selecting a square results in an answer being revealed and the contestant must provide an appropriate question for that answer (i.e., the "questions" from the board should be presented in the form of an answer and the "answers" provided by the participants should be phrased as questions). Once the answer is revealed by the proctor, the learner who buzzes in first has the first chance to answer. An electronic buzzer system can be used, or the learner can say his or her name out loud. The winner is determined to be the player with the most money at the end of the game. (Of note, the learners can play as teams or independently.)

Hollywood Squares can also be easily adapted to a classroom environment. Select nine participants (residents, faculty, or a mix of both) to serve as the "celebrities." Predetermined questions are posed to the celebrities. Two individuals (or perhaps two teams) hear a question, select a celebrity to answer the question, and then choose to agree or disagree with the response. If the team provides the correct response, the square occupied by that celebrity converts to the team's mark (either X or O). The object is to win a game of Tic-Tac-Toe by having three of your team's marks aligned horizontally, vertically, or diagonally. The game can be extremely low-tech simply using a whiteboard display of the names of the celebrities in the nine boxes of a Tic-Tac-Toe board and placing the Xs and Os on the board.

Regardless of the format utilized, it is important to ensure that the students understand the material as the game is played. After each question is answered, whether correctly or incorrectly, an explanation should be provided. This can be done by the learners to encourage peer teaching or can be done by the proctor. (If using Hollywood Squares the "celebrity" can provide the explanation.)

Barriers

There are a few potential barriers in the utilization of games in anesthesiology education. One of the biggest barriers is the time necessary to develop the game. In addition to writing good questions with varying degrees of difficulty, the actual game board must be developed. This time requirement will be a one-time occurrence as the game can be reused for different groups of learners.

Another potential issue is the number of learners who can participate in the game simultaneously.

Spinal anesthesia	Epidural anesthesia	Complications	Spine anatomy	This, that and the other
$100	$100	$100	$100	$100
$200	$200	$200	$200	$200
$300	$300	$300	$300	$300
$400	$400	$400	$400	$400
$500	$500	$500	$500	$500

Figure 15.5 Pain Jeopardy! game board. Developed by Dr. Brooke Chidgey.

Generally speaking, this format may be better utilized for small group learning sessions. However, the learners can be organized into teams. The team format may be beneficial as it will encourage peer teaching, communication, and teamwork.

Conclusion

Educational games have a place in anesthesiology education. They bring a sense of fun and competition into the learning environment. They also allow for the educator to bring creativity and excitement into their material. Although the literature hasn't demonstrated a significant increase in knowledge gain relative to more traditional educational methods, the learners have demonstrated a preference for playing games. The time required to develop a worthwhile educational game may be prohibitive to some educators, but perhaps some of these games can be shared across departments in the future to offset that issue.

Peer Teaching

The Merriam-Webster dictionary defines *peer* as "one that is of equal standing with another." Based on that literal interpretation, a peer teacher should be someone of equal rank with the learners. *Peer teaching* is generally defined as having students provide instruction to one another. Implicit in this situation is that the students who are teaching have less knowledge than a faculty member and generally have little didactic teaching experience.[35] Perhaps the best example of this form of teaching involves second-year medical students teaching anatomy to first-year medical students – a practice that has been in place for decades if not centuries. Technically, this should be considered "near peer teaching" because the student doing the teaching is a year ahead of the students being taught. For the purposes of this chapter, we will consider "peer teaching" to involve one resident teaching one or more other residents. A circumstance in which a fellow is doing the teaching will be considered "near-peer teaching." Putative advantages of peer teaching include:

- Decreased cost (fewer faculty members required);
- Decreased faculty burden (more time for faculty members to be engaged in other activities, e.g., research or clinical care);
- Increased knowledge acquisition by learners;
- Increased knowledge acquisition by peer teachers; and

- Increased teamwork skills (from working in small groups).

Peer teaching may occur in many didactic formats. (Although a lecture delivered by a resident to classmates is a form of peer teaching, it is not considered in this section because it is not a form of interactive learning.) Probably the most commonly used format is having a peer lead all or parts of a PBL session. Other methods include team-based learning (TBL) and "think, pair, share," which will be discussed separately in subsequent sections.

Evidence

Peer teaching is common in medical schools; in 2010 Soriano reported that approximately 50 percent of US medical schools use peer teachers in some capacity.[36] Especially when considering articles relating to teaching gross anatomy, there is a plethora of publications on the use of medical students to teach other medical students. Because the literature on peer teaching of residents by other residents is almost nonexistent, most of this section will be based on evidence from studies involving medical students as peer teachers.

Increased Knowledge Acquisition by Peer Teachers

> No one learns as much about a subject as one who is forced to teach it.
>
> – Peter F. Drucker

Logically, peer teachers would be expected to increase their knowledge of the area in which they are teaching by virtue of:

- Increased motivation to learn the material (presumably so they would be perceived as effective and not be embarrassed by an inability to answer a question from the learners);
- Spending more time on the material they are teaching (presumably a reflection of the increased motivation to learn the material);
- Processing the information more deeply (resulting in organizing and integrating the knowledge more completely); and
- Retrieving the information during teaching episodes.

Studies on the knowledge acquisition of medical student peer teachers are mixed. Some studies show a greater improvement in areas a student is asked to teach than in other areas. For example, in a study by Gregory, senior medical students were asked to prepare to teach two subjects to junior medical students: Advanced Cardiovascular Life Support (ACLS) algorithms and interpretation of electrocardiograms (ECGs).[37] After students completed preparation for teaching both subjects, they were randomized to teach either ACLS algorithms or ECG interpretation. Although peer teachers demonstrated increased knowledge in both subjects, the effect size was greater for the subject for which they provided instruction. Other studies fail to document this effect. For example, although peer-teacher senior medical students who taught patient interviewing skills to first-year medical students reported more confidence in their interviewing skills, objective assessment by observers failed to demonstrate any difference between the peer teachers and their classmates.[38] Overall, the majority of studies reporting on the impact of peer teachers indicate that students functioning as peer teachers increase their fund of knowledge in the areas in which they teach. Analysis of this literature must consider the nonrandom selection of peer teachers (i.e., only higher-performing students are offered the opportunity to function as a peer teacher and only those students with an interest in the area are likely to accept the offer) and the potential for selection bias (i.e., preferential publishing of studies that demonstrate a beneficial effect). Because no publications report that peer teachers' test scores are lower in the area being taught, at the very least it can be assumed that peer teaching was not detrimental to the teachers' fund of knowledge in that area.

Increased Knowledge Acquisition by Learners

Multiple studies have objectively compared knowledge acquisition of learners taught by peers with those taught by faculty members. While some results show no difference whether teaching was by peers or faculty, others report improved scores for content taught by peers. Studies have not reported higher test scores for classes taught by faculty. Clearly, faculty members have more experience and more knowledge to transfer than medical students. At least two hypotheses have been advanced to explain the fact that peer teaching is just as effective (or perhaps even more effective) than that provided by faculty members:

- **Cognitive Congruence**: By virtue of being more closely associated with the students, peers are hypothesized to have a better understanding of the learners' existing fund of knowledge and

challenges they are facing. In addition, they may be better able to describe techniques that worked for them to learn the material.

- **Social Congruence**: Because peer teachers rarely provide grades for the learners, they are perceived to be less threatening and to provide a more comfortable learning environment. As a result, learners may be more willing to ask questions that help them achieve a better grasp of the information.

Implementation

Most programs already have some elements of peer teaching incorporated into their didactic schedule. Examples would include:

- Residents presenting cases and discussing relevant issues at case discussion conferences;
- Residents presenting results of quality assurance/ quality improvement projects; and
- Residents presenting results of research or other activities to fulfill the "scholarly activities" element of the core program requirements.

Additionally, there are methods of peer teaching that can be utilized to activate a classroom. In a PBL session, specific residents may be assigned an aspect of a case in advance of class that they then teach their peers in class. There can also be informal peer teaching such as TPS questions (which will be further described in the following text) and peer teaching that occurs in team learning through social/cooperative games (as described in the preceding text).

Barriers

Because one of the major advantages of peer teaching, as perceived by medical schools, is freeing up faculty for other pursuits, use of this modality would not be expected to require additional resources. But it may be worthwhile to provide specific instruction in educational modalities to residents if the program plans to use them to fulfill a major role in residency education through peer teaching (see Chapter 21).

Assigning responsibility for all, or a major portion, of the regularly scheduled didactic presentations to residents who function as peer teachers may create problems. It is unlikely that the Anesthesiology Review Committee of the Accreditation Council for Graduate Medical Education (ACGME) would look favorably on a program in which a majority of the didactic presentations are the responsibility of the residents. Additionally, the residents may resent having to prepare a significant number of full-length didactic presentations every year. Furthermore, residents may believe they will learn more from the expert faculty members than from their peers (regardless of the evidence).

Conclusion

Peer teaching, which should decrease faculty burden for educational activities, has been used extensively in medical school. Although there is essentially no literature on the efficacy of peer teaching in graduate medical education, most studies involving medical students show that knowledge acquisition by learners is the same or better when peer teaching is used. There is also a potential benefit to the peer teachers, who may have a better understanding of the material they teach. Most anesthesiology residency training programs already incorporate some element of peer teaching in a variety of didactic settings.

Team-Based Learning

TBL is a process in which small groups of students (usually three to five) are assigned a task. As initially described, there are three phases to TBL (Box 15.2).

Because commonly there are various acceptable answers to a question (e.g., anesthetic technique for a cesarean section for failure to progress), it is expected that the different techniques will provide the basis for a discussion of the merits of each solution. When initially described, TBL was intended for classes where the teacher:student ratio was at least 1:6 (i.e., where there would be at least two groups of three students/group). It has subsequently been adapted to larger groups, including situations in which the teams remained constant throughout a year of medical school.[39]

Authors, including the originator of TBL, have developed the following list of seven elements to TBL (Box 15.3).

The elements of incentive and peer evaluation are probably not applicable to TBL for residents, especially if teams are constituted for a single didactic presentation.

Evidence

Beginning in 2003, Thompson et al. studied the effect of TBL in ten medical schools. Two years later use of TBL persisted in nine of the ten schools, and over that period TBL was added to more courses in the schools that continued its use; however, no effort was made to assess the efficacy of TBL.[40] Two different one-year studies in a single medical school evaluated the performance of second-year medical students who were randomized to receive instruction in pathology using either case-based discussion or TBL; analysis of final exam scores failed to demonstrate a difference in scores between the two groups.[41] When

---

Box 15.2 Phases of team-based learning

- **Phase I**: Learners individually complete assigned work before class.
- **Phase II**: Initial individual readiness assurance test (iRAT) administered followed by group working together to establish consensus answers (group readiness assurance test, gRAT).
- **Phase III**: Learners complete group assignment requiring application of concepts based on information in preclass work assignments, results of which will be presented in class.

Box 15.3 Elements of team-based learning

1. Team formation;
2. Readiness assurance;
3. Immediate feedback;
4. Sequencing of problems;
5. Use of "4S Principle" (all groups work on a **S**ignificant problem, the **S**ame problem, provide **S**pecific recommendations, and **S**imultaneously complete report to the group);
6. Establish an incentive structure (e.g., grades);
7. Peer review (members of each team "grade" other members of their team).

the study was repeated several years later using TBL to teach only part of the course content, the authors found that the students demonstrated a statistically significant increase in standardized test scores for content taught using TBL; interestingly, the effect size was greater for students in the lower quartile of the class.[42] In a study involving 156 medical students in Saudi Arabia, teaching neurosciences using TBL resulted in a higher percentage of students with a grade of B or higher (51 percent) compared to the prior year (25 percent).[43]

When TBL was implemented at noon conferences for a group of internal medicine residents (n = 27), it was associated with greater resident engagement, decreased number of residents leaving before the end of the conference, and a high degree of self-reported interest in the content. No effort was made to test knowledge acquisition or retention.[44]

In 2011 Fatmi et al. performed a systematic review of publications relating to TBL use in the education of health professionals (defined as physicians, nurses, pharmacists, veterinarians, physical therapists, occupational therapists, psychologists, and dentists). Of the 330 articles reviewed, 14 met their inclusion criteria. Seven of those studies, representing about 50 percent of the more than 3,000 students who were involved in the 14 studies, reported that use of TBL was associated with a better improvement in test scores compared to students in the control groups. Only half of the included studies assessed learner preferences; in one study the learners favored TBL, in one study learners favored the alternative, and there were no differences in the remaining five studies. Notably only 1 of the 14 studies utilized residents. That study, a prospective cohort study performed on internal medicine residents evaluating teaching fundamentals of rheumatology, found no difference in test scores on rheumatology-related questions on the In-Training Exam between the two groups as a whole. When broken into subgroups, postgraduate year 1 (PGY-1) residents taught using TBL had a greater improvement in scores than PGY-1 residents taught using traditional lectures. This finding is consistent with other reports demonstrating that individuals with lower test scores improved more with TBL than individuals with higher test scores.[45] The study involving 111 internal medicine residents documented that the average gRAT score was higher than the average iRAT score and that more than 67 percent of faculty and almost 90 percent of residents believed

that residents were actively involved, contributed in a meaningful, fair manner, and were perceived as learners during TBL sessions.

Implementation

Faculty members should review the material to be completed by the residents prior to the TBL session. If Readiness Assessment Tests are to be used, appropriate questions must be constructed. The exercises to be used in classroom discussion must also be developed.

Because no unique resources are necessary, implementation of TBL merely requires the willingness to try the method and to inform the residents in advance what will be expected of them. TBL sessions may be most successful if residents understand the format of this learning technique and expect its use. Constituting teams in advance offers several possible advantages:

1. Members of the team tend to feel a sense of responsibility to other members of the team, thereby encouraging attendance.
2. Members of teams can sit together at the beginning of the conference, thereby avoiding the need to consume class time by rearranging individuals.
3. Membership in teams can be balanced to include individuals of varying academic strengths.
4. Designation of a leader for each team places an additional sense of responsibility on that individual and may encourage previously unrecognized leadership talents.

Barriers

Just as with medical students who have commented on their first experience with TBL, residents who have never experienced this mode of teaching may not understand what is expected of them.[46]

Faculty members may be reluctant to depart from the comfortable and familiar lecture format in which the faculty member has complete control of the class. A faculty development session on TBL may facilitate implementation, but even under those circumstances faculty members using TBL for medical students have indicated that they had problems adapting to the different role (as facilitator as opposed to lecturer), anticipating (and therefore being prepared for) the direction some discussions took, managing the discussions to allow multiple viewpoints to be presented, and preventing one individual or group from dominating the conversation.[39]

Conclusions

TBL is best utilized with learners who are committed and functioning on a high level. In that environment TBL combines elements of the FC (residents are given assignments before class) and peer teaching resulting in active learning. In the short time normally allocated to didactic sessions for residents, it may be wise to consider omitting the readiness assurance tests to allow more time for teams to work together and for discussion of the conclusions.

Think-Pair-Share

TPS is effectively a form of peer instruction. (Students, who have less knowledge than the faculty member and little experience teaching, provide instruction to one another.) Box 15.4 outlines the usual format of a TPS session.

Typically, learners from some, but not all, teams are asked to provide their answers to the class. With a heterogeneous group of residents, it may be beneficial to pair learners at varying learning levels (e.g., pair a PGY-2 resident with a PGY-3 or PGY-4 resident). One advantage of this approach is that it tends to keep all residents engaged. (Not only because no team knows which will be called on to provide an answer, but also because the two members of the team must discuss the question between themselves.)

Evidence

The literature regarding the use of TPS in healthcare education is almost nonexistent. Kaddoura analyzed critical-thinking skills in two groups of nursing students. Compared to the students learning in a traditional lecture format, those students for whom TPS was incorporated as an educational element

> **Box 15.4 Elements of think-pair-share strategy**
>
> **Think**: Learners independently consider the question and develop an answer or alternatives.
>
> **Pair**: Pairs of learners discuss each other's answers and discuss the merits of each.
>
> **Share**: Learners present their answers to the class.

experienced a greater increase in all five subsets of critical thinking (defined as analysis, arguments, prioritization, problem solving, and resolution).[47] A group of graduate students in psychology indicated that using TPS in conjunction with Google Docs, which permits users to add content, allowed them to learn beyond the specified course content.[48] Compared to conventional teaching, use of TPS did not result in an improvement in test scores for undergraduate biology students.[49]

Implementation

Implementation does not require special equipment. Although most authors recommend using open-ended questions, TPS can also be used with multiple-choice questions, for example, in a board review format. TPS can be incorporated into a wide variety of educational activities from large lecture formats to small group FC environments. TPS can also be used in conjunction with an audience response system (ARS).

Barriers

Other than familiarizing faculty and residents with the TPS process there are no known barriers to implementation.

Conclusions

TPS can create an interactive learning environment with less effort than some of the other methods. Data on the benefits from the use of TPS in healthcare students over other modalities are essentially nonexistent.

Role Play

Role play (RP) is an active learning technique that can be considered a form of simulation in which the learner can either play themselves or another person in a scripted scenario. The scenario can be entirely scripted (in which the participants are given a thoroughly developed role) or it can be partially scripted (in which the participants are given a general overview of their role and they further develop it as they see fit). The level of scripting does not have to be consistent across all participants. Some participants might even play themselves with no script.[50]

The most common utilization of RP in medical education is to assist learners in the development of communication and interpersonal skills. This skill set not only applies to patient interactions, but can benefit the learner in relations with colleagues and peers as well.[51] Learners may gain insight into their body language, empathy, personal communication skills, fears, and tendency to avoid challenging situations, emotions, and others' perceptions of what was said (or not said).[51]

Evidence

Bosse and colleagues conducted a randomized controlled trial comparing the utilization of RP and standardized patients for medical students learning to counsel parents with sick children. The use of both standardized patients and RP improved the learners' self-assessment with regard to communication and objective structured clinical examination (OSCE) performance compared to coursework alone (the control group). In addition, RP led to a self-reported better understanding of the patient's perspective than use of standardized patients alone.[52] A separate study conducted by the same authors also demonstrated cost-effectiveness with the utilization of RP versus standardized patients.[53]

Nestrel and colleagues did a questionnaire study with first-year medical students to determine their attitude toward the use of RP in education regarding communication. Prior to the experience, students' responses to a questionnaire indicated that 77 percent felt that RP would be a valuable way to practice communication skills and provide insight into the behavior of themselves and others; 22 percent felt that it would not be helpful but would be embarrassing, intimidating, anxiety provoking, and unrealistic. Following the RP intervention, however, 96 percent of students reported that RP was helpful in their learning.[50] A similar attitudinal survey was done within a group of second-year medical students who used RP to practice delivering bad news. Ninety-seven percent of these students felt that RP helped them to learn different approaches in communication and 63 percent felt that it improved their comfort in this skill.[54]

Implementation

It is important to ensure a safe environment when using RP in education. It may be necessary to set ground rules to ensure that confidentiality is maintained on sensitive matters and that respect is shown to all participants. If possible, involve all the learners and allow them some choice in their role assignment.

RP may be best suited for education in the communication and professionalism realms. There are multiple situations in anesthesiology education in which RP may be helpful including consenting patients for an anesthetic, disclosing adverse events, addressing ethical issues involving patient care, delivering feedback, and conflict resolution. Of note, these topics are all considered necessary traits of an anesthesiologist by the American Board of Anesthesiology as they can be found in various forms in the Anesthesiology Milestones.[1] When doing teamwork training, it might be helpful for the learners to play the role of another team member to better understand the perspective of that individual.

To implement RP into education, a scenario and associated roles must be developed. Each role can be scripted to various desired levels. (The more scripted a role is, the more lead time you may want to give the learner playing the role for the learner to gain comfort in the role.) To decrease preparatory time for learners, consider minimizing the scripted level of a role. To keep the scenario on track, the facilitator may hand one of the actors a cue card with a suggestion of how to behave (i.e., disengage by playing on your phone).

Although RP scenarios can be done with only a select few members of the class, it is encouraged for everyone in the class to have a role. If only a couple of people are put in the hot seat, this may lead to anxiety and pressure of those involved. One method to utilize the entire class is the Trio RP method described by Stobbs. Learners are grouped in threes. Two of the learners are the actors (anesthesiologist, patient, family member, surgeon, nurse, etc.) The third learner is the observer and is tasked with providing feedback to the actors.[55]

Specific Example

RP can be utilized in teaching residents how to give feedback. First provide some foundational knowledge on feedback to the resident learners. (This can be in the form of a lecture, video, reading assignment, etc.) During the in-class time, show the group a brief (five-minute) video of a scenario involving two intensive

---

1 www.acgme.org/Portals/0/PDFs/Milestones/AnesthesiologyMilestones.pdf (accessed November 15, 2017).

care unit residents. One of the residents is signing out the service to the other resident. This scenario should be scripted to be flawed. (The resident giving report can be rushed, miss important details, dismiss questions, etc. The resident receiving report may not ask enough questions, accept the deficient report without resistance, etc.) The resident learners will then be broken into groups of two. Learner A will play the role of the resident giving report from the video. Learner B will give feedback to Learner A on his or her sign-out report. The roles will then reverse with Learner B playing the role of the resident accepting sign out and Learner A providing feedback to Learner B on his or her acceptance of sign out. Prior to viewing the video, the resident learners should break into groups of two and choose whether they will be Learner A or Learner B. These roles of each learner should be explained prior to viewing the video. (Please see Video 15.4 in the supplemental online content for example.)

Barriers

A prominent concern regarding the utilization of RP with our learners is their preconceived feelings toward this educational method. The idea of RP may induce anxiety amongst learners,[56] regardless if they have had previous experience with this teaching method. There may be fear of being judged by colleagues and having to play a role with which they are uncomfortable or for which they feel unprepared. Establishing a safe environment and setting ground rules may help make the learners more comfortable. An additional barrier to this educational method may be faculty comfort with the utilization of RP. Education about utilizing RP may assist faculty to overcome this barrier.[57]

Conclusion

RP is an educational method that may best be suited for teaching anesthesiology residents communication skills and professionalism. Although not studied in graduate medical education, it has been shown to lead to self-reported benefits by medical students. When implementing this method, it is important to develop a safe environment and provide a role for each learner.

Audience Response System

ARSs trace their history back to the 1950s when hard-wired systems were only capable of accepting input to respond to multiple-choice questions and displaying overall responses to teachers using needle gauges. Although a discussion of modern systems is beyond the scope of this chapter, systems that are currently available generally incorporate a handheld device ("clicker") capable of two-way communication through infrared or radiofrequency signals to a dongle attached to a laptop. Systems based on radiofrequency signals have been more expensive but do not require line-of-sight to communicate with the dongle and are less subject to interference. Most ARS software is an add-on for Microsoft PowerPoint and not only presents questions but is also capable of displaying histograms of each response (Figure 15.6).

Responses are anonymous to the audience but, depending on the configuration, may allow the presenter to attribute responses to specific individuals.

Some systems use smart devices (e.g., mobile phones) to connect wirelessly through Wi-Fi directly to the software on the presenter's laptop. Smart devices and some clickers allow free text input. (It should be noted that, because the responses are not categorized, free text responses may result in similar answers being placed into different categories, e.g., "subarachnoid block," "SAB," "spinal," and "spinal anesthesia" would each be treated as a different response by the ARS [Figure 15.7], making interpretation of the results more complex.)

Throughout recent history, each new technological innovation (e.g., radio, filmstrips, films, television, laser discs, computers) has been touted as a means to improve educational outcomes. Reality has never matched hype, and educational outcomes have remained essentially unchanged.[58] By now the message should be clear – if the goal is to increase learning, using technology for the sake of technology is likely to be a futile exercise. Instead, improvements in educational outcome are a result of using technology in a manner that enhances learning, that is, by making the learners become more active participants. The value of an ARS is not in the specific technology, but the way that the information is used to facilitate interaction between the teacher and the learners. In fact, some authors have described using an ARS that consists simply of color-coded cards held up by students in response to a multiple-choice question.[59]

Mayer, who distinguishes between information (which constitutes facts) and knowledge (which is the

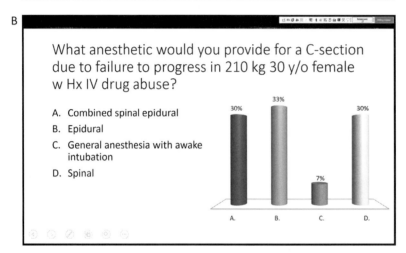

Figure 15.6 Turning Point™ ARS software is an add-on for Microsoft PowerPoint. (A) Using Turning Point in conjunction with Microsoft PowerPoint, the presenter displays a question to which learners respond using clickers. (B) When the presenter advances to the next slide, Turning Point displays a histogram of the responses.

ability to apply the factual information), has described three metaphors of multimedia learning[58] (Box 15.5).

As a learning tool, an ARS functions primarily either as a response-strengthening device (when used in a board review prep session) or as a knowledge construction device (when used to stimulate discussion by the audience).

Examples of Ways to Use an Audience Response System

Different authors have reported multiple ways to incorporate an ARS into a didactic presentation (Box 15.6).

Attendance Taking

Using an ARS to take attendance is arguably the best example of a waste of the technology. In this system, the students were assigned a specific clicker so the teacher could retrospectively determine who was present for the class. Although this application has been reported to be associated with an increase in undergraduate attendance at lectures, that occurred only when attendance resulted in credit toward final grades. In addition, it was reported that students resented the association between grades and use of the ARS.[60] Obviously, this application does not result in an increase in interactivity.

Lecture Pacing

Perhaps the easiest use of an ARS is to assess resident learning of material that has been presented and to use the ARS responses to determine if material needs to be repeated. For example, a lecture on neonatal surgical emergencies might be divided into several parts (gastroschisis, omphalocele, tracheoesophageal

A

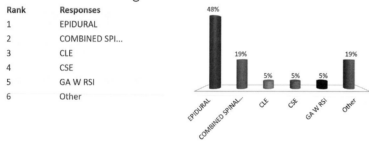

What anesthetic would you provide for a C-section due to failure to progress in 210 kg 30 y/o female with Hx of IV drug abuse?

COMBINED SPINAL EPIDURAL

EPIDURAL CSE

SAB CLE SINGLE SHOT SAB SPINAL GA W RSI
SINGLE SHOT SPINAL

B

What anesthetic would you provide for a C-section due to failure to progress in 210 kg 30 y/o female with Hx of IV drug abuse?

Rank	Responses
1	EPIDURAL
2	COMBINED SPI...
3	CLE
4	CSE
5	GA W RSI
6	Other

48% 19% 5% 5% 5% 19%

EPIDURAL COMBINED SPINAL... CLE CSE GA W RSI Other

Figure 15.7 ARS responses using smart devices in Turning Point. Using Turning Point with smart devices allows users to enter free text as the response. (A) Responses displayed using Word Cloud©. Because there are no constraints on the way the text is entered, multiple responses may mean the same thing (e.g., "SAB," for subarachnoid block and "spinal," or "single shot spinal"). The size of the font and the location of the response on the screen reflect the frequency with which the response was given. (In this example, the "Epidural" was the most common response, followed by "Combined Spinal Epidural." If "Spinal," "Single Shot Spinal," and "SAB" had been combined, that would have been the third most common response, but that fact is not evident because each word or phrase was considered as a different response.) This may make interpretation of the responses more difficult. (B) Responses displayed as a histogram. In this example none of "SAB," "spinal," or "single shot spinal" are displayed. All are grouped in the "Other" category making it impossible for the presenter to realize that this was the third most common response.

Box 15.5 Mayer's metaphors for multimedia learning

Information Acquisition: the objective is to facilitate movement of information from one place (i.e., a PowerPoint slide) to another (the minds of the learners).

Response Strengthening: the objective is to provide positive feedback for a correct response, thereby making it more likely that a specific response will occur in response to a stimulus; useful for drill and practice exercises to reinforce knowledge (e.g., board preparation questions).

Knowledge Construction: the objective is to facilitate the learner's acquisition of knowledge (individualized construction of a coherent mental model, see Chapter 3).

---

fistula, diaphragmatic hernia). After a mini-lecture of 8–10 minutes on gastroschisis the faculty member might ask one or two questions about that condition. If enough of the residents indicate understanding by correctly responding to the questions, the faculty member progresses to the next condition. If the faculty member determines that there were too many incorrect responses, the salient points may be repeated. This also helps to activate a lecture by bringing the audience in as participants.

Box 15.6 Examples of ways to use an ARS

- Attendance taking;
- Lecture pacing;
- Contingent teaching;
- Stimulate peer discussion;
- Assessment of didactic presentation.

Contingent Teaching

Another easily developed use of an ARS is to allocate time during a didactic presentation based on learner responses. Continuing the example of neonatal surgical emergencies, if more than 90 percent of the residents correctly answer a question regarding the congenital anomalies associated with omphalocele prior to presenting material on the subject, there is little value in spending time presenting that content.

Stimulate Peer Discussion

Displaying a histogram of all learner responses allows learners to see how others responded to the question. Individuals can be asked to defend the options they selected. For example, learners who select awake intubation as the preferred airway management technique for a neonate with a tracheoesophageal fistula can describe the potential advantages of that technique compared to a mask induction with maintenance of spontaneous ventilation. Learners may also be paired or grouped to discuss the results.

Assessment of Didactic Presentation

Some authors report that a higher return rate occurs when medical students[61] or emergency medicine residents[62] are asked to use an ARS to evaluate a didactic presentation at the end of each session compared with an online assessment.[61] Education would likely be improved if the presenter used the results of the assessment to alter future presentations on the same or similar subjects.

Students place a high value on the anonymity provided by an ARS[63] – they are not afraid of making a mistake in an answer. In addition, if the histogram of responses is not displayed until all voting is complete, students will not be swayed by other students' answers. An ARS is also an excellent way to present ethics questions that often have no single correct answer.

Evidence

There are few reports in the literature regarding the use of ARS in graduate medical education, but multiple studies have been performed with other groups of learners.

Numerous authors have attributed several advantages to the use of an ARS (Box 15.7), but the majority of these results are simply reports of preferences by students or teachers. Few articles report objective data (e.g., test scores).

Box 15.7 Perceived advantages of an ARS

Perceptions by students:

- Increased learning;
- Increased engagement during lecture;
- Increased participation during lecture;
- Increased interest in course material;
- Increased scores on tests;
- Compared individual performance with rest of class;
- Anonymity;
- Feedback;
- Reinforcement of content.

Perceptions by instructors:

- Improved understanding of course material;
- Identified students' misperceptions about content;
- Adapted didactic session to address misconceptions;
- Improved peer interactions;
- Increased interactivity;
- Increased discussions.

Learner Acceptance

Most studies report that learners see value in the use of ARS-based presentations. Use of an ARS for teaching graduate students has been reported to result in keeping the learners engaged,[64] increasing participation,[63,65] and stimulating beneficial discussions[65] that help clarify topics.[63] Dental students report that use of an ARS was motivating[66,67] and considered it useful to be able to assess their level of knowledge at the outset of the session.[67]

Studies document medical students expressed a preference for classes using an ARS,[68] but indicated it had no impact on their decision about whether to attend a class.[69] Students also perceived the ARS as being easy to use, providing useful feedback, and stimulating them to study the material in advance.[69] Uhari reported that the majority of medical students believed ARS classes increased their interactivity during lectures and enhanced their learning.[70]

Two-thirds of neurology residents believed that pairing reading assignments with an ARS quiz was more effective than a paper-based test, and more than three-fourths of those residents believed it was a strong motivator to read the articles and believed it helped with learning and retention.[71]

Faculty Acceptance

By using student responses to ARS questions, instructors in a pharmacy course reported they could optimize the pace of lectures by spending more time on areas in which students struggled and skipping material if more than 90 percent of the class correctly answered questions prior to presentation of material.[65] In that same study, faculty members expressed concern about not having as much time to cover the material because of the time consumed by the ARS questions. More than 85 percent of faculty members using clickers in lectures to dental students reported their use was dynamic and resulted in increased student motivation and learning.[66] Alexander et al. reported that faculty found an ARS easy to use and allowed the lecturer to adapt the presentation based on responses from the first-year medical students.[69]

Improved Test Scores

Literature on the impact of an ARS on test scores is mixed. Slain et al. documented that pharmacy students achieved higher test scores, higher scores on questions requiring analytical thinking, and higher final exam scores on segments taught using an ARS.[72] When an ARS was used in pharmacy classes with a historically low pass rate, grades were higher than the three prior years.[65] In two separate studies, first-year[67] and second-year[73] dental students were randomized to receive either traditional lectures or ARS presentations; both studies reported that there was no significant difference in exam scores between the groups. In a study randomizing medical students to either traditional lecture or presentation with an ARS, no difference was found in test scores either immediately after the lectures or 8–12 weeks later.[74] Hettinger et al. reported that the use of an ARS in review sessions for

the psychiatry In-Training Exam was associated with a greater increase in scores than prior to the use of the ARS.[75] When comparing posttest scores, family medicine residents who were taught using an ARS scored significantly higher than those receiving a traditional lecture.[76] Pradhan et al. randomized residents in an obstetrics and gynecology program to receive either a traditional lecture or a case discussion class incorporating an ARS; six weeks following the presentations students in the ARS group had a higher posttest score than those who were randomized to the traditional presentation.[77]

Because the ultimate objective is to increase learning, student support is of secondary interest unless it has an indirect effect on learning, for example, making the sessions more enjoyable may stimulate a student's desire for self-directed learning. Ultimately, as noted previously, most improvements reported for classes using an ARS are almost certainly less likely attributable to the technology and more likely due to an increase in interactivity produced by use of the ARS.

Implementation

One of the keys to optimal use of an ARS is the quality of the questions. Questions may be written for a variety of reasons (Box 15.8).[78]

If multiple-choice questions are used, distractors should be plausible. Because the objective is to engage learners with the material, presenting questions with more than one "correct" answer may initiate a discussion regarding the options.

There are multiple ways beyond simply presenting questions to integrate an ARS into a didactic session (Box 15.9).

Think-Pair-Share

Using the same principles as conventional TPS, one clicker can be assigned to two residents. The same processes should apply, that is, residents are expected to consider the options independently before discussing their selections with their partners. Each pair then decides on the response to submit.

Team-Based Learning

Teams can be constituted using a variety of mechanisms. Each team is given one clicker. After the question is presented, teams are given an opportunity to consider the options. It would be expected that some

Box 15.8 Some reasons for ARS questions

- To assess students:
  - Assess preparation (e.g., questions about reading assignments);
  - Assess understanding of lecture material (and adapt presentation);
  - Complete practice problems;
  - High-stakes assessment;
  - Compare performance before and after lecture.

- To determine audience:
  - Assess demographics of audience;
  - Assess level of understanding of subject to be covered.

- To guide audience:
  - Focus attention on material by asking question(s) prior to presentation;
  - Review material at end of presentation.

- To stimulate interaction:
  - Audience participation;
  - Discuss rationale behind different responses;
  - Create peer instruction opportunities.

- To determine outcome of a "debate."

Box 15.9 Some suggestions on way to use an ARS

Unique to an individual – one clicker per resident;
Think-pair-share – one clicker per pair of residents;
Team-based learning – one clicker per team;
Team competition – each team member has an individual clicker; team scores are determined by responses of all team members.

element of peer instruction would occur before each team selects a response.

Team Competition

If an ARS presentation is anonymous, there are no consequences for selecting an incorrect response. Dividing the audience into groups to constitute teams (e.g., males vs. females) creates a sense of competition. In this scenario, no TBL is used. Every member of each team has a clicker. By inserting a demographic slide at the start of the session, the ARS software automatically tracks the answers for all members of each team and can provide a score after each ARS slide. (Figure 15.8 and Video 15.5 in the supplemental online material.)

The team score depends on the responses of each individual on that team. Feedback from participants indicates that they perceive an increased sense of responsibility to their team to provide a correct response (and based on personal experience in many instances the losing team has requested a rematch).

Blank Slate

If the presenter is using a tablet with a touch screen that accepts handwritten input from a stylus, it is possible to pose a question, solicit responses from the audience, write those responses on the ARS slide, and then have learners vote on the best response (Figure 15.9 and Video 15.6 in the supplemental online material).

This permits the learners to provide input essentially equivalent to the free text response but maintains categorization to facilitate interpretation. This technique has the advantage of making the session even more interactive by soliciting answers from the audience. In addition, making the residents provide four or five responses forces them to develop alternatives to diagnosis or management. (See Chapter 3 for a discussion of the importance of not focusing on a limited number of diagnoses.)

Barriers

The cost of an ARS is not insignificant. After the initial purchase of the system, it must be anticipated that some clickers will disappear sporadically so replacement costs must be considered as well. If a web-based system is utilized, it will be contingent on Wi-Fi, which may not be dependable in all learning environments.

Most systems are designed to integrate with the Microsoft PowerPoint program, so instructors only need to learn how to use the specific ARS system. Given the simplicity of most systems, the time required to acquire this skill is extremely short.

Concerns are listed in Box 15.10, appearing on page 182.

As ARSs are being used more frequently in undergraduate and medical school courses, residents likely have experience with this technique. Unless working in an environment where participants can be essentially forced to download an application on a smart device, the use of clickers is probably preferable. Participants in a didactic presentation may be reluctant to download an application onto their smart devices to be able to participate. In addition, the download will take a finite amount of time, so the learners may be requested to complete this step prior to class.

A

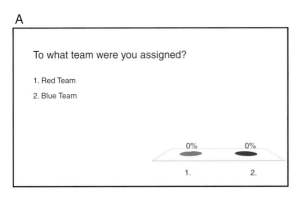

B

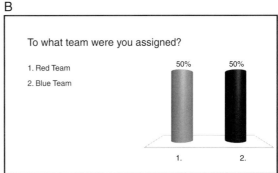

C

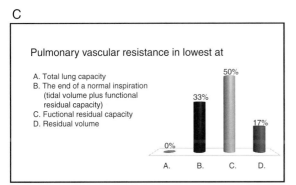

D

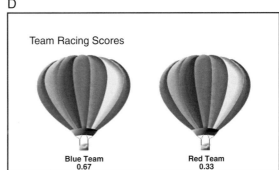

Figure 15.8 ARS using teams. Turning Point software constitutes teams based on a demographic slide at the beginning of the presentation. (A) Demographic slide. Learners can be assigned to a team randomly, for example, based on sequence of arrival as in this example, or through a specific characteristic, for example, sex, year of training, etc. (B) ARS slide showing the distribution of the participants. (C) ARS question with histogram for responses. Responses can be assigned different point values within a question, for example, the correct response could be assigned five points and the other responses could each be assigned one point thereby penalizing a team for individuals who do not submit a response. Questions can also be assigned different point values, for example, the correct response to an easy question may be assigned one point while the correct response to a difficult question could be assigned five points. (D) Team scores are displayed numerically and with an animation; the higher score for a team the further the balloon ascends. Turning Point also provides an option to simply display the scores numerically.

Conclusion

As previously described, interactive sessions are associated with increased learning, comprehension, and ability to integrate information to solve problems. Used correctly, an ARS can facilitate interactions between instructors and learners. In contrast to the conventional method of soliciting volunteers to answer a question (which usually results in the most confident individuals raising their hands) or calling on an individual to answer a question in front of the class (which puts pressure on the individual selected), use of an ARS allows all participants to commit to an answer.[72] When asking a fact-based question with an ARS, each student who responds is forced to commit to an answer (one of the elements of One Minute Preceptor teaching modes discussed in Chapter 3).

This makes them take responsibility for their answer and prevents them from passively listening to another resident's response and saying to themselves, "I knew that."[77] Use of ARS slides for questions without a single correct answer (e.g., an ethics question) can be used to stimulate discussion. Having the residents provide the distractors for a multiple-choice question makes the session even more interactive.

Consider alternatives beyond the simple "one resident, one clicker" approach. Peer instruction can be used by issuing one clicker to two residents to establish the TPS approach or TBL can occur if four or five residents are aggregated into a team and given one clicker. Competition among groups, for example, males versus females, stimulates a sense of rivalry that may result in learners being more concerned about providing a correct response.

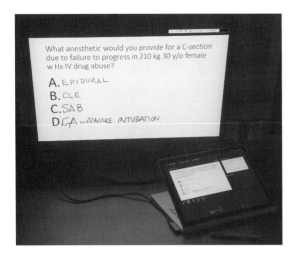

Figure 15.9 Blank slate. An example of a setup for having learners provide the responses to the question. This arrangement consists of a Microsoft Surface Book™ connected to a desktop monitor, the latter representing the image that will be projected on the screen during a presentation. The Surface Book is running PowerPoint in Presenter View©. The screen of the Surface Book has been tilted to display what the leader would see during the presentation but it's easier to write on the screen during the presentation if the screen is flat. The leader presents a question with the responses left blank. As responses are provided by the learners, the leader writes the responses on the screen of the Surface Book and the learners select the preferred response. The results are displayed in a histogram.

Box 15.10 Concerns of using an ARS

- Instructor concerns:
  - Time required to set up the system;
  - Decreased content covered (due to time for students to respond).
- Student concerns:
  - Loss of classroom time for setting up the system.

Conclusions

The superiority of active learning over traditional teaching methods has been well established in other settings. Educators generally accept the fact that meaningful learning, that is, construction of a mental model that can be used to solve problems, is determined by the cognitive activity of the learner during the learning session. Documenting an actual benefit from active learning in graduate medical education is difficult, not only because testing for problem-solving skills is more difficult than testing for transfer of factual information, but also because the small class sizes associated with graduate medical education programs makes it difficult acquire a study sample size large enough to demonstrate statistical differences in outcomes. Active learning is thought to have additional benefits such as fostering teamwork and communication skills, and engaging learners in the classroom.

We have described a variety of techniques that can be utilized to activate a classroom.

Because learners vary in their preferred educational techniques, it may be optimal to incorporate a variety of these active learning techniques in addition to some more traditional learning techniques into anesthesia resident curriculum.

References

1. J. Michael. Where's the evidence that active learning works? *Adv Physiol Leduc* 2006; 30: 159–67.

2. J. K. Knight, W. B. Wood. Teaching more by lecturing less. *Cell Biology Education* 2005; 4: 298–310.

3. National Research Council. *How People Learn: Brain, Mind, Experience and School*. Washington, DC: National Academies Press, 1999.

4. R. R. Wilke. The effect of active learning on student characteristics in a human physiology course for nonmajors. *Advances in Physiology Education* 2003; 27: 207–23.

5. History.com Staff. History in the Headlines: A Taste of Lobster History. 2011. www.history.com/news/a-taste-of-lobster-history (accessed November 15, 2017).

6. K. H. Evans, E. Ozdalga, N. Ahuja. The medical education of generation Y. *Acad Psychiatry* 2016; 40: 382–5.

7. M. M. LaBan. A late Y2K Phenomenon: Responding to the learning preferences of generation Y – bridging the digital divide by improving generational dialogue. *PMR* 2013; 5: 596–601.

8. B. L. Gleason, M. J. Peeters, B. H. Resman-Targoff et al. An active-learning strategies primer for achieving ability-based educational outcomes. *Am J Pharm Educ* 2011; 75: 186.

9. J. E. Thistlethwaite, D. Davies, S. Ekeocha et al. The effectiveness of case-based learning in health professional education. *Med Teach* 2012; 34: e421–44.

10. R. W. Jones. Problem-based learning: description, advantages, disadvantages, scenarios and facilitation. *Anaesth Intensive Care* 2006; 34: 485–8.

11. C. Onyon. Problem-based learning: A review of the educational and psychological theory. *Clin Teach* 2012; 9: 22–6.

12. M. A. Rosenblatt. The educational effectiveness of problem-based learning discussions as evaluated by learner-assessed satisfaction and practice change. *J Clin Anesth* 2004; 16: 596–601.

13. H. Al-azri, S. Ratnapalan. Problem-based learning in continuing medical education: Review of randomized controlled studies. *Can Fam Physician* 2014; 60: 157–65.

14. E. Carrero, C. Gomar, W. Penzo, M. Rull. Comparison between lecture-based approach and case/problem-based learning discussion for teaching preanaesthetic assessment. *Eur J Anaesthesiol* 2007; 24: 1008–15.

15. J. A. Colliver. Effectiveness of PBL curricula. *Med Educ* 2000; 34: 959–60.

16. S. Rajan, A. Khanna, M. Argalious et al. Comparison of two resident learning tools-interactive screen-based simulated case scenarios versus problem-based learning discussions: A prospective quasi-crossover study. *J Clin Anesth* 2016; 28: 4–11.

17. T. Sakai, P. L. Karausky, S. L. Valenti et al. Use of a problem-based learning discussion format to teach anesthesiology residents research fundamentals. *J Clin Anesth* 2013; 25: 434–8.

18. T. Korin, J. B. Thode, S. Kakar, B. Blatt. Caffeinating the PBL return session: Curriculum innovations to engage students at two medical schools. *Acad Med* 2014; 89: 1452–7.

19. T. H. Wong, E. P. Ip, I. Lopes, V. Rajagopalan. Pharmacy students' performance and perceptions in a flipped teaching pilot on cardiac arrhythmias. *Am J Pharm Educ* 2014; 78: 185

20. J. E. McLaughlin, D. H. Rhoney. Comparison of an interactive e-learning preparatory tool and a conventional downloadable handout used within a flipped neurologic pharmacotherapy lecture. *Curr Pharm Teach Learn* 2015; 7: 12–9

21. R. Pierce, J. Fox. Vodcasts and active-learning exercises in a "flipped classroom" model of a renal pharmacotherapy module. *Am J Pharm Educ* 2012; 76: 196

22. F. Chen, M. A. Lui, S. M. Martinelli. A systematic review of the effectiveness of flipped classroom in medical education. *Med Educ* 2017; 51(6): 565–670.

23. S. M. Martinelli, F. Chen, A. N. DiLorenzo, et al. Results of a flipped classroom teaching approach in anesthesiology residents. *J Grad Med Educ* 2017 Aug; 9(4): 485–90.

24. D. A. Morton, J. M. Colbert-Getz. Measuring the impact of the flipped anatomy classroom: The importance of categorizing an assessment by Bloom's taxonomy. *Anat Sci Educ* 2017; 10: 170–5.

25. J. E. McLaughlin, L. M. Griffin, D. Esserman et al. Pharmacy student engagement, performance, and perception in a flipped satellite classroom. *Am J Pharm Educ* 2013; 77: 196.

26. J. E. McLaughlin, M. T. Roth, D. M. Glatt et al. The flipped classroom: A course redesign to foster learning and engagement in a health professions school. *Acad Med* 2014; 89: 236–43.

27. C. M. Critz, D. Knight. Using the flipped classroom in graduate nursing education. *Nurse Educ* 2013; 38: 210–13.

28. K. M. Kapp. *The Gamification of Learning and Instruction: Game-Based Methods and Strategies for Training and Education.* San Francisco: Pfeiffer, 2012.

29. P. Yunyongying. Gamification: Implications for curricular design. *J Grad Med Educ* 2014; 6: 410–12.

30. E. A. Akl, R. W. Pretorius, K. Sackett et al. The effect of educational games on medical students' learning outcomes: A systematic review: BEME Guide No 14. *Med Teach* 2010; 32: 16–27.

31. P. R. Shiroma, A. A. Massa, R. D. Alarcon. Using game format to teach psychopharmacology to medical students. *Med Teach* 2011; 33: 156–60.

32. S. O'Leary, L. Diepenhorst, R. Churley-Storm, D. Magrane. Educational games in an obstetrics and gynecology core curriculum. *Am J Obstet Gynecol* 2005; 193: 1848–51.

33. D. Telnar, M. Bujas-Bobanovic, D. Chan et al. Gabe-based versus traditional case-based learning: Comparing effectiveness in stroke continuing medical education. *Can Fam Physician* 2010; 56: e345–51.

34. E. A. Akl, V. F. Kairouz, K. M. Sackett et al. Educational games for health professionals. *Cochrane Database Syst Rev* 2013; 28: CD006411.

35. K. L. Bene, G. Bergus. When learners become teachers: A review of peer teaching in medical student education. *Fam Med* 2014; 46: 783–7.

36. R. P. Soriano, B. Blatt, L. Copit et al. Teaching medical students how to teach: A national survey of students-as-teachers programs in US medical schools. *Acad Med* 2010; 11: 1725–31.

37. A. Gregory, I. Walker, K. Mclaughlin et al. Both preparing to teach and teaching positively impact learning outcomes for peer teachers. *Med Teach* 2011; 33: e417–22.

38. D. Nestel, J. Kidd. Peer assisted learning in patient-centered interviewing: The impact on student tutors. *Med Teach* 2005; 27: 439–44.

39. J. D. Kibble, C. Bellew, A. Asmar et al. Team-based learning in large enrollment classes. *Adv Physiol Educ* 2016; 40: 435–42.

40. B. M. Thompson, V. F. Schneider, P. Haidet et al. Team-based learning at ten medical schools: Two years later. *Med Educ* 2007; 41: 250–7.

41. P. Koles, S. Nelson, A. Stolfi et al. Active learning in a year 2 pathology curriculum. *Med Educ* 2005; 39: 1045–55.

42. P. G. Koles, A. Stolfi, N. J. Borges et al. The impact of team-based learning on medical students' academic performance. *Acad Med* 2010; 85: 1739–45.

43. K. Anwas, A. A. Shaikh, M. R. Sajid et al. Tackling student neurophobia in neurosciences with team-based learning. *Med Educ Online* 2015; 20: 28461

44. P. Haidet, K. J. O'Malley, B. Richards. An initial experience with "Team Learning" in medical education. *Acad Med* 2002; 77: 40–4.

45. M. Fatmi, L. Hartling, T. Hillier et al. The effectiveness of team-based learning on learning outcomes in health professions education: BEME Guide No. 30. *Med Teach* 2013; 35: e1608–24.

46. D. Parmlee, L. K. Michaelsen, S. Cook et al. Team-based learning: A practical guide: AMEE guide no 65. *Med Teach* 2012; 34: e275–87.

47. M. Kaddoura. Think pair share: A teaching learning strategy to enhances students' critical thinking. *Educ Res Quart* 2013; 36: 3–24.

48. N. C. Slone, N. G. Mitchell. Technology-based adaptation of think-pair-share utilizing Google drive. *JoTLT* 2014; 3: 102–4.

49. K. Prahl. Best practices for think-pair-share active-learning technique. *Am Bio Teach* 2017; 79: 3–8.

50. D. Nestrel, T. Tierney. Role-play for medical students learning about communication: Guidelines for maximizing benefits. *BMC Med Educ* 2007; 7: 3.

51. W. F. Baile, A. Blatner. Teaching commination skills: Using action methods to enhance role-play in problem-based learning. *Simul Healthc* 2014; 9: 220–7.

52. H. M. Bosse, J. H. Schultz, M. Nickel et al. The effect of using standardized patients or peer role play on ratings of undergraduate communication training: A randomized controlled trial. *Patient Educ Couns* 2012; 87: 300–6.

53. H. M. Bosse, M. Nickel, S. Huwendiek et al. Cost-effectiveness of peer role play and standardized patients in undergraduate communication training. *BMC Med Educ* 2015; 15: 183–8.

54. E. P. Skye, H. Wagenschutz, J. A. Steiger, A. K. Kumagai. Use of interactive theater and role play to develop medical students' skills in breaking bad news. *J Cancer Educ* 2014; 29: 704–8.

55. N. Stobbs. Role-play without humiliation: Is it possible. *Clin Teach* 2015; 12: 128–30.

56. C. Lane, S. Rollnick. The use of simulated patients and role-play in communication skills training: A review of the literature to August 2005. *Med Educ* 2008; 42: 637–44.

57. C. L. Bylund, R. F. Brown, B. L. di Ciccone et al. Training faculty to facilitate communication skills training: Development and evaluation of a workshop. *Patient Educ Couns* 2008; 70: 430–6.

58. R. E. Mayer. Introduction to multimedia learning. In R. E. Mayer, ed. *The Cambridge Handbook of Multimedia Learning.* Cambridge: Cambridge University Press, 2005; 1–16.

59. D. E. Meltzer, K. Manivannan. Transforming the lecture hall environment: The fully interactive physics lecture. *Am J Phys* 2002; 70: 639–54.

60. L. Greer, P. J. Heaney. Real-time analysis of student comprehension: An assessment of electronic student response technology in an introductory earth science course. *J Geosci Educ* 2004; 52: 345–51.

61. S. Felix, N. Bode, C. Straub et al. Audience-response systems for evaluation of pediatric lectures – comparison with a classic end-of-term online-based evaluation. *GMS Zeitschrift fur Medizinische Ausbildung* 2015; 32(2): 1860–3572.

62. L. R. Stoneking, K. H. Grall, A. Min et al. Role of an audience response system in didactic attendance and assessment. *J Grad Med Educ* 2014; 6: 335–7.

63. K. A. Clauson, F. M. Alkhateeb, D. Sing-Franco. Concurrent use of an audience response system at a multi-campus college of pharmacy. *Am J Pharm Educ* 2012; 76: Article 6.

64. M. V. DiVall, M. S. Hayney, W. March et al. Perceptions of pharmacy students, faculty members, and administrator on the use of technology in the classroom. *Am J Pharm Educ* 2013; 77: Article 48.

65. J. Cain, E. P. Black, J. Rohr. An audience response system strategy to improve student motivation, attention, and feedback. *Am J Pharm Educ* 2009; 73: Article 21.

66. C. Llena, L. Forner, R. Cueva. Student evaluations of clickers in a dental pathology course. *J Clin Exp Dent* 2015; 7: e369–73.

67. A. Rahman, S. Jacker-Guhr, I. Staufenbiel et al. Use of elaborate feedback and an audience-response-system in dental education. *GMS Zeitschrift fur Medizinische Ausbildung* 2013; 30(3): 1860–3572.

68. S. W. Draper, M. I. Brown. Increasing interactivity in lectures using an electronic voting system. *JCAL* 2004; 20: 81–94.

69. C. J. Alexander, W. M. Cerscini, J. E. Juskewitch et al. Assess the integration of audience response system technology in teaching of anatomical sciences. *Anat Sci Educ* 2009; 2: 160–6.

70. M. Uhari, M. Renko, H. Soini. Experiences of using an interactive audience response system in lectures. *BMC Med Educ* 2003; 17: 12.

71. R. Hasan, J. Fry, J. DeToledo et al. Effectiveness of pairing weekly reading assignments and quiz with audience response system for neurology resident learning (P1.315). *Neurology* 2014; 82 (Suppl. 10): P1.315. www.neurology.org/content/82/10_Supplement/P1.315 (accessed November 15, 2017).

72. D. Slain, M. Abate, B. M. Hodges et al. An interactive response system to promote active learning in the doctor of pharmacy curriculum. *Am J Pharm Educ* 2004; 68: 1–9.

73. N. Robson, H. Popat, S. Richmond et al. Effectiveness of an audience response system on orthodontic knowledge retention of undergraduate dental students. *J Orthod* 2015; 42: 307–14.

74. P. M. Duggan, E. Palmer, P. Devitt. Electronic voting to encourage interactive lectures: A randomized trial. *BMC Med Educ* 2007; 7: 25.

75. A. Hettinger, J. Spurgeon, R. El-Mallakh et al. Using audience response system technology and PRITE questions to improve psychiatric residents' medical knowledge. *Acad Psychiatry* 2014; 38: 205–8.

76. T. E. Shackow, M. Chavez, L. Loya et al. Audience response system: Effect on learning in family medicine residents. *Fam Med* 2004; 36: 496–504.

77. A. Pradhan, D. Sparano, C. V. Ananth. The influence of an audience response system on knowledge retention. *Am J Obstet Gynecol* 2005; 193: 1827–30.

78. J. E. Caldwell. Clickers in the large classroom: Current research and best-practice tips. *CBE Life Sci Educ* 2007; 6: 9–20.

Chapter

16

E-Learning in Anesthesiology

Amy N. DiLorenzo and Randall M. Schell

Introduction

Traditional learning in anesthesiology was characterized by residents reading the literature and attending lectures, while learning from faculty daily in the perioperative environment. Changes in anesthesiology graduate education, exponential advances in technology, changes in expectations of learners (e.g., for the use of technology in education),[1] and increased evidence and understanding of how people learn have all led to the development of, and increase in, electronic learning (e-learning) in anesthesiology education. E-learning is the use of technology to access educational content and to provide education beyond the traditional classroom. E-learning is increasingly used as a tool in graduate medical education. This chapter describes multiple types of e-learning resources available to anesthesiology teachers and learners, as well as considerations regarding benefits and challenges to using e-learning, and a discussion of the evidence for the value of e-learning.

Types of E-Learning

A wide variety of e-learning options are available for use in teaching anesthesiology residents. Following is a description of several types of e-learning resources available to teachers, as well as learners for self-study. E-learning may be used in both active learning formats as well as more passive learning experiences (Table 16.1).

Synchronous vs. Asynchronous

Synchronous e-learning consists of learners engaging in the learning process together in real-time. Examples of synchronous e-learning include facilitated web-based courses where students engage in real-time interactions with the teacher and their peers. In asynchronous e-learning, web-based materials are provided for students who engage with the

Table 16.1 Examples of active and passive e-learning

Passive	E-books
	Podcasts
	Videocasts
Active	Question banks
	Collaborative wikis
	E-flashcards
	Adaptive learning

materials at a time of their choosing.[1] Asynchronous does not necessarily imply that there are no interactive components to the learning. For example, an asynchronous web-based course may include a discussion board where learners and the teacher can communicate, share ideas, and conduct peer-review of work products.

Web 2.0

Web 2.0, a term coined in 1999 but popularized at a conference in 2004, refers to the second stage of development of the World Wide Web, where users have the ability to generate and add content at any time. YouTube and Twitter are examples of Web 2.0. In education, Web 2.0 is characterized by the ability of users (both teachers and learners) to engage with the instructional content and collaborate with others. Web 2.0 platforms such as YouTube often provide useful information,[2] but the content is not peer-reviewed in the same manner as more traditional sources of anesthesiology education (e.g., textbooks, journal articles). Wikis (websites that allow collaborative

---

[1] E.g., American Society of Anesthesiologists Practice Management for Residents. www.asahq.org/quality-and-practice-management/practice-management (accessed November 18, 2017).

[2] E.g., the anatomy of an anesthesia machine. www.youtube.com/watch?v=BGSDpZdYh28 (accessed November 18, 2017).

editing) are another example of Web 2.0; Wikipedia, the online encyclopedia, is probably the best-known example of a wiki. By definition, Web 2.0 allows anyone to post anything with the expectation that incorrect or inappropriate postings are modified by other users. Many wikis used in education are password protected so that a defined group of invited users (e.g., a department, school, or class) have access to view and edit the content, to prevent inappropriate postings or deletions. Studies suggest that widely used wikis such as Wikipedia rapidly corrected or deleted incorrect information.[2] Twitter (messages initially limited to no more than 140 characters) is another example of Web 2.0 social media technology used in education. In this platform, students may use Twitter to tweet comments or questions to broaden participation during a lecture.

Web 2.0 technology is predicated on ease of use and the inclusion and encouragement of user-generated content.[3] Instead of simply reading content on a website, learners are encouraged and able to add to the content, ask questions, provide opinions, and tag content (i.e., provide descriptive labeling to enhance search functions). Open Anesthesia,[3] sponsored by the International Anesthesia Research Society (IARS), is an example of a wiki designed specifically for anesthesiology residents. The wiki includes a growing body of content including a question of the day, keyword of the day, transesophageal echocardiography rounds, subspecialty podcasts, articles of the month, and virtual grand rounds.

Podcasts and Videocasts

Podcasts are typically digital audio files (most commonly MP3) hosted on the Internet for downloading to a computer or mobile device. Videocasts (aka "videos") combine audio with visual files, for example a slide presentation with voice-over. Another option is to video record a procedure, lecture, or simulation scenario and provide the video for viewing. Anesthesiology podcasts and videocasts are produced by groups (e.g., Open Anesthesia), departments (e.g., the University of Kentucky produces an anesthesiology YouTube Channel), or individuals. Some podcasts and videos are publicly available (e.g., iTunes University, YouTube), while others are recorded and accessible only by learners with a log-in for the material (e.g., content provided at a university only for its

own students). Common applications of podcasts and videos include the ability of faculty to record a topic previously delivered as a live lecture so learners can access the materials anytime, anywhere in a just-in-time learning fashion. For example, a lecture on cardiac anesthesia may be of little current relevance to a new CA-1 anesthesiology resident, but a recorded lecture could be accessed directly before and during the first cardiothoracic anesthesia rotation. There are multiple potential uses for videos including providing visual instructions of the proper way to perform a procedure,[4] providing instructions on how to properly use new equipment, and depicting simulated patient events illustrating crisis-management techniques. In addition, brief introductory videos of foundational content have been used effectively in the flipped-classroom teaching methodology.

Electronic Books

Most major textbooks now have electronic versions (e-books) available for use either as an alternative to a traditional printed textbook or as a supplement with additional content. More than 270 anesthesiology titles are available in e-book format, including "major" textbooks (e.g., *Clinical Anesthesia*, 8th edn.; *Miller's Anesthesia*, 8th edn.) as well as multiple subspecialty textbooks, pharmacology texts, and anesthesiology boards review texts. E-books typically have tables of contents, figures, and tables just like traditional textbooks. While some e-books allow downloading content so the information remains present on the device and can be used even when the device is offline, for others the device must be online to access the material.

Advantages of e-books over traditional volumes include the ability to store and access many books on a single device; portability to take the book anywhere a mobile device is accessible; and enhancements to the learner experience including the ability to increase font size, the ability to update the content after original publication, and electronic note-taking capability. Additionally, e-books are searchable for content and references, adding efficiency to the reading experience, eliminating the need for a traditional index, and even providing the ability to search multiple books simultaneously. Bonus materials (for example, additional

---

[3] www.openanesthesia.org (accessed November 18, 2017).

[4] E.g., Procedures Consult, www.proceduresconsult.com/medical-procedures/anesthesia-specialty.aspx (accessed November 18, 2017).

illustrations, video clips, and audio content) are often included with e-books.

E-books are not without disadvantages. Limited duration of availability is a significant concern; while there is no "expiration date" on a conventional book, a user will be left without access to the content of an e-book when the publisher stops providing support. Platform compatibility is another consideration; it has historically been difficult or impossible to access books purchased through Apple's iBooks on a Windows device. In contrast, the issue of platform compatibility is resolved when chapters are made available using Adobe's Portable Document Format (pdf); documents in this format can be read by multiple applications, including Adobe's free Acrobat Reader DC, which allows the user to add notes as well as to highlight and underline text. The field of e-publishing is relatively new, and it is logical to assume that there will be some formats that will disappear while others, although not eliminated, may not be used by publishers of medical textbooks in the future. (Example: Lippincott e-published the seventh edition of Barash's *Clinical Anesthesia* on the Inkling platform but e-published the eighth edition on VitalSource.)

Some educators extol the virtues of the paper book over e-books, citing such issues as "screen fatigue" related to our nearly constant visual connection to screens; the possibility of distractions from social media and Internet browsing; the ability to tangibly mark progress by turning the pages of a book and taking notes; and some research connecting the heavy use of cell phones and computers with an increase in stress, sleep disorders, and depression.[4]

Further research weighing the benefits of e-books with traditional texts is warranted.

Electronic Flashcards

Technology has provided easily accessible development and use of electronic flashcards (e-flashcards) for use in education and self-study. E-flashcards utilize the evidence-based educational principles of active recall and spaced repetition. With active recall, when given a prompt on an e-flashcard (a question or keyword), the learner is challenged to recall the definition or answer. Spaced repetition is a teaching and learning technique whereby information is presented at increasing intervals of time to increase long-term memory and recall of facts and concepts (for more information see Chapter 18).[5,6] E-flashcards hold

potential educational advantages over traditional paper flashcards and notes due to accessibility, portability, and the ability for e-flashcards to contain programming that allows automatic spaced repetition of content. Multiple websites and apps are available for teachers and learners to create their own flashcard sets, including for example Quizlet (www.quizlet.com; accessed November 18, 2017).

Assessments

Test-enhanced learning (the potential for testing to promote learning gains and the subject of Chapter 18) may be provided with the use of electronic question banks. Electronic question sets may be developed locally for use in conjunction with subspecialty rotations or progress assessments of residents' acquisition of core anesthesiology content. Alternatively, commercially available question banks are available for resident assessment, self-assessment, and study for certification examinations. Examples of self-guided question banks for anesthesiology residents are SelfStudy Plus (www.selfstudy.plus; accessed November 18, 2017) and True Learn (www.truelearn.com/anesthesiology/; accessed November 18, 2017). The SelfStudy products, sponsored by the IARS, are designed to incorporate personalized learning with adaptive testing and interval repetition of topics to accelerate learning. True Learn Anesthesiology is designed specifically for learners preparing for the American Board of Anesthesiology (ABA) Basic and Advanced exams, and seeks to create a test environment that replicates the experience of taking these exams. Advantages of electronic versions of assessments include the ability:

- Of residents to self-assess their knowledge quickly and on their own time;
- For residents and teachers to receive immediate feedback on resident knowledge acquisition;
- Of residents to have instant access to detailed explanations and illustrations explaining answers and distractors; and
- Of the program to adjust to the learner's knowledge level (i.e., adaptive or tailored testing).

E-Learning Curricula

E-learning curricula encompass many of the aforementioned resources to provide a comprehensive set of materials for learning. As an example, the

Anesthesia Toolbox[5] provides a growing collaborative, shared, peer-reviewed curriculum inclusive of subspecialty areas such as regional anesthesia, obstetric anesthesia, and neuroanesthesia. For each curricular area, content is provided for resident self-study (e.g., readings and video-recorded lectures) as well as to facilitate faculty teaching (e.g., simulation scenarios and problem-based learning discussions). As an assessment of learning, questions related to the curricular topics are provided at the end of each section.

Mobile Learning

A subset of e-learning is mobile learning (m-learning). As technology has become increasingly mobile with smartphones and tablets, likewise, e-learning is increasingly available and delivered through these mobile platforms. M-learning is defined as "learning across multiple contexts, through social and content interactions, using personal electronic devices."[7,8] M-learning further widens the opportunities for location, timing, and context of learning, as it is accessible to teachers and learners anywhere that a mobile device may be used. As processing speeds and device storage have increased, the capability gap has narrowed between mobile devices and desktop or laptop computers.

A practical application of m-learning is as an enhancement to intraoperative teaching (Chapter 7). Checklists related to patient care (e.g., anesthesia machine checkout) and cognitive aids (e.g., guidelines for the cardiac evaluation of noncardiac surgical patients) may be easily accessed using a mobile device.

Analysis of E-Learning Benefits and Challenges

The use of e-learning presents multiple benefits and challenges to take into consideration (Table 16.2). A significant benefit is the ability for residents to engage in learning anytime, in virtually any location, and to engage in self-paced learning. As the time available for classroom learning decreases and as additional content is constantly being added, e-learning may help educators with providing content efficiently. Likewise, learners have the ability to be self-paced in their learning. Podcasts may be played at double speed or paused to reflect on a concept or look up related information. Question banks may be completed at the learner's pace. As residents have increasingly been exposed to e-learning throughout their education, they expect to have these learning platforms available for use. E-learning, with its multiple dynamic platforms, has the potential to be more engaging to learners. A comparative reduction in cost may be a benefit to residency training programs using e-learning. For example, when a faculty member records a videocast of a lecture, the availability of this resource allows the learner to access it at any time and to listen to it multiple times. The podcast would be accessible to the residents as a "just-in-time" learning tool (i.e., when the information is most relevant and needed). Likewise, the faculty member will not need to provide the same lecture multiple times once the initial time is invested in developing and recording the video.

An additional benefit of e-learning is its potential to assist residents in their ability to study for important exams. Question banks delivered in an electronic format, rather than paper-and-pencil format, are closer to replicating the genuine testing conditions of the ABA In-Training Exam, ABA Basic Exam, and ABA Advanced Exam. Question banks equipped with computerized adaptive testing (CAT) capabilities are able to adjust subsequent test questions based upon the correct and incorrect answers, thus adjusting to the appropriate level of the individual learner. Additionally, some question banks with CAT ask for a response from test takers of how sure they are of their answer before they respond. Depending upon the response, the program will recycle the same questions or similar questions on the topic later if the test taker was unsure of their answer choice, thus providing further individualization of the question bank experience.

The ability for instructors to utilize adaptive learning technology is a considerable benefit of e-learning. Adaptive learning technologies are web-based systems that modify the presentation of materials in response to the learner's individualized performance and learning needs. The previously discussed examples of e-flashcards and computerized adaptive testing systems are two illustrations of the way this technology can be effectively used to tailor the learning experience. Multiple options exist for teachers to use existing adaptive learning technologies or even to design their own. The options range in complexity, capabilities, and price. In early 2017, one of the most

---

[5] https://toolboxlms.collectedmed.com/ (accessed November 17, 2017).

Table 16.2 Benefits and challenges of e-learning

Benefits of E-Learning	Challenges of E-Learning
• Anytime/anywhere learning	• Technical challenges
• Potentially more engaging to learners	• Security and copyright issues
• Cost (may be less expensive than face to face)	• Cost (may be expensive to purchase or develop)
• Ability to deliver multimedia dynamic content	• Risk of distraction to learners
• Ability for just-in-time learning	• Risk of disengagement with patients
• Ability for computer adaptive testing	• Risk of technology becoming obsolete
• Simulates more realistic testing conditions	
• Self-paced learning activities	

full-featured authoring platforms is Adobe Captivate.[6] Captivate 2017 allows a user to import a preexisting set of PowerPoint slides as a starting point for a robust experience that can include full motion video as well as audio and can automatically be configured for a wide variety of devices (desktop, tablet, smartphone) of virtually any brand. The almost limitless capabilities come at the expense of complexity (resulting in a relatively flat learning curve) and a high acquisition cost. In contrast, Google Scholar offers a functional platform that is easy to learn and free but is not easily adapted to various devices thereby limiting the applicability of the course for m-learning. The recommendations regarding multimedia learning (Chapter 14) are just as applicable to the creation of an e-learning experience as to a traditional classroom presentation.

Some of the challenges of providing e-learning mirror the challenges of any Internet content. For example, e-learning is web-based and thus dependent upon reliable and user-friendly technology. Creation of electronic resources may be daunting to some teachers unfamiliar with providing content in this manner. Likewise, security and copyright issues are potentially problematic when developing and utilizing web-based content. Although cost may potentially be an advantage (less expensive than providing education face to face), the initial development of e-learning resources, the cost of software and hardware, the cost of support from technology staff, the cost of storage space, and the purchase of commercially available resources may be a barrier in some teaching environments. The speed of technology development ensures that educational platforms continue to be refined, improved, and

expanded. However, the rapid development of technology also leads to the risk that e-learning products developed or purchased may soon be outdated and obsolete; factors that need to be considered in the cost analysis.

While part of the significant attraction and benefit of e-learning is its ability to be delivered and accessed anywhere and anytime, this can also pose potential problems. The use of mobile devices such as smartphones and tablets in the operating room or intensive care unit for teaching purposes is convenient. However, it is unknown how patients and other medical providers may perceive the use of these devices in the patient care setting. In addition, the use of e-learning on mobile technology in the patient care setting has the potential to distract from patient care and monitoring. The issue of distractions in the operating room has been widely discussed in the popular media and should be the subject for further study.

Evidence for E-Learning

As e-learning methods and technologies continue to develop, so does the growing body of research regarding its effectiveness in learner outcomes. Although a meta-analysis of online learning revealed similar learning outcomes between online and face-to-face instruction, it also revealed that a blend of online and face-to-face instruction (blended learning), on average, had stronger learning outcomes than did either modality alone.[9] Specifically, the flipped-classroom technique, in which in-class interactive learning is preceded by learners watching video content of foundational information, has shown promise including learners being more engaged with course material and performing better on exams than with traditional lecture alone.[10]

---

[6] www.adobe.com/products/captivate.html (accessed November 18, 2017).

Conclusion and Future of E-Learning

As technology continues to advance, the growth of e-learning options is anticipated. E-learning represents a potentially effective supplement to traditional teaching techniques for anesthesiology residents. Multiple formats for e-learning are available for social learning, and technology currently utilized in gaming (including 3D holographic images, augmented reality, and virtual reality) represent potential areas of future development in medical education e-learning methods. Further research investigating learning outcomes using e-learning, as well as investigation of student experiences using e-learning, is needed.

References

1. P. G. Boysen, L. Daste, T. Northern. Multigenerational challenges and the future of graduate medical education. *Ochsner J* 2016 Spring; 16(10): 101–7.

2. J. Giles. Internet encyclopedias go head to head. *Nature* 2005; 438(7070): 900–1.

3. L. F. Chu, C. Young, A. Zamora, V. Kurup, A. Macario. Anesthesia 2.0: Internet-based information resources and Web 2.0 application in anesthesia education. *Curr Opin Anaesthesiol* 2010 Apr; 23(2): 218–27.

4. A. M. Grandner, R. A. L. Gallagher, N. S. Gooneratne. The use of technology at night: Impact on sleep and health. *J Clin Sleep Med* 2013; 9(12): 1301–2.

5. J. D. Karpicke, H. L. Roediger. Expanding retrieval practice promotes short-term retention, but equally spaced retrieval enhances long-term retention. *J Exp Psychol Learn Mem Cogn* 2007; 33(4): 704–19.

6. F. Deng, J. A. Gluckstein, D. P. Larsen. Student-directed retrieval practice is a predictor of medical licensing examination performance. *Perspect Med Educ* 2015 Dec; 4(6): 308–13.

7. E. Ozdalga, A. Ozdalga, N. Ahuja. The smartphone in medicine: A review of current and potential use among physicians and students. *J Med Internet Res* 2012 Sep–Oct; 14(5): e128.

8. H. Crompton. A historical overview of mobile learning: Toward learner-centered education. In Z. L. Berge and L. Y. Muilenburg, eds. *Handbook of Mobile Learning*. Florence, KY: Routledge, 2013; 3–14.

9. B. Means, Y. Toyama, R. Murphy, M. Bakia, K. Jones. *Evaluation of Evidence-Based Practiced in Online Learning: A Meta-Analysis and Review of Online Learning Studies*. Washington, DC: US Department of Education, 2010.

10. D. Gross, E. Pietri, G. Anderson et al. Increased pre-class preparation underlies student outcome improvement in the flipped classroom. *Life Sci Educ* 2015; 14: 1–8.

11. S. M. Martinelli, D. Chen, A. N. DiLorenzo et al. Results of a flipped classroom teaching approach in anesthesiology residents. *J Grad Med Educ* 2017 Aug; 9(4): 485–90.

The Role of Simulation in Anesthesiology Education

Amanda R. Burden

Introduction

The Society for Simulation in Healthcare defines *simulation* as "the imitation or representation of one act or system by another."[1] Using an orange to have a student practice administering intramuscular injections is an example of simulation in its most rudimentary form. Aside from the use of fruit for certain task simulations (e.g., a banana as an epidural simulator),[2] the earliest widespread adoption of simulation in healthcare education began in 1960 with the development of Resusci Anne®, the life-sized mannequin that has been used in training healthcare workers, first responders, and eventually the general public in cardiopulmonary resuscitation.[3] More recently, there has been increased development of simulation devices to teach specific tasks (task trainers). Most compelling for the purposes of anesthesia education has been the appearance of high-fidelity, programmable, patient-simulation devices that can replicate an accurate physiologic response in clinical situations. These devices are commonly used not only to teach physiology and pharmacology, but additionally to teach clinical reasoning. When used with multiple providers from different disciplines, they have also been used to teach teamwork and crisis resource management (CRM).

Anatomy of Simulation

As David Gaba, MD, who is regarded as the father of modern simulation, notes, "Simulation is a technique, not a technology."[4] Simulation sessions should primarily consist of and focus on the educational elements (Box 17.1) rather than the tools (e.g., the mannequins, task trainers) used in simulation sessions.

This process, which should be led by an experienced facilitator, commences prior to initiation of the scenario, includes the scenario, and concludes with an assessment of performance.

Preparatory Element

Sometimes described as the "prebrief," the preparatory element should make certain that the participants are familiar with the "etiquette" associated with simulation.[5] For example, in a simulation, the session should be a safe, respectful environment in which the learners are allowed to voice their opinions without being concerned that either performance or opinions will have an impact on grades.[6] The objectives of the session and any didactics necessary to complete the simulation should be provided at this time. In many sessions, especially those with new residents or where the objective is to teach a specific technique (e.g., ultrasound guidance for a transversus abdominis plane block), some form of didactic presentation might precede the scenario. Research suggests that this period may have an impact not only on the behavior of the participants, but also on the quality of the learning resulting from the entire session.[7,8] (Anesthesia providers who were prebriefed prior to participating in a simulation exercise for management of difficult mask ventilation in infants resolved the problem significantly faster than those who were not prebriefed.[7]) The performance of individuals and the scenario should remain confidential. Creating a good scenario is very time consuming.

Scenario Element

The simulation scenario may range from using task trainers for providing experience to novices (e.g., intubation skills to new residents) to complex, team-based experiences (e.g., an *in situ* simulation of obstetric hemorrhage involving nurses, obstetricians, pediatricians, and anesthesiologists).

Debriefing Element

Debriefing is a critical component of simulation education. Because the period of debriefing is the time

> **Box 17.1** Anatomy of a simulation session
>
> 1. **Preparatory element**: informs participants of objectives of session; provides participants with content relevant to scenario element.
> 2. **Scenario element**: provides experience with clinical circumstances.
> 3. **Debriefing element**: assessment of performance and suggestions for improvements.

when the focus is on getting the participants to reflect on their performance and understand what improvements can be made, most experts say that the debriefing period should be at least twice as long as the simulation scenario. The facilitator should assume that the learners are trying to do their best. The learners will readily pick up on the facilitator's perceptions of them and respond accordingly (e.g., openness, defensiveness, ambivalence). Whatever mode of debriefing is used (*vide infra*, Table 17.5 ["Modes of Debriefing"]), there must be some determination of how the participants fulfilled the objectives of the session.

The debrief should allow the participants to consider their performance and analyze their own behaviors through guided feedback. Ideally, this will allow them to develop the skills for reflection on their own performance as their training evolves. During the debrief session, the participants discuss what occurred and reflect on the case. They can identify points where an individual did things well or where the team worked well together; opportunities for improvement should also be discussed. Debriefing sessions can also uncover what led to different management decisions.

Simulation: Anesthesiology at the Forefront

Work on Resusci Anne began in the late 1950s following Dr. Peter Safar's work that demonstrated the efficacy of mouth-to-mouth ventilation. By 1960, Asmund Laerdal had developed a functioning model of Resusci Anne that allowed learners to practice the cardiopulmonary resuscitation techniques being championed by Dr. Safar and others. In the 1980s, Dr. David Gaba developed a patient simulator that he used in the training of anesthesia residents.[9] The expansion of simulation-based education was led largely through the efforts of anesthesiologists to improve patient safety. The recognition of the value of simulation has resulted in the development of different types of devices; competition among manufacturers

has resulted in a decrease in price resulting in more widespread adoption of the technology. Educational institutions are creating simulation programs while hospitals are creating programs not only for trainees in graduate medical education but also for established practitioners in an effort to enhance teamwork and improve patient safety (Table 17.1).

Furthermore, governing bodies are beginning to require the addition of simulation to educational, certification, and recertification processes.[1,4] This chapter discusses the best practices for using simulation to teach and learn in anesthesiology education.

Adult Learning Theory and Simulation

Adult learners are self-directed, are goal-oriented, and desire to learn timely, relevant, and practical information. Effective adult learning is primarily experiential in nature and characterized by a cycle of experiences, reflection, conceptualization, and experimentation (i.e., feeling, reflecting, thinking, doing).[10] Adults develop expertise through deliberate practice (see Chapter 3). The elements of deliberate practice include:

- A learner fully devoted to his or her own education and improvement who is fully devoted to the practice session designed to achieve explicit goals;
- An experienced coach providing precise feedback regarding whether the goals are being achieved; and
- A coach and learner working together to decide what can be done to improve performance.

Simulation is ideally suited to provide each of the elements of deliberate practice. The person conducting the simulation session (the facilitator), guides the learners to reflect on their performance (addressing skills, clinical reasoning, or both) and discusses what worked well and where there is room to improve. The learners and the facilitator then identify a plan for improvement.

Table 17.1 Simulation report card for patient safety

Through the process of expert consensus and literature review, a system was employed to define the potential of simulation-based medical education to train each of the seven desired competencies within the CanMEDs (Canadian Medical Education Directives for Specialists) framework.[10]

	Competency	Description
Simulation has documented efficacy in this area	Medical Expert	Strong evidence base for the use of simulation to teach procedural skills; emerging evidence suggests that this decreases patient risk. Opportunities to routinely teach healthcare practitioners by simulation remain rare in many settings.
	Communicator	Strong evidence of the use of simulation to teach and assess communication skills. While objective structured clinical examinations are often used to assess these skills, simulation is still underused to teach communication skills in medical schools and residency training programs.
	Collaborator	Strong evidence for the use of simulation to teach skills involving teamwork. These scenarios are expensive and time consuming to run, so are seldom used in practice.
Simulation has potential to be used in this area, but is either underused or its evidence base remains weak	Scholar	Simulation may be used to promote reflective practice, and encourage learning by observing and reflection. The evidence base for its use remains poor.
	Professionalism (see Chapter 19)	Simulation is increasingly seen as a means to assess professionalism. As simulation is grounded in scenarios, which are observed and discussed, rather than didactic classroom lessons, it provides a rich opportunity for teaching professionalism that is currently underused.
	Manager	Simulation has potential to be used to teach management and leadership skills, which are important for patient safety, but the evidence base is weak.
	Health Advocate	Simulation has potential to be used to train patient safety advocates, but its use in this area has not been developed.

Task trainers are ideal for allowing learners, especially novices, to practice a skill, make repeated attempts at a procedure, and experiment with different ways of performing a task while receiving immediate and constructive feedback. This process has been shown to be extremely important in the development of technical expertise.[11] Through the process of repeated practice and experimentation, learners should ultimately be able to master skills.

Based on adult learning theory, simulation is ideally suited for knowledge acquisition and retention. In addition to the elements of deliberate practice already described, simulation puts the teaching in a clinical context. This makes it obvious that the content being taught is practical and clinically relevant. As with any educational exercise, the first step should be to establish the educational objective. Once that is determined, an attempt should be made to determine what teaching modality, with simulation being one of the potential modalities, is best suited to achieving this objective. With task trainers, the objective is usually obvious – a new resident working on an airway simulator needs to be able to provide adequate mask ventilation, to insert a laryngeal mask airway, and to perform tracheal intubation with reasonable facility. The goals for an immersive simulation experience may not be as obvious. (Example: What are the learning objectives and who are the learners in an *in situ* simulation scenario of obstetric hemorrhage?)

Anesthesiologists must learn from mistakes, build on prior knowledge, and reflect on performance to promote safe, effective patient care. Anesthesiology uses the full spectrum of simulation tools including task trainers, virtual reality, standardized patients (SPs), and high-fidelity mannequins[1–2,9,13,14] to achieve these learning goals. High-fidelity simulation provides a controlled environment with immersive scenarios that activate emotions to help enhance learning and memory. Simulation also allows facilitators to immediately provide feedback that helps guide learners and fosters reflection on the experience without the responsibility of patient care. Effective simulation-based education programs adhere to several best practice features (Table 17.2).[15]

Simulation allows the instructor to pause the session at particularly difficult segments so the learner can practice and master each segment separately (Figure 17.1).

Table 17.2 Best-practice features of effective simulation education

Feature	Benefits
Feedback	Allows for reflection so learner can reinforce positive performance and correct mistakes
Deliberate practice	Allows learner to repeatedly practice skills to gain expertise and improve
Curriculum	Simulation sessions must be integrated into the larger curriculum. Allows for a cohesive learning approach
Outcome measurement	Learners need defined outcomes that are achievable and measurable
Simulator validity and fidelity	Choose the best simulator or simulation tool to fit learning objectives
Skill acquisition and maintenance	Sessions should allow learners to build on and develop skills to increase retention
Mastery learning	Simulation sessions should allow learners to address errors and repeatedly practice skills
Transfer to practice	Sessions should allow learners to transfer skills to patient care
Team training	Simulation provides an ideal environment for team training
High-stakes testing	Simulation allows for standardized environments for testing
Instructor training	Faculty needs development and education in reflective learning techniques and debriefing
Educational and professional context	Sessions must be relevant to practice and authentic representations of patient environment

Source: Adapted from McGaghie.[15]

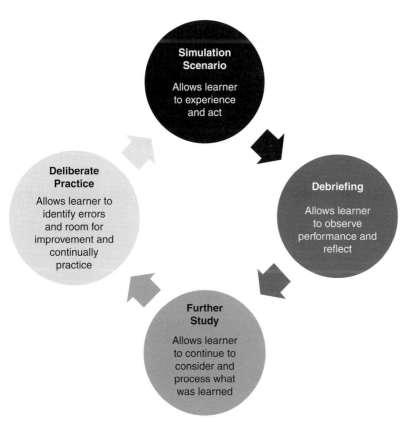

Figure 17.1 Simulation and experiential learning. Elements of simulation that correspond to the adult learning cycle (adapted from Kolb).[10]

Simulation also provides an opportunity for learners to experience rare cases that they may not have previously encountered, but that they must be able to rapidly identify and manage (e.g., malignant hyperthermia, local anesthetic systemic toxicity, airway fire).[4,11,16]

How to Teach Procedures Using Simulation

Using task trainers designed to teach specific skills, learners may work through the essential steps in a safe setting. Although the tendency of most novices is to focus on how to accomplish the specific task, an effective simulation session should put the task in the context of patient care. Indications, contraindications, risks, benefits, alternatives, and justification for the procedure are as important as the physical steps necessary to accomplish the task. For example, an effective simulation session for a resident who wants to learn how to place a central line is not limited to teaching the resident where to place the needle. The session should include instruction in other elements of central line placement beyond the physical task such as advantages and disadvantages of different types of catheters and different insertion sites; patient preparation and positioning; sterile precautions; identification of landmarks; and confirmation of correct placement. A central line task trainer allows the learner to engage in deliberate practice. Teaching when to do the procedure (i.e., under what circumstances the procedure should be done) is at least as important as teaching how to do the procedure.

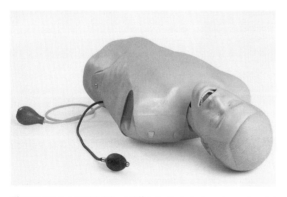

Figure 17.2 Laerdal deluxe difficult airway trainer. (www.laerdal.com/us/doc/160/Deluxe-Difficult-Airway-Trainer; accessed November 14, 2017).

Airway Trainers

Airway trainers (Figure 17.2) may be used to teach bag and mask ventilation, orotracheal intubation, nasotracheal intubation, placement of supraglottic airway devices, retrograde intubation, fiberoptic intubation, one-lung ventilation with conventional double lumen tubes or bronchial blockers, and surgical airway skills including surgical and needle cricothyrotomy. (See Chapter 10.) Some of these task trainers also allow manipulation of the airway (e.g., inflation of the tongue) to replicate difficult airways. Some devices have been modified to allow practice of superior laryngeal and recurrent laryngeal nerve blocks.

Fiberoptic Bronchoscopy Trainers

Bronchoscopy trainers are available as either models (Figure 17.3) or virtual reality devices (Figures 17.4 and 17.5).

Models may vary from highly realistic to highly stylized devices, the latter of which are essentially valuable only for teaching the resident how to manipulate the bronchoscope. Virtual-reality devices consist of a controller resembling a bronchoscope and a screen. Virtual-reality trainers allow learners to practice driving the bronchoscope while learning detailed anatomy. Most devices incorporate scenarios that advance in difficulty as the learner becomes more skilled. In general, virtual-reality devices are intended more for teaching pulmonary medicine procedures (e.g., transbronchial needle biopsy, endobronchial ultrasound) and are much more robust (and comparably more expensive) than needed for most anesthesia-related training.

Echocardiography Trainers

The use of simulators for training in echocardiography is addressed in more detail in Chapter 12. Echocardiography requires manual skills to manipulate the probe while obtaining images and the knowledge to interpret the images. Trainers such as those offered by CAE (https://caehealthcare.com/ultrasound-simulation/vimedix; accessed November 14, 2017) or HeartWorks (www.medaphor.com/heartworks/; accessed November 14, 2017) have controllers that resemble a transesophageal echocardiography (TEE) probe that interact with a computer model to provide simulated views (Figure 17.6).

These trainers also include tutorials, provide the ability to see the TEE image side by side with an

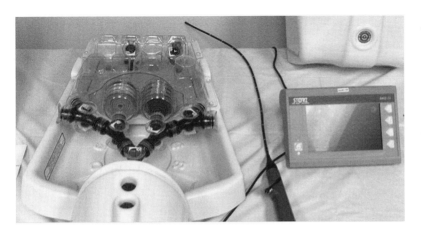

Figure 17.3 Dexter Bronchoscopy Training System (www.dexterendoscopy.com/website/home; accessed November 14, 2017).

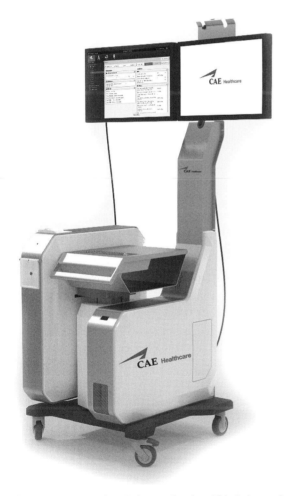

Figure 17.4 CAE EndoVR Endoscopy Simulator. This device can be used to train advanced bronchoscopic and upper gastrointestinal procedures (https://caehealthcare.com/surgical-simulation/endovr; accessed November 14, 2017).

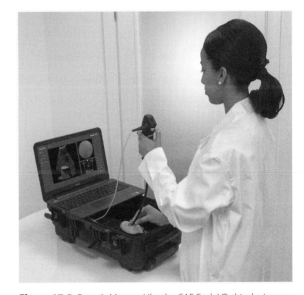

Figure 17.5 Bronch Mentor. Like the CAE EndoVR, this device can be used for more than simple training regarding bronchoscopic training (http://simbionix.com/simulators/bronch-mentor/; accessed November 14, 2017).

anatomic correlate, and provide pathophysiologic scenarios. (See Video 17.1 for supplemental online content.)

Epidural and Spinal Anesthesia Trainers

In addition to using a banana and rolled up towels (Figure 17.7) simulators are available for epidural anesthesia (Figure 17.8) or spinal and epidural anesthesia (Figures 17.8, 17.9, and 17.10) techniques.

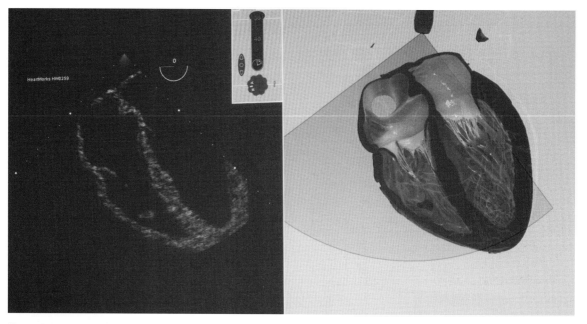

Figure 17.6 HeartWorks screen image. Photograph of screen from HeartWorks simulation monitor. TEE image is displayed side by side with illustrated anatomic cutaway of the heart. The gray fan on cutaway image shows that portion of the heart that is being displayed on the TEE image.

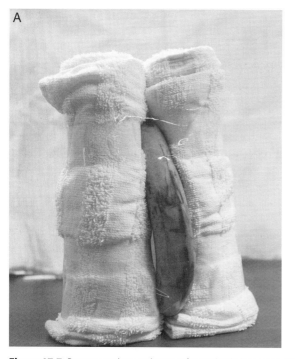
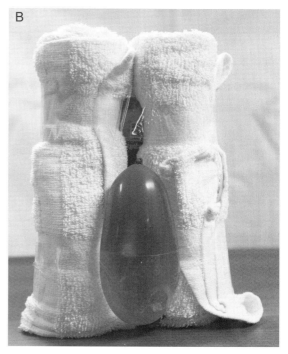

Figure 17.7 Banana used as a task trainer for epidural placement. (A) Front of simulator showing banana taped between two towels. (B) Back of simulator showing a balloon taped in place to replicate the thecal space. A balloon filled with water or air can be positioned behind the banana. Popping the balloon is an indication that too much pressure was exerted on the needle during insertion[17] (http://upennanesthesiology.typepad.com/upenn_anesthesiology/2007/11/the-greengrocer.html; accessed November 14, 2017).

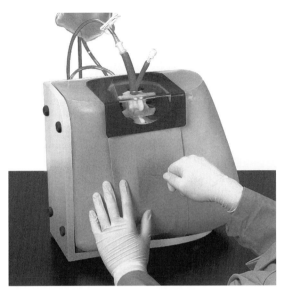

Figure 17.8 Epidural simulator by 3-Dmed. The simulator allows the learner to practice thoracic, lumbar, or caudal epidurals as well as lumbar puncture. The simulator permits thoracic and lumbar midline or paramedian approaches (www.3-dmed.com/product/epidural-anesthesia-simulator; (accessed November 14, 2017).

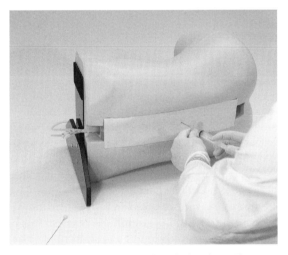

Figure 17.9 Spinal injection simulator by Simulution. The simulator allows learner to practice epidural, caudal, and spinal anesthesia. (Fluid in simulator indicates correct placement of needle for spinal anesthesia or a "wet tap" when attempting epidural anesthesia.) (www.simulution.com/sites/default/files/lf01036%20spinal%20injection%20simulator.pdf; accessed November 14, 2017).

The commercial simulators consist of a torso with an imbedded synthetic spinal column that includes ligamentum flavum and spinal cord in a fluid-filled thecal sac. Some models can be positioned in both

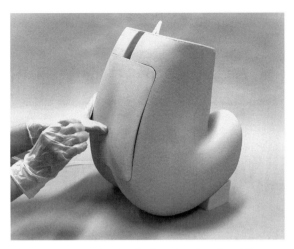

Figure 17.10 Spinal and epidural simulator by 3-Dmed. The simulator allows the learner to practice lumbar epidural and lumbar puncture (including measurement of cerebrospinal fluid pressure) (www.3-dmed.com/product/lumbar-puncture-simulator-ii; (accessed November 14, 2017).

the upright and lateral decubitus positions and can be used to practice midline and paramedian approaches. These trainers reasonably recreate the feel and consistency of the structures involved in neuraxial techniques.

Regional Anesthesia Trainers

Ultrasound guidance is a key element in the performance of regional anesthesia. Simulators provide an opportunity to teach the hand-eye coordination required to maneuver the needle and the ultrasound probe to obtain an appropriate target image of the anatomic structures. Realistic ultrasound simulation has been reported using a pork loin penetrated by a Category 5 (CAT 5) cable and IV tubing filled with ultrasound gel.[18] Commercially available options allow use of a dummy probe connected to a laptop (Figure 17.11) or torso models that allow for the use of any ultrasound probe to demonstrate nerves and blood vessels (Figure 17.12).

Some models may be used for both regional anesthesia and central line training (Figure 17.13).

Vascular Access Trainers

These models provide palpable anatomy and arterial and venous systems (e.g., central venous, peripheral venous) that can be cannulated. It is important to determine the level of realism required to provide an

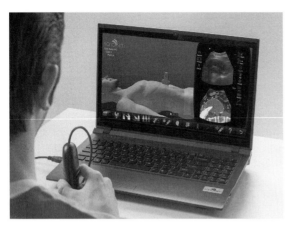

Figure 17.11 SONOSIM ultrasound simulator. A dummy probe connected to a laptop allows the learner to practice a multitude of ultrasound techniques. Options also exist to track learner performance and to present pathology as well as normal anatomy. (https://sonosim.com; accessed November 14, 2017).

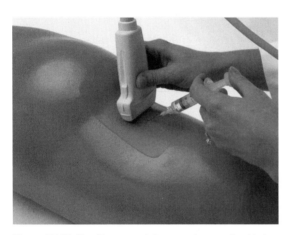

Figure 17.12 Blue Phantom sciatic nerve ultrasound-guided regional anesthesia simulator by CAE Healthcare. Simulators also exist to permit practicing for transverus abdominis plane blocks and femoral nerve blocks (www.bluephantom.com/product/Sciatic-Nerve-Regional-Anesthesia-Ultrasound-Training-Model.aspx?cid=394; accessed November 14, 2017).

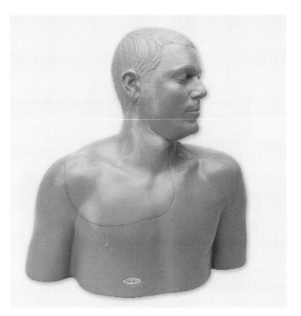

Figure 17.13 Blue Phantom upper extremity regional anesthesia and central line simulator by CAE Healthcare. The simulator allows learners to practice supraclavicular, interscalene, and infraclavicular nerve blocks either using an anatomic ("blind") approach or with ultrasound guidance. The device also includes internal jugular, brachiocephalic, subclavian, and axillary veins as well as carotid, subclavian, and axillary artery and allows learners to practice central line insertion (www.bluephantom.com/product/Regional-Anesthesia-and-Ultrasound-Central-Line-Training-Model_NEW.aspx?cid=394; accessed November 14, 2017).

appropriate instructional environment for the skill and which vessels should be cannulated during the task simulation because there are a variety of trainers available for this purpose.

Integrating Simulation into an Anesthesiology Residency Program

Simulation may be integrated into the educational curriculum from the beginning of anesthesiology residency training. The educational leadership in each department must determine what residents should initially learn and experience in a simulated environment, prior to working with patients. Simulation is a powerful patient safety tool. It allows learners to practice and improve their skills in a place where patients can't be harmed and where they have time to explore mistakes and improve their knowledge base. The following section discusses strategies for introducing various topics and skills to anesthesiology residents.

Examples of Courses

The following are examples of simulation sessions/courses used by some residency training programs.

Anesthesiology Clerkship Boot Camp

An anesthesiology clerkship "boot camp" can introduce medical students to select aspects of anesthesia care prior to their clinical assignments. Short didactic classroom sessions can be combined with high-quality, highly realistic simulation scenarios and facilitated debriefing sessions allowing students to learn and practice skills. Students can be led through preoperative assessment, anesthetic planning, and the induction sequence, including drug selection and titration, and airway management.

Introduction to Anesthesiology Residency

Simulation sessions for anesthesia residents who are just beginning training can be utilized to prepare them for the operating room (OR) environment. Residents can be oriented to the OR setting allowing them to safely learn a variety of induction techniques without the distractions of time pressure.

Objectives

At the conclusion of the experience, the resident should be able to complete and chart a preoperative evaluation, prepare for an anesthetic, conduct all phases (induction, maintenance, and emergence) of a routine anesthetic, and conclude an anesthetic.

Didactics

Depending on what phase(s) are being addressed, lectures may be provided on topics such as preoperative evaluation, anesthesia machine checkout, and airway management.

Simulation Techniques

These objectives may be achieved in a variety of ways, for example, a series of workstations (Figure 17.14) including:

- Preoperative evaluation (using simulated patients to make certain all necessary information is obtained and appropriately entered in the institution's electronic or paper preoperative evaluation form);
- Preparation for anesthesia (using an anesthesia machine to complete a machine check protocol and an anesthesia cart to prepare the necessary equipment, e.g., laryngoscope and drugs);
- Anesthesia induction (using a mannequin and an anesthesia machine to familiarize residents with denitrogenation, drug doses, and sequencing);

Preoperative evaluation • Using simulated patients to make certain all necessary information is obtained and appropriately entered in the institution's electronic or paper preoperative evaluation form.

Preparation for anesthesia • Using an anesthesia machine to complete a machine check protocol and an anesthesia cart to prepare the necessary equipment (e.g., laryngoscope, and drugs).

Anesthesia induction • Using a mannequin and an anesthesia machine to familiarize residents with denitrogenation, drug doses, and sequencing.

Airway management • Using a task trainer or a mannequin to practice manual ventilation, tracheal intubation, placement of a supraglottic airway device, and settings for mechanical ventilation.

Intraoperative management • Using a mannequin and anesthesia machine to appropriately adjust depth of anesthesia, adjust infusion pumps, and use an electronic anesthesia record or paper record to accurately record intraoperative events.

Emergence • Using a mannequin to understand when to discontinue anesthetic agents, reversal of neuromuscular blockade, and extubation criteria.

Transport to PACU • Using a combination of a mannequin and equipment from the OR (i.e., a self inflating bag and mask ventilation, and a portable monitor) along with confederates playing the roles of nurses, respiratory therapists, etc. to teach transitions of care including handoffs.

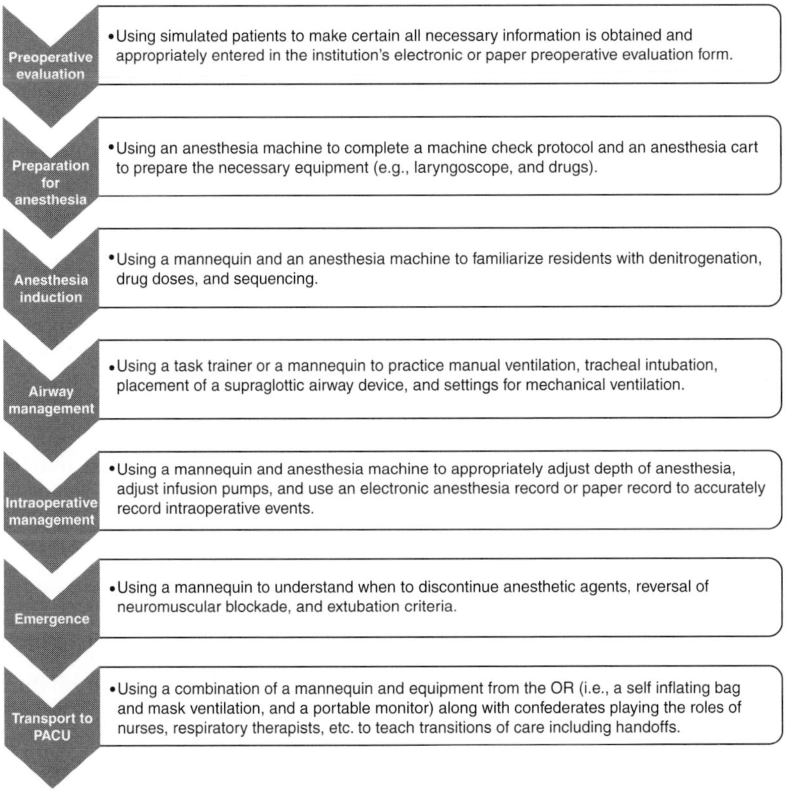

Figure 17.14 Simulation workstations. Examples of workstations that may be used for an "Introduction to Anesthesiology Residency" course.

- Airway management (using a task trainer or a mannequin to practice manual ventilation, tracheal intubation, placement of a supraglottic airway device, and settings for mechanical ventilation);
- Routine intraoperative anesthetic management (using a mannequin and anesthesia machine to appropriately adjust depth of anesthesia, adjust infusion pumps, and use an electronic or paper anesthesia record to accurately record intraoperative events);
- Emergence (using a mannequin to understand when to discontinue anesthetic agents, reversal of neuromuscular blockade, and extubation criteria); and
- Transport to the Post Anesthesia Care Unit (using a combination of a mannequin and equipment from the OR, i.e., a self-inflating ventilation bag and a portable monitor) along with confederates playing the roles of nurses, respiratory therapists, and so forth to teach transitions of care including handoffs.

Similarly, simulation can be used to familiarize residents with recognition and management of common hemodynamic and respiratory complications (e.g., esophageal intubation, intubation of a mainstem bronchus, laryngospasm, dysrhythmias, and hypotension/hypertension following induction of anesthesia). In this situation, the scenario can focus on temporizing measures, differential diagnosis, and CRM skills. The simulation environment permits the resident full autonomy to recognize and address the problems without any time constraints and while not exposing any patient to risk.

Summary

Presenting these sessions in the simulation center gives new residents the opportunity to "slow the process down," ask questions, learn procedures and techniques using deliberate practice, discuss their performance with faculty, receive feedback, and ease their introduction into clinical anesthesia assignments.

Difficult Airway Course

The simulation center is an ideal place to conduct difficult airway sessions for anesthesiology residents or experienced anesthesiologists.

Objectives

At the conclusion of the course participants should have had an opportunity to practice airway management techniques with a variety of devices and should demonstrate an improved understanding of the management of difficult airways and failed intubation, that is, the cannot intubate, cannot ventilate scenario.

Didactics

These courses often begin with didactic lectures where the evidence-based approach to identifying and managing the difficult airway is presented. The American Society of Anesthesiologists' Difficult Airway Algorithm[1] should be discussed along with physiology and pathophysiology of different patient populations (e.g., parturients, morbidly obese patients, or patients with obstructive sleep apnea).

Simulation Techniques

The course may include difficult airway task trainer stations that permit the use of video laryngoscopes, placement of supraglottic airway devices, intubation using fiberoptic scopes, and surgical or needle cricothyrotomy. Ideally, each participant can use this opportunity as a refresher course on skills that they rarely use as well as acquire skills that may have been lacking from their repertoire. Although the tendency is to focus on the high-fidelity technical devices, lower cost alternatives have also been used successfully (e.g., an excised pig trachea to teach cricothyrotomy).[16]

Some courses include immersive, high-fidelity simulation sessions where the participants are required to identify and manage a difficult airway while also managing the patient's deteriorating physiology and leading the resuscitation team.

Summary

Performing this course in the simulation center provides a unique and valuable opportunity to learn these critically important concepts in an environment that is safe for patients.

Central Line Course

Participants should understand that the goals and objectives of a central line insertion simulation course extend beyond the mechanics of placing a central line.

---

[1] http://anesthesiology.pubs.asahq.org/article.aspx?articleid=1918684 (accessed November 15, 2017).

Policies vary between institutions, but many hospitals require a simulation experience followed by a specific number of central lines placed under the direct supervision/observation of someone already credentialed in this task before residents are deemed capable of independently placing central lines.

Objectives

Participants should understand the indications, contraindications, and complications associated with placement of a central line. At the end of the experience, the learners should be able to demonstrate their competence when placing a central line.

Didactics

In addition to the preceding factors, the didactic sessions should emphasize adherence to sterile technique, use of barrier precautions, use of ultrasound, and use of a checklist during line insertion. The significance of removing the line as soon as feasible should also be emphasized. The values, risks, and benefits of different insertion sites and types of lines should also be discussed.

Simulation Techniques

Line placement can be performed in a variety of sites (internal jugular, external jugular, subclavian, femoral) using task trainers (see Figure 17.13). Video review helps the learners view their actual performance and allows them to more readily correct mistakes.[11]

Summary

Debriefing following the experience should include an assessment of all aspects of the resident's performance. Particular attention should be given not only to the physical process of placing the line but also adherence to the issues discussed in the initial didactic presentation (e.g., sterile technique).

Neuraxial Anesthesia Simulation

Historically anesthesiology residents have been introduced to neuraxial anesthetic techniques in the clinical setting (OR, acute pain service, obstetric anesthesia service). A variety of programs incorporate some form of introductory course before a resident begins performing these procedures on patients.

Objectives

At the end of the session, the resident should demonstrate familiarity with sterile technique and should be able to demonstrate the appropriate process for placing a neuraxial block. The resident should demonstrate understanding of the relevant anatomic relationships and be able to describe the complications and initial treatment of those complications associated with each technique.

Didactics

A presentation may describe the anatomic relationships, appropriate techniques (including sterile technique), and common complications.

Simulation Techniques

In some situations, residents have used low-fidelity devices to simulate the haptics of placing a needle in the epidural or thecal space. In others, commercial task trainers have been incorporated in the introductory course.

Summary

The efficacy of some of these high-fidelity devices is open to question. One study showed that there was no difference in manual skills or global rating scale in epidural placement between two groups of second-year anesthesia residents, one group that used a high-fidelity simulator while the other group placed an epidural needle into a banana.[20] A second study compared two groups of residents instructed on how to perform a spinal anesthetic. Both groups were introduced to the equipment and had a didactic session on spinal anesthesia. One group practiced the technique using an orange while the other group practiced on a virtual-reality simulator. The group that practiced using an orange performed better on a global assessment scale than the group that practiced using the virtual-reality simulator.[21]

Critical Event Simulation

A program in critical event simulation should be designed to allow residents to practice the management of potentially catastrophic critical events (Box 17.2) in anesthesiology practice.

These simulation sessions should involve both the medical treatment of these problems as well as leading a team to manage the problem. An additional element of working with the healthcare system (e.g., identifying the disaster plan for the institution in the circumstance of a power failure) is present in some of these situations. The resident who is acting as the

Box 17.2 Examples of some common or catastrophic critical events

- Airway fire;
- Amniotic fluid embolism;
- Anaphylaxis;
- Atrial fibrillation with rapid ventricular response;
- Bronchospasm;
- Cardiac tamponade;
- Electrical power failure;
- Local anesthetic systemic toxicity;
- Malignant hyperthermia;
- Massive transfusion;
- Myocardial ischemia/infarction;
- Pneumothorax;
- Postpartum hemorrhage;
- Power failure;
- Pulmonary edema;
- Pulmonary embolism;
- Stroke;
- Venous gas embolism;
- Ventricular fibrillation/ventricular tachycardia.

lead anesthesiologist can be allowed to work through issues involving supervision of other residents, certified registered nurse anesthetists, or anesthesia assistants. These sessions allow the residents to explore challenges of transitioning to independent practice. The faculty leaders must be able to debrief both the medical elements of the scenarios and the crisis management elements.

Subspecialty Simulations

Simulation scenarios in subspecialty areas can serve as an introduction to the service or as an opportunity to deal with problems unique to that service.

Obstetric Anesthesia Simulation

These sessions can serve as an introduction of residents to the labor and delivery floor. The sessions can include didactic lectures to discuss challenges and critical topics in obstetric anesthesia. Simulation scenarios can address procedural skills (e.g., continuous lumbar epidural, combined spinal epidural, spinal anesthesia) and clinically important scenarios (e.g., prolapsed umbilical cord leading to emergent

cesarean section, retained placenta, total spinal). Because obstetric anesthesia is a subspecialty actively involved in team training, the anesthesiology residents can work through these challenges from both the anesthesia perspective and an interdisciplinary approach.

Pediatric Anesthesia Simulation

Prior to beginning their pediatric rotations, residents can participate in a series of simulation sessions designed to help them provide anesthesia for pediatric patients. Examples include:

- For residents before their first rotations on pediatric anesthesia: A lecture on the differences between adult and pediatric airways can be followed by a session with pediatric airway trainers to practice tracheal intubation or placement of a laryngeal mask airway.
- For residents with limited experience in pediatric anesthesia: A lecture on common situations in pediatric anesthesia can be followed by sessions to diagnose and manage laryngospasm or to place a caudal block.
- For residents preparing to anesthetize neonates: A lecture on fetal/neonatal circulation can be followed by a session managing a neonatal mannequin which experiences reversion to fetal circulation.

In addition, a progression of increasingly complex cases can be created to expose the residents to critical pediatric emergencies (e.g., bradycardia, masseter muscle rigidity, foreign body in the airway, cardiac arrest). Simulation sessions provide an ideal environment to learn and practice the management of these crises using Pediatric Advanced Life Support algorithms. The scenarios can take place in a simulated OR and may include nurses, scrub technicians, and surgeons.

Thoracic Anesthesia Simulation

Residents new to thoracic anesthesia would likely benefit from a lecture on lung isolation techniques followed by a session with an airway management device to practice placement of double lumen tracheal tubes and bronchial blockers. Sessions may involve management of hypoxemia during one lung ventilation and loss of lung isolation in the middle of an anesthetic.

Cardiac Anesthesia Simulation

Residents on their first rotation on cardiac anesthesia can familiarize themselves with transesophageal echocardiography, the process of instituting and terminating cardiopulmonary bypass, placement and interpretation of a pulmonary artery catheter, and management of common problems (e.g., hypotension) on cardiopulmonary bypass. For residents with more experience on cardiac anesthesia, these sessions can present scenarios such as failure to successfully separate from cardiopulmonary bypass or initiation and management of extracorporeal membrane oxygenation (ECMO).

Chronic Pain Simulation

Teaching the management of chronic pain is the subject of Chapter 9, but immersive simulation sessions can be created using SPs, or different members of the pain team to focus on conducting difficult interviews, performing a physical exam focused on pain problems, and teaching communication skills. Sessions with task trainers can also be used in teaching ultrasound guidance and performing specific blocks.

Critical Care Medicine Simulation

Teaching critical care medicine is discussed in Chapter 8. Using a combination of short didactic sessions and simulation sessions can focus on subjects such as:

- Different modes of mechanical ventilation under simulated pathophysiologic conditions using a test lung;
- Ventricular fibrillation following cardiac surgery;
- Cardiac tamponade following cardiac surgery;
- Various methods of mechanical cardiac support (e.g., ventricular assist devices, ECMO);
- Discussing end-of-life care with simulated patients/family members;
- Pacemaker malfunction; and
- Withdrawal of life support.

Multidisciplinary immersive simulation sessions (e.g., displaced tracheostomy tube, donation after cardiac death) are particularly useful in allowing residents to work with the multidisciplinary team including critical care fellows, residents from other services, surgeons, nurses, respiratory therapists, and pharmacists.

Ultrasound-Guided Regional Anesthesia Simulation

Teaching regional anesthesia is discussed in Chapter 11. Simulation sessions on this subject can also incorporate didactic lectures with hands-on workshops. Working in small groups, residents can practice using ultrasound guidance to place various regional anesthesia blocks. All the commonly performed ultrasound-guided blocks (e.g., supraclavicular, sciatic, and femoral blocks) can be reviewed. Each year, new techniques can be incorporated into the workshop, such as ultrasound-guided neuraxial block and transversus abdominis plane block. These sessions can allow for review of the relevant anatomy as well as practice of the requisite hand-eye coordination.

Simulation to Teach Crisis Resource Management

CRM was first developed in an effort to improve aviation safety by helping crews prepare for and mitigate serious events in flight. (Notably, Captain Chesley Sullenberger, "Sully," attributes his successful landing on the Hudson River in January 2007 in part to the time spent in simulation training for different catastrophic events.) CRM specifically focuses on interpersonal communication, leadership, and decision-making. Gaba and his team adapted CRM to anesthesiology in the 1990s and incorporated simulation education in an effort to teach the skills.[4,16] CRM is designed to focus the attention of individuals and the entire team on factors aimed at improving patient safety by reducing the causes of adverse events and improving responses to evolving events. While medical knowledge and technical skills are essential components to patient care in a crisis, nontechnical skills such as leadership, communication, and situational awareness are equally critical for the safe care of the patient. To manage the crisis effectively, the anesthesiologist must understand and apply the principles and actions that comprise effective CRM (Table 17.3). It is expected that many of these principles, for example, effective communication, will carry over to routine activities in ways that will prevent the development of a crisis.

Components of Crisis Resource Management

Table 17.3 presents the fundamental elements of Anesthesia Crisis Resource Management as defined by David Gaba.

Know the Environment

The environment includes not only the equipment and supplies, but also the individuals available, including the anesthesia provider. (The support for resuscitation

Table 17.3 Key points of Anesthesia Crisis Resource Management

Cognitive Components of Dynamic Decision-Making	Team Management Components
Know the environment	Call for help early enough to make a difference
Anticipate and plan	Designate leadership
Use all available information and cross-check it	Establish role clarity
Allocate attention wisely	Distribute the workload
Mobilize resources	Communicate effectively
Use cognitive aids	

Source: Table 2-1 from D. M. Gaba, K. J. Fish, S. K. Howard, A. R. Burden. *Crisis Management in Anesthesiology,* 2nd edn. Philadelphia: Elsevier Saunders, 2014.[16]

of a patient in the radiation medicine suite or pain clinic is undoubtedly dramatically different than the support available in a cardiac OR.)

Allocate Attention Wisely

The variability of workload during an anesthetic results in changing demands for attention. (See Chapter 5.) This needs to be considered not only for the conduct of an anesthetic but also for intraoperative teaching. (It is unreasonable to expect a resident to be maximally attentive to a mini-lecture during or immediately after induction of anesthesia; in most cases, there are times that, when task load is reduced, offer ideal opportunities for resident education.)

Call for Help Early

Calling for help is not a sign of weakness; in most catastrophic situations, the patient can be salvaged if the right people are available early enough and have the necessary tools.

Designate Leadership

Leadership and seniority are not synonymous; the person best able to make decisions about what needs to be done in what order and to assign those responsibilities should be the leader. Having too many individuals competing for that responsibility and having no individual in charge are both likely to result in problems and result in a suboptimal outcome. The command authority of the leader is important, but the leader must also accept information and listen to suggestions from other members of the team.

Establish Role Clarity

The leader should assess the entire situation and then articulate a plan of action for the team.

Communicate Effectively

In addition to making precise commands or requests, specific individuals should be identified to perform these tasks as opposed to making these statements into thin air. The communication loop should be closed with the designated individual acknowledging and "reading back" the instructions. As noted in the preceding text, input from all team members should be received and evaluated by the leader.

CRM skills are difficult to incorporate into practice. To make CRM part of the clinical culture, these behaviors must be practiced repeatedly in situations that closely and realistically approximate the actual conditions under which the behaviors would be used.[4,16] Being conversant with the principles means more than just knowing about them or being able to answer multiple-choice questions about them. It means being able to use them to care for patients. Training interdisciplinary patient care teams (e.g., resuscitation teams) in CRM is an example of a suggested use of simulation. Benefits of simulation to teach CRM skills are described in Table 17.4.

The CRM simulations can be performed as prescheduled activities or they can be conducted unannounced. The simulation can be set up and a code paged as if it were a real patient event. When done this way, the participants do not know that it is a simulation until they enter the door of the patient's room. This can be done in a real OR or in the simulation center. The main advantage to a surprise event, especially if conducted *in situ*, is that it allows the team to behave as they would in the real event and allows for investigation of systems challenges and potential quality improvement issues.

Table 17.4 Benefits of using simulation to teach CRM skills

- Encourages learners to perform required skills
- Allows practice in a controlled, safe, environment
- Allows situations that challenge the behavioral aspects such as communication or leadership as well as the medical and diagnostic elements
- Allows for feedback from peers and experts as well as self-reflection
- Allows team members to discuss plans for care outside of caring for real patients
- Allows for discussions of hierarchy

Characteristics of Scenarios for Use in CRM Training

To be useful for CRM training, simulation scenarios usually have special requirements:

- **Interaction with the team is required**: Members of the rest of the clinical team should be fully interactive, whether played by real clinicians in combined-team training or by actors or SPs acting in the roles.
- **Interpersonal challenges are presented**: Scenarios should be created that require handling interpersonal issues (e.g., unprofessional conduct, difficult or belligerent surgeons, angry family members), whether between clinical team members, with patients, or with the patient's family.
- **Learners must look beyond an initial tentative diagnosis:** It is important for learners to explore differential diagnoses beyond their initial impression (see Chapter 3). Simulation allows for the presentation of confounding information that suggests several possible etiologies for the patient's problem.
- **Requires operationalizing backup plans:** It is important to present scenarios where trainees need to move beyond their expected plan to "plan B" or other alternatives, for example, plan C, D, or even E. For the scenario, the usual initial responses should not be sufficient to solve the problem.
- **Scenarios cover a variety of different problems**: Some scenarios may be primarily about technical and environmental challenges such as power failure, oxygen failure, or faulty equipment. Some may be about ethical challenges. Others can relate to specific infrequently faced clinical conditions requiring special responses (e.g., cardiac arrest scenarios).

How to Create a Simulation

The effectiveness of learning environments depends less on the tools and technology or even the facilities than it does on the preparation of these and the guidance offered by the faculty. Before creating a scenario for any purpose, the intended goals should be identified and articulated; they should be simple, attainable, and prioritized. The learning objectives should be specific, measurable behaviors that the learners can achieve and demonstrate. A prebrief before the scenario begins establishes standards for the conduct of the session and includes policies, protocols, and role expectations; introduces the participants to the setting and simulation equipment; and sets the rules for debriefing prior to the simulation.

Creating Appropriate Realism

While no simulation can match all the elements of real life, experience with simulation shows that once a critical mass of realism is created and the clinical experience of the participants has been tapped, the dynamic challenge of problem solving that is presented is sufficient and participants behave as if it is a real patient event.

Debriefing

Anesthesiologists require an in-depth understanding of physiology and pathophysiology to make decisions in dynamic clinical settings. It is critical that anesthesiologists be able to diagnose and treat problems in an extremely short period. A particular hallmark of anesthesiology is that the decision-maker does not just determine what action is required but also directly implements those actions. Development of a broad base of clinical knowledge, procedural skills, judgment, adaptability, and ability to respond to emergency situations is required. These skills, along with the ability to communicate with individuals and lead a team, must be developed during training and continually improved throughout one's career. Mastering and honing the skills of proficient anesthesia care requires hours of hands-on practice. Some practice can occur during patient care, but immersive simulation provides an opportunity in which to initially learn and practice key elements of requisite skills.[4,16]

In the majority of simulation sessions, debriefing is the period when most learning occurs and when summarization of the actions and learning results in changes to long-term behavior. Accordingly, the general consensus is that the period of debriefing should be at least twice as long as the scenario and potentially three times the length of the scenario (i.e., a 20-minute scenario should be debriefed for one hour). Generally speaking, the debriefing occurs somewhere other than the room where the simulation occurred. (Among other things, this provides access to the expensive equipment for a different group of learners.)

Although several different modes of debriefing have been described, with few exceptions, all have essentially three phases:

- **Reactions phase**: Used to review the facts of the scenario. Any technical malfunctions that might have had an impact on the scenario should be addressed in this phase. Most participants are still emotionally invested in the scenario and may tend to focus on concrete issues (e.g., drug dosages or selection of specific agents from the same class of drugs). In many scenarios, these issues will be superficial, but the consensus is that the participants must be given this time to absorb what occurred during the scenario before they are ready to progress to the next phase. The reactions phase is largely driven by the participants; the facilitator may provide direction, but the participants essentially determine what is discussed.
- **Analysis phase**: This phase is used to address specific events of the scenario and how they relate to the learning objectives. The facilitator plays a larger role in this phase of the debriefing. Teaching in relation to the scenario occurs in the analysis phase. Beyond simple teaching regarding the events of the specific scenario, attention should be directed to creating an understanding of the

implications for daily practice. The objective is to provide a generalization that the participants can transfer to their specific practices.
- **Summary phase**: This phase is used to make certain that all important concepts, especially those related to the goals of the simulation, have been addressed. Some educators advocate that the participants, not the facilitator, should create the summary of the session. Whoever does the work, at the conclusion of the summary phase (and therefore at the conclusion of the debriefing and the simulation session), the objective should be to reinforce the most important concepts, provide a context for those concepts (including developing links to prior knowledge), and develop a list of action items for a commitment to change.

Several modes of debriefing have been described in the literature (Table 17.5). With few exceptions, all contain the elements of reaction, analysis, and summary described in the preceding text.

The process of naming the modes implies that each mode is distinct. The reality is that individuals experienced with debriefing may use one mode for one simulation session and another for a different session. Furthermore, there are times when a single debriefing session may use more than one mode. The important points are described by the three phases of debriefing outlined in the preceding text and summarized as allowing the participants to reflect on what transpired during the scenario, teaching in a way that emphasizes opportunities for improvement, and developing a synopsis of what was learned along with a commitment to change on the part of the participants.

Debriefing with Good Judgment – Advocacy Inquiry

This mode is typically described as consisting of three actions:

1. Determine the learner's basis for actions and decisions, i.e., the mental models (scripts or frames) used by the participant (see Chapter 3);
2. Express genuine curiosity on the part of the facilitator about why the participant took specific actions; and
3. Make an observation, express a point of view, and then inquire about how the participant's mental model compares with that of the facilitator's.

Advocacy is a type of speech where the facilitator identifies a specific behavior through observation of

Table 17.5 Modes of debriefing

Good Judgment – Advocacy Debriefing – The goal of this approach is to uncover the participant's knowledge, assumptions, and feelings allowing the facilitator to "reframe" and improve future actions and behavior.

GAS (Gather, Analyze, Summarize) Debriefing – The goal of this approach is to encourage participant self-reflection through a standardized process for learners and facilitators.

Plus Delta Debriefing – The goal of this approach is to determine opportunities for improvement by tabulating actions taken, the effectiveness of those actions, and opportunities for improvement.

4Es Debriefing – The goal of this approach is to consider the events and performance of all members of the team, including their perceptions of what was transpiring.

Technical-Only Debriefing – The goal of this approach is to identify deviations of performance from recommended guidelines.

Alternatives and Their Pros and Cons Debriefing – The goal of this approach is to discuss the advantages and disadvantages of different alternatives.

the trainees' actions and makes an objective statement about their behaviors. Inquiry is a genuinely curious question posed by the facilitator that attempts to illuminate the trainees' frame (i.e., what they were thinking) in relation to the action described in the instructor's advocacy. This technique pairs advocacy and inquiry. It is assumed that participants strive to do their best and that their actions constituted the best actions as they understood the scenario. Good Judgment – Advocacy Inquiry debriefing is intended to help participants revise their frames (i.e., mental models, illness scripts). Essential elements of this approach include creating an atmosphere of curiosity, avoiding the "guess what I'm thinking" approach, and avoiding either lecturing or humiliating the learner. [22,23]

Advocates of this technique posit that it is necessary to understand the frame of reference of the participant to understand why a particular course of action was selected. Once that is accomplished, the objective is to help the participant revise their mental model to improve management in future cases.

GAS (Gather, Analyze, Summarize) Debriefing

This method of debriefing, developed for the American Heart Association (AHA), consists of three phases:

1. **Gather**: Participants discuss their perspectives on the scenario;
2. **Analyze:** Facilitator objectively compares actual actions with those that were expected or optimal; and
3. **Summarize**: Participants outline what they intend to modify in their practices.

As with the Good Judgment – Advocacy method, an attempt should be made to understand the actions of the participants as a function of their assumptions,

fund of knowledge, situational awareness, and so forth. Perhaps because this mode was developed for use in situations in which there are unambiguous expectations, for example, compliance with the AHA guidelines for cardiopulmonary resuscitation, the technique tends to seem more judgmental than some other modes and specific performance gaps are identified.

Plus Delta Debriefing

This method of debriefing uses a table with three columns. The first column lists the actions taken during the scenario. The second column lists the effective outcomes from the actions that were taken. The third column (the "delta" column) lists opportunities for improvement.

Unlike some other methods of debriefing, Plus Delta is easily learned with a minimum amount of training. This technique offers several advantages:

- Applicable to most scenarios;
- Provides a written record;
- Can be used in a variety of settings (e.g., bedside).

4Es Debriefing

There are four phases to 4Es debriefing:

1. **Events**: Participants are encouraged to describe their perspective of what transpired during the scenario;
2. **Emotions:** The facilitator attempts to get the participants to explain the emotions and ideas they experienced;
3. **Empathy:** Participants are encouraged to consider the challenges faced by other participants as well as their efforts during the scenario; and
4. **Explanation:** Used to summarize the most important points of the scenario.

This form of debriefing may be particularly useful in a team training situation in which participants come from a variety of backgrounds. (Consider a team training exercise with a scenario involving an intraoperative case of MH. The individuals should function as a team, e.g., the circulating nurse obtaining the MH cart in a timely manner, individuals assisting in the reconstituting of the dantrolene.)

The Alternatives and Their Pros and Cons Debriefing

This approach encourages participants to consider the various alternatives that were available and the pros and cons of each. As in clinical practice, there is rarely a single option; this technique allows the participants to practice considering different approaches. This challenges participants to think about how they arrived at different decisions and to consider the relative merits of choices the team made. Reviewing these different options can yield new insights and can also mitigate hindsight bias.

Technical-Only Debriefing

For some debriefing sessions, it may be necessary to focus almost entirely on the medical or technical content and concentrate on diagnoses, treatments, and procedures. These approaches often compare the medical and technical steps that were followed to what is recommended for specific patient problems. Examples include a new resident practicing airway management techniques or a more experienced learner's adherence to the MHAUS guidelines when managing a scenario in which the diagnosis of MH has been established. Even during more involved debriefing sessions, it can be appropriate to explicitly identify time to focus only on some medical/technical issues.

The Pause and Teach Technique

Pause and teach is another method of communicating information to participants. Because it occurs during the simulation, it is an atypical form of debriefing. In this mode, the facilitator is in the simulation room throughout the scenario. When the scenario arrives at a decision point, the scenario pauses while the instructor and learners discuss options and determine the best action. Another variation is to allow the participant(s) to make a decision and then pause the scenario to discuss options. The scenario may then be continued to present the consequences of the decision. This technique is often used with medical students and other novice learners who have minimally developed clinical skills.

The debriefing period is the time when the greatest amount of information is transmitted to the learners. It is also the time when participants should reflect on their actions and refine their mental models for the scenario presented. Guiding learners through this process requires an experienced facilitator.

Summary

Simulation is ideally suited for adult learners who are best educated through a cycle of experiences, reflection, conceptualization, and experimentation (feeling, reflecting, thinking, doing).[10] Simulation provides a safe environment that allows participants to learn and practice without production pressure or patient consequences. Once it has been determined that simulation is an appropriate way to teach the desired content, as with any educational endeavor, the first step is to determine the objectives of the experience. The simulation process, led by an experienced facilitator, commences prior to initiation of the scenario with a prebriefing session in which the ground rules and the objectives are outlined. The scenario may involve the use of task trainers, virtual reality, SPs, or high-fidelity mannequins. The focus, however, should be on the experience rather than the technology. The debriefing session is the most important part of the simulation experience. Because the majority of learning occurs in the debriefing session, most authorities recommend that the period of debriefing be two to three times the duration of the actual simulation session. Debriefing generally consists of three phases: a reaction phase (in which learners react to their experiences), an analysis phase (in which attention is directed to creating an understanding of the implications for daily practice and to providing a generalization that the participants can transfer to their specific practices), and a summary phase (which is used to ensure that all important concepts, especially those relate to the goals of the simulation, have been addressed).

There are multiple potential ways to integrate simulation into the curriculum of an anesthesiology residency training program. Simulation may be used to prepare novices prior to providing patient care (e.g., teach preoperative evaluation techniques), teach new skills (e.g., transthoracic echocardiography), provide an opportunity for learners to experience rare cases that they may not have previously encountered but that they must be able to rapidly identify and manage (e.g., recognition and treatment of malignant hyperthermia), train individuals in techniques (e.g., ultrasound-guided regional anesthesia), or practice CRM with a multidisciplinary team.

A focus on patient quality and safety suggests that simulation should be used for teaching, learning, and deliberate practice prior to actual performance of important aspects of patient care.

References

1. Society for Simulation in Healthcare. About Simulation. www.ssih.org/About-Simulation (accessed April 19, 2017).

2. University of Pennsylvania Department of Anesthesiology and Critical Care. The Greengrocer epidural simulator. http://upennanesthesiology.typepad.com/upenn_anesthesiology/2007/11/the-greengrocer.html (accessed April 19, 2017).

3. Laerdal Medical. The story of Resusci Anne and the beginnings of modern CPR. www.laerdal.com/gb/doc/2738/The-Story-of-Resusci-Anne-and-the-beginnings-of-Modern-CPR (accessed April 19, 2017).

4. D. M. Gaba. The future vision of simulation in healthcare. *Qual Saf Health Care* 2004; 13 (Suppl 1): i2–10.

5. D. M. Gaba, A. DeAnda. A comprehensive anesthesia simulation environment: Re-creating the operating room for research and training. *Anesthesiology* 1988; 69: 387–94.

6. J. W. Rudolph, D. B. Raemer, R. Simon. Establishing a safe container for learning in simulation the role of the pre-simulation briefing. *Simul Healthc* 2014; 9: 339–49.

7. M. St. Pierre, G. Breuer, D. Strembski et al. Briefing improves the management of a difficult mask ventilation in infants: Simulator study using web-based decision support. *Anaesthesist* 2016; 65: 681–9.

8. S. Steinemann, A. Bhatt, G. Suares et al. Trauma team discord and the role of briefing. *J Trauma Acute Care Surg* 2016; 81: 184–9.

9. R. Aggarwal, O. T. Mytton, M. Derbrew et al. Training and simulation for patient safety. *Qual Saf Health Care* 2010; 19(Suppl 2): i34–43.

10. D. Kolb. *Experiential Learning: Experience as the Source of Learning and Development*. Englewood Cliffs, NJ: Prentice-Hall, 1984.

11. K. A. Ericsson. Deliberate practice and the acquisition and maintenance of expert performance in medicine and related domains. *Acad Med* 2004; 79(Suppl 10): S70–81.

12. J. B. Cooper, V. R. Taqueti. A brief history of the development of mannequin simulators for clinical education and training. *Postgrad Med J* 2008; 84: 563–70.

13. A. I. Levine, M. H. Swartz. Standardized patients: The "other" simulation. *J Crit Care* 2008; 23: 179–84.

14. E. Sinz. Simulation-based education for cardiac, thoracic, and vascular anesthesiology. *Semin Cardiothorac Vasc Anesth* 2005; 9: 291–307.

15. W. C. McGaghie, S. B. Issenberg, E. R. Petrusa et al. A critical review of simulation based medical education research: 2003–2009. *Med Educ* 2010; 44: 50–63.

16. D. M. Gaba, K. J. Fish, S. K. Howard, A. R. Burden. *Crisis Management in Anesthesiology,* 2nd edn. Philadelphia: Elsevier Saunders, 2014.

17. B. L. Leighton, J. B. Gross. Air: An effective indicator of intravenously located epidural catheters. *Anesthesiology* 1989; 71: 848–51.

18. S. Sparks, D. Evans, D. Byars. A low cost, high fidelity nerve block model. *Crit Ultrasound J* 2014; 6: 12.

19. K. R. Stringer, S. Bajenov, S. M. Yentis. Training in airway management. *Anaesthesia* 2002; 57: 967–83.

20. Z. Friedman, N. Siddiqui, R. Katznelson et al. Clinical impact of epidural anesthesia simulation on short- and long-term learning curve: High- versus low-fidelity model training. *Reg Anesth Pain Med* 2009; 34: 229–32.

21. Z. Kulcsar, E. O'Manony, E. Lovquist et al. Preliminary evaluation of a virtual reality-based simulator for learning spinal anesthesia. *J Clin Anesth* 2013; 25: 98–105.

22. J. W. Rudolph, R. Simon, R. L. Dufresne, D. B. Raemer. There's no such thing as "nonjudgmental" debriefing: A theory and method for debriefing with good judgment. *Simul Healthc* 2006; 1: 49–55.

23. J. N. Van Heukelom, T. Begaz, R. Treat. Comparison of postsimulation vs. in-simulation debriefing in medical simulation. *Simul Healthc* 2010; 5: 91–7.

Test-Enhanced Learning: Using Retrieval Practice via Testing to Enhance Long-Term Retention of Knowledge

Randall M. Schell and Amy N. DiLorenzo

Introduction

If you were preparing a learner for a high-stakes examination and she was struggling to retain information, what would be your suggested method of study? Would you suggest rereading what she had previously highlighted in a textbook, rereading her notes on a topic, reading from a new comprehensive textbook to make sure that she didn't miss any concepts, listening to an expert lecturer (i.e., podcast) review the topic, or taking practice test questions?

A goal in anesthesiology education is to help learners acquire knowledge, retain it, and be able to recall and apply it at some time in the future. Unfortunately, a consequence of learning is forgetting. Ebbinghaus, a nineteenth-century psychologist, described the forgetting curve trajectory where large amounts of forgetting occur quickly after learning and then with a slower but steady decline with time. How can we beat the forgetting curve? Cognitive science suggests that we take information (e.g., audio, visual) into our limited short-term memory and then must encode that information into our "unlimited" long-term memory, and eventually retrieve it from long-term memory when needed. Retrieval practice is the act of calling information to mind rather than rereading or rehearsing it. Long-term retention substantially increases the more often items are retrieved from memory.[1,2] When information is recalled from memory during testing (doing questions and receiving feedback), retention is better than if the material is simply restudied.[3] This is called the testing effect and using tests to enhance learning is an evidence-based approach that promotes retrieval practice through testing as a way to enhance retention of knowledge.[3–6] Simply, the act of retrieving a memory changes the memory, making it easier to retrieve again later (Figure 18.1).

Testing (and Spacing) Effect

Although Aristotle told us that "Exercise in repeatedly *recalling* a thing strengthens the memory"

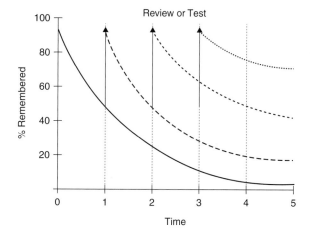

Figure 18.1 Ebbinghaus forgetting curve.

(emphasis added), it wasn't until just more than 100 years ago that the first empirical evidence of the testing effect was demonstrated. Since that time, and with an increasing interest over the last decade, the effects of testing and spacing have become two of the most well-studied learning principles in cognitive psychology.[3–5] The testing effect is the principle that when information is recalled from memory during testing, retention is better than if the material was simply studied. The spacing effect is the principle that when testing (or studying) is distributed over time, information is more likely to be retained than if studying or testing is massed over a short period (i.e., cramming).[7,8] Although cognitive psychology is replete with evidence supporting these two principles of learning, a search of PubMed using the search term *test-enhanced learning and anesthesiology* resulted in few citations. This chapter will discuss the current understanding of test-enhanced learning and provide suggestions on how this evidence-based principle of learning might be further incorporated into the education of anesthesiologists.

Misconceptions About Testing and Learning

The testing and spacing effects are evidence-based principles of learning. There are, however, misconceptions about tests and learning:

1. *Tests are only for summative assessment. Sampling of one's knowledge is neutral with regard to learning and does not alter it.* Most can probably remember a time they struggled with recall of answers to questions on a test and then remembered those topics well for some time afterward. The word *test* often has a negative connotation. However, testing that is formative, low stakes, or no stakes (quizzing, self-testing), and utilized as a recall activity, promotes learning. The act of retrieving information from memory promotes long-term retention. Interestingly, learners often don't believe that testing is an effective way to learn. They also don't feel like they are learning as much as when they reread or rehear a topic, and frequently complain that self-testing is tedious even when better long-term retention with testing is conclusively demonstrated.

2. *Lectures are an effective way to deliver didactics in graduate medical education and are associated with long-term retention of knowledge.* In fact, a passive lecture format often utilized in graduate medical education and continuing medical education courses is associated with very little if any long-term knowledge retention. The Ebbinghaus forgetting curve trajectory is steep, and without effortful recall/retrieval, what was learned is not retained.

3. *Performance during learning or immediately afterward will be maintained. Objective measures like tests can measure how well information has been stored in memory.* In fact, objective tests measure how well knowledge has been stored in memory only at that moment in time. For example, massed learning (cramming) may have been utilized by the learner immediately before a factual test and is not associated with long-term retention of information.

4. *When people emphasize rereading material as their major study method and estimate how well they know individual facts, they are quite good at predicting performance on subsequent tests.* In fact, their estimates show little correlation with subsequent performance on a test. By contrast, when they are tested (e.g., quizzing with feedback), their estimates become much more accurate. Students tend to read the same passages over and over from their textbooks or their notes and may develop a false comfort with the material, or an illusion of knowing. The learners whose study strategies emphasize self-testing have a more accurate sense of what they don't know (and what they do know) and the act of retrieval practice strengthens their learning.

5. *Retaining factual knowledge is unimportant; you can Google anything nowadays.* The ability to recall facts and basic concepts is the foundation of Bloom's Taxonomy and without knowledge you don't have the requisite foundation for higher-level skills such as application of knowledge and problem solving. Both the learning of basic knowledge and the development of creative thinking need to be encouraged. However, "One cannot apply what one knows in a practical manner if one does not know anything to apply" (R. Sternberg).

History of Evidence in Support of Retrieval Practice

Early studies of the testing effect (1917, 1939) were in elementary school students and demonstrated that testing decreased forgetting and that silent recitation (recall) resulted in better performance on recall tests than did rereading.[4] In the 1960s, repeated testing resulted in as much learning as studying when research subjects were trying to remember a list of words. In the 1970s, cramming for a test was demonstrated to lead to higher scores on immediate tests but as most learners know, rapid forgetting. Practicing retrieval leads to longer retention of knowledge. In 2006, adding no-stakes quizzes to sixth-grade social studies classes without adding additional learning time and over a three-semester duration resulted in students scoring a full letter grade higher on the material that had been quizzed. This research was extended to eighth-grade science classes in 2007 and at the end of three semesters the eighth graders averaged 79 percent correct on the material that had not been quizzed versus 92 percent correct on the material that had been quizzed. This was a dramatic increase in letter grade from C+ to A-. Moreover, this testing effect persisted on year-end examinations demonstrating the long-term benefit of retrieval practice.

Rapid accumulation of studies since that time has demonstrated the generalizability of test-enhanced learning across the age spectrum, with medical students and residents, and across many types of materials (e.g., texts, lectures, multimedia) and knowledge domains (e.g., science, history, medicine).[3] Most studies on testing effect have compared retrieval practice with restudy, a passive practice. However, when retrieval practice has been compared with more active learning strategies, such as concept mapping, the benefits of testing relative to the other learning strategies has remained.[9]

Why Does Retrieval Practice Promote Knowledge Retention?

Several theories[3,10] that are not mutually exclusive (and each with supporting evidence) have been developed to explain the direct effects of why retrieval practice promotes knowledge retention: (1) When a memory is retrieved, the memory trace is elaborated and new retrieval routes are created, making it more likely it will be successfully retrieved in the future; and (2) memory performance is enhanced when the cognitive processes that are engaged during learning match the processes that are required during retrieval (retrieval practice with test questions and then taking criterion tests). Indirect benefits of testing and retrieval practice include (1) helping students assess what they know while providing feedback to guide learning in future study; and (2) motivating students to study and avoid postponing studying until the last minute (mass study, cramming).

Factors That Influence Test-Enhanced Learning; Types of Questions, Repetition, Spacing, and Feedback

Test Type: What type of questions?

Tests that require generation of information (short answer, essay, fill in the blank) as opposed to tests that involve recognizing and selecting a response from information provided (multiple choice, true/false), generally produce better long-term retention benefits although both types of questions are helpful (see Figure 18.2). The more mental effort (retrieval effort) put forth, the greater appear to be the benefits. One example of questioning that requires generation of information would be a free recall test asking the anesthesiology learner the sensory and motor innervation of the larynx.

Repetition: How often should testing be repeated?

Although a single test is better than no test, improved long-term retention of information is possible with repeated retrieval practice. Repetition, spaced over time, allows the learner to take advantage of feedback and practice to correct errors.

Spacing: How much time between testing?

Spacing practice (distributed practice) over time improves retention of information (and motor skills) compared with massed practice (cramming). There is, however, a considerable amount of uncertainty regarding optimal spacing intervals. Some have suggested that if you are going to do a "single" repetition, the best interval tends to be 10–20 percent of the testing interval. For example, if you want to know something for six months, the single repetition after learning should be at one month. What is most important to understand, is that if information is to be retained over long periods of time (months to years), then the learner must space practice over weeks and months, and expanding intervals between repetitions is recommended.[7,8]

Feedback: Should it be given and when?

Testing improves retention even without feedback. There is evidence that retrieval has a direct effect on memory even when no further study or exposure to information is accomplished. However, feedback enhances the benefits of testing and should be provided to help the learner close the gap between what they desire to learn and what they learned. The timing of feedback, whether immediate or delayed, may have an influence on retention with some evidence that delaying feedback is more beneficial.

Applying Test-Enhanced Learning in Anesthesiology Education

Anesthesiology educators should identify what they want their learners to know (learning objectives, facts,

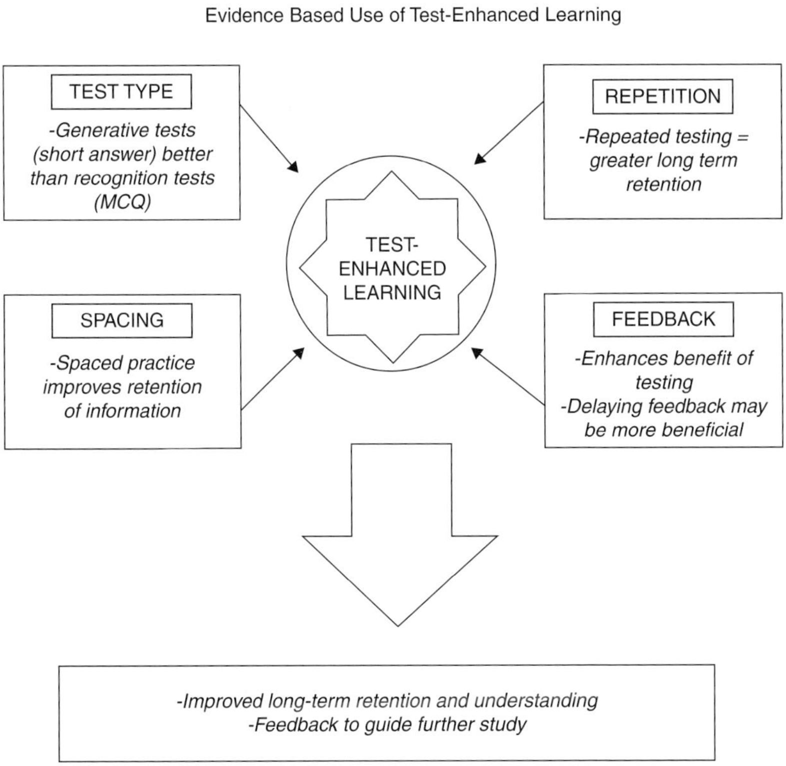

Evidence Based Use of Test-Enhanced Learning

Figure 18.2 Factors involved in designing and optimizing test-enhanced learning in an attempt to improve long-term retention of knowledge (figure by R. Schell).

concepts) or do, and match the form of retrieval practice to the desired type of learning (see Table 18.1).

Faculty development sessions and resident orientation time might be used to explain the benefits of test-enhanced learning. All would benefit from an understanding of the role of "tests" as formative and as an opportunity to utilize the evidence-based educational principle of retrieval practice. All would also profit from an understanding that quizzing/testing can provide a reliable measure of what we learned, and improve long-term retention of information despite the fact that effortful retrieval practice such as doing questions with feedback may not feel as productive as rereading notes and highlighted passages of texts.

The test-enhanced learning principles of types of questions, repetition, spacing, and feedback (Figure 18.2) should be utilized when possible. Pretests, aligned with learning objectives, can enhance and alert memory. They can prime the learner to focus on key information and cognitive activities encountered during study. Pretests can be used before

rotations (e.g., pediatric anesthesia) and before didactic sessions (IRAT, GRAT). Quizzes during didactic sessions (using an ARS) and after didactics (podcasts or videocasts, active learning sessions) may be utilized. However, recall is relatively easy immediately after study, and level of performance immediately after learning is not a good indicator of future retention. Other examples of retrieval practice include departmentally developed tests after a didactic series, purchased examinations (AKT), and the annual ABA ITE. There are multiple online question banks that mainly utilize recall (multiple choice) rather than generative questions. The "MOCA Minute" program utilized by the ABA is an example of retrieval practice using quizzing with feedback and a response by the test taker of their confidence in their answer to help determine the presentation of further questions. A formative oral examination is an example of retrieval practice. How ably a learner can explain (quiz, short answer, peer teaching) a concept is also an excellent cue for judging comprehension.

Table 18.1 Factors to consider when utilizing test-enhanced learning and retrieval practice for knowledge acquisition and retention in anesthesiology education

1. Explain	• Make sure anesthesiology educators understand the role and value of formative testing in helping learners retain knowledge (faculty development) • Make sure anesthesiology learners understand the value of test-enhanced learning and orient them to how educators plan to utilize formative testing in their education
2. Align	• Alignment of educational learning objectives with retrieval practice ◦ Determine what you want your students to know ◦ Align retrieval practice with the desired way in which knowledge and skills will need to be retrieved
3. Evidence	• Use generative questions when possible • Use repeated testing for greater long-term retention • Space out the retrieval practice over weeks to months if desired retention is months to years • Provide feedback to enhance the benefits of testing
4. Apply	• Consider using pretests (aligned with learning objectives) to enhance and alert memory. Prime students to focus on key information and cognitive activities encountered during study ◦ Before rotations, before didactic sessions (Individualized Readiness Assessment Test [IRAT], Group Readiness Assessment Test [GRAT]) • Utilize quizzes during didactic sessions (Audience Response System [ARS]) and questions after in-person or online didactics (self-assessment questions) • Utilize departmental formative tests after portions of the core curriculum have been presented • Utilize American Board of Anesthesiology (ABA) In-Training Examination (ITE) ◦ Multiple-choice question format without correct answer feedback; published keywords and most frequently missed concepts can be utilized • Utilize Anesthesia Knowledge Test (AKT) ◦ Multiple-choice question format, without correct answer feedback; report to learner and program can be used as feedback • Utilize question banks (OpenAnesthesia SelfStudy Plus, https://selfstudyplus.openanesthesia.org/ [accessed November 15, 2017]; TrueLearn, www.truelearn.com/anesthesiology/ [accessed November 15, 2017]; M5, https://m5boardreview.com/ [accessed November 15, 2017]) ◦ Multiple-choice questions with correct answer feedback and explanations • Utilize oral examinations

Beyond Facts and Knowledge

Evidence is building that the principle of retrieval practice can be applied beyond simple written tests to psychomotor skills (e.g., cardiopulmonary resuscitation) or procedures (e.g., sciatic nerve block) that are retrieved from memory. The type of retrieval that is practiced during learning needs to be a good match for the way in which the information will need to be retrieved (oral examinations, mannequin simulation scenarios, standardized patient encounters) and used in the future.

Educators in anesthesiology should consider the abundant evidence for test-enhanced learning, and as part of a rich multimodal educational system, leverage these principles to promote long-term retention of knowledge in their learners.

Summary Points

- **We are poor judges** of when we are learning well and when we are not. The level of performance immediately after learning (studying) is a poor indicator of future retention of knowledge.
- **The forgetting curve trajectory** after learning is initially very steep, with large amounts of forgetting occurring quickly and then a slower steady decline with time.
- **Retrieval practice** is the act of recalling information to mind rather than rereading or rehearing it. The act of retrieving a memory changes the memory, making it easier to retrieve again later and thus improving long-term retention.

- **Testing effect:** When information is recalled from memory during testing, retention is better than if the material is simply restudied.
- **Test-enhanced learning** is an approach that promotes retrieval practice through testing as a way to enhance retention of knowledge.
- **Tests should not be used just for assessment**, but also to promote learning by increasing retention of information. Learners should quit rereading the material attempting to be mastered; taking a test is associated with superior long-term retention relative to restudying for an equivalent amount of time.
- Questions that require **effortful recall and generation** of information (short answer, oral answer) have potential benefits versus questions that require recognition, that is, multiple-choice questions.
- **Repeated testing** is better for improving long-term retention than taking a single test.
- **Spacing effect:** When testing (or studying) is distributed over time, information is more likely to be retained than if studying or testing is massed over a short period (cramming).
- Spacing and testing are **evidence-based educational methods** of increasing long-term retention without known boundary conditions and are effective for many types of learners.
- Testing with **feedback** leads to greater benefits than taking practice tests without feedback.
- **Retrieval practice** can be **applied beyond written tests** to other aspects of learning. The key is that the information, procedure (e.g., how to perform a sciatic nerve block), or skill is retrieved from memory.

References

1. H. L. Roediger, A. C. Butler. The critical role of retrieval practice in long-term retention. *Trends Cogn Sci* 2011; 15(1): 20–7.
2. J. D. Karpicke, H. L. Roediger III. The critical importance of retrieval for learning. *Science* 2008; 15: 966–8.
3. D. P. Larsen, A. C. Butler. Test-enhanced learning. In K. Walsh, ed. *Oxford Textbook of Medical Education.* Oxford: Oxford University Press, 2013; 443–52.
4. R. P. Phelps. The effect of testing on student achievement, 1910–2010. *Int J Testing* 2012; 12: 21–43.
5. D. P. Larsen, A. C. Butler, H. L. Roediger III. Test-enhanced learning in medical education. *Med Educ* 2008; 42: 959–66.
6. P. C. Brown, H. L. Roediger IIII, M. A. McDaniel. *Make It Stick: The Science of Successful Learning.* Cambridge, MA: The Belknap Press of Harvard University Press, 2014.
7. D. P. Larsen. Picking the right dose: The challenges of applying spaced testing to education. *J Grad Med Educ* 2014 Jun; 349–50.
8. N. J. Cepeda, E. Vul, D. Rohrer, J. T. Wixted, H. Pashler. Spacing effect in learning: A temporal ridgeline of optimal retention. *Psychol Sci* 2008; 19: 1095–102.
9. J. D. Karpicke, J. R. Blunt. Retrieval practice produces more learning than elaborative studying with concept mapping. *Science* 2011; 331: 772–5.
10. A. Keresztes, D. Kaiser, G. Kovacs, M. Racsmany. Testing promotes long-term learning via stabilizing activation patterns in a large network of brain areas. *Cerebral Cortex* 2014; 24: 3025–35.

Chapter 19

Teaching Professionalism during Anesthesiology Residency

John E. Tetzlaff and Edwin A. Bowe

The customary approach to medical education places emphasis on teaching clinical care through the apprenticeship model and increasing medical knowledge using traditional didactics. Historically, teaching in anesthesiology residency follows the model of topic-based passive lectures with success measured by high-stakes written examinations, including the In-Training Exam[1] as well as the American Board of Anesthesiology (ABA) Basic Exam,[2] the Advanced Exam,[3] and the Applied Exam.[4] In the Next Accreditation System (NAS), the Accreditation Council for Graduate Medical Education (ACGME) has implemented a competency-based system. In a competency-based accreditation system what is important is what is learned by the resident, as opposed to what is taught. Professionalism (see Box 19.1), one of the behaviorally based competencies, is described by the Anesthesiology Milestones (Figure 19.1).

For behaviorally based competencies such as professionalism, residents are limited in their ability to become competent through traditional didactic tools, such as lectures. As a result, residents must learn professionalism by alternate approaches. The challenges are to construct a curriculum that drives learning of professionalism and to develop assessment tools that measure what is learned while encouraging competency-based learning.

> **Box 19.1** Elements of professionalism
>
> - Accountability – patient needs supersede self-interest.
> - Humanism – integrity, compassion, dependability, collegiality, understanding/acceptance of diversity.
> - Ethical behavior – honesty, highest level of moral behavior, tolerance and respect.
> - Physician well-being – physical and mental health for themselves and their colleagues.

Theoretical professionalism comes into contrast with the day-to-day experiences of residents. Evidence suggests that there is a linkage between excellence in the professionalism competency and other markers of good performance. Residents who are regarded as highly professional by faculty are also independently rated highly in assessments of clinical performance.[1] A resident who is highly rated in the area of professionalism is likely to place more emphasis on acquiring the necessary knowledge and skills, thereby achieving a high rating in the clinical arena. Clearly, if the best residents in the clinical arena are also those rated most highly for professionalism, and the two may be linked (an assumption, but reasonable), then anesthesiology residency programs should strive to structure their curricula and assessment tools to achieve the best performance in professionalism for all their residents to encourage overall excellence.

What is most relevant is not what is taught by the faculty, but rather what is learned by the residents, including elements of the "hidden curriculum," for professionalism. Observed actions are contrasted with ideals and, at times, this contrast is more like conflict. This learning from observation, particularly from less than ideal role models, has been referred to as the hidden curriculum.[2] Although the hidden curriculum directly impacts what residents learn about

---

[1] www.theaba.org/TRAINING-PROGRAMS/In-training-Exam/About-the-In-Training-Exam (accessed November 17, 2017).

[2] www.theaba.org/Exams/BASIC-(Staged-Exam)/About-BASIC-(Staged-Exam) (accessed November 17, 2017).

[3] www.theaba.org/Exams/ADVANCED-(Staged-Exam)/About-ADVANCED-(Staged-Exam) (accessed November 17, 2017).

[4] www.theaba.org/Exams/APPLIED-(Staged-Exam)/About-APPLIED-(Staged-Exam) (accessed Noember 17, 2017).

Has not Achieved Level 1	Level 1	Level 2	Level 3	Level 4	Level 5
	Acts responsibly and reliably with commitment to patient care as expected for level of experience	Completes routine tasks reliably in uncomplicated circumstances with indirect supervision	Completes tasks reliably in complex clinical situations or unfamiliar environments, utilizing available resources, with indirect supervision	Completes all work assignments reliably and supports other providers to ensure patient care is optimized; supervises and advises junior residents on time and task management with conditional independence	Manages the health care team to ensure patient care is the first priority while considering the needs of team members
	Completes most assigned clinical tasks on time, but may occasionally require direct supervision	Identifies issues of importance to diverse patient populations and how limited resources may impact patient care and resource allocation	Identifies options to address issues of importance to diverse patient populations, and creates strategies to provide care when patient access or resources are limited		Completes all work assignments reliably, and independently supports other providers to ensure patient care is optimized
	Recognizes a patient's right to confidentiality, privacy, and autonomy, and treats patients and their families with compassion and respect				Demonstrates leadership in managing multiple competing tasks
	Seeks assistance appropriate to the needs of the clinical situation while taking into consideration one's own experience and knowledge				Manages the health care team in a manner that is respectful of patient confidentiality, privacy, and autonomy, and ensures that patients and their families are treated with compassion and respect
	Displays sensitivity and respect for the needs of diverse patient populations and challenges associated with limited access to health care				Demonstrates mentorship and role modeling regarding responsibilities to diverse patient populations and optimizing patient care when resources are limited

Figure 19.1 Professionalism 1: Responsibility to patients, families, and society. Milestone definition of levels (from the Anesthesiology Milestone Project).

professional behavior, its role is generally underrecognized. This means that programs need to create a curriculum that matches the behavioral elements of the competency and, equally (or more) importantly, create an environment that encourages the best in professional behavior in the context of anesthesiology.

The Hidden Curriculum for Professionalism in Anesthesiology

Do as we say, not as we do.

Giovanni Boccaccio[3]

This quote, which has morphed into the idiom "Do as I say, not as I do," captures the essence of the educational conflict between the stated objectives and the lessons that are learned but not openly intended (i.e., the hidden curriculum). Just as children learn by observing the actions of their parents and other adults, when it comes to professionalism, medical students and residents learn at least as much by observing the actions of their faculty mentors as from didactic presentations on the subject. Accordingly, the hidden curriculum plays a vital role in what residents learn about professionalism and is an important

factor in determining how they are likely to behave in the future.

The hidden curriculum is defined as values that are learned implicitly in the workplace. A case has been made that exposure to the hidden curriculum begins in the process of submitting applications to medical school.[4] Applicants report writing essays in applications and answering questions during medical school interviews in ways that magnify their successes and glorify their accomplishments in an effort to meet the standards and expectations that they perceive to be inherent in the admissions process. The consequences of these actions have been described by some as the "vanquishing of virtue."[5]

Although elements of the hidden curriculum may either support or undermine the formal curriculum,[6] research and writings on the subject tend to focus almost exclusively on its negative aspects. Perhaps the hidden curriculum is most evident in the oft-heard phrase, "Page me if you need me." Although the words indicate the availability of the supervising individual, the real message is more, "I'm leaving. You're on your own. Don't bother me." A study of internal medicine residents revealed that almost 50 percent of residents would "rarely" or "never" call their attending after having been told, "Page me if you need me," and the responses of the attending physicians indicated they were aware that this statement would result in the particular behavior of the residents.[7] On occasion, this is accompanied by the supposedly tongue-in-cheek addendum, "But if you page me it's a sign of weakness." The addendum captures the real message communicated by the primary instructions.

The hidden curriculum is described as associated with medical students transitioning to

- Being closed-minded instead of open-minded;
- Being focused on facts instead of intellectually curious;
- Being emotionally detached instead of empathetic; and
- Being arrogant and irritable instead of civil and caring.[8]

Box 19.2 shows some of the negative aspects commonly modeled in the hidden curriculum.[9]

Learning professionalism from the hidden curriculum falls into experiences within subcategories for medical professional behavior. Hilton[10] has divided the elements of medical professionalism into six main domains:

- Ethics;
- Reflection;
- Responsibility;
- Teamwork;
- Respect for patients; and
- Social responsibility.

While didactic presentations may emphasize these domains, the hidden curriculum may respond to these concepts with derogatory comments (e.g., encouraging a student to skip a lecture on ethics to care for a patient and learn "real" medicine) and/or actions (e.g., rolling the eyes). The result is that which is communicated is contrary to the content of the formal curriculum (see Box 19.2).

The institutional hierarchy may protect a physician, especially one who is particularly productive, by ignoring allegations of unprofessional behavior,[11] sometimes promoting the physician in question,[12] or dismissing individuals who raise concerns.[13] The message to medical students and residents is obvious.

Within anesthesiology, [14] there are specialty-specific elements of professionalism that are found in unique interactions with patients, with surgeons, within the residency program/department, and with

---

Box 19.2 Examples of the hidden curriculum

Examples of values relating to healthcare workers commonly part of the hidden curriculum:

- Doctors know more than nurses.
- Individuals junior to you may be treated with less respect than those senior to you.
- Specialists are superior to generalists.
- Female physicians are expected to prioritize a family above a career.

Examples of values relating to patients commonly part of the hidden curriculum:

- Obese patients are obese because they lack self-control.
- Patients from lower socioeconomic classes are not interested in their health.
- Homosexual couples should not raise a child.

---

support personnel. Recognition within the specialty of the unique expectations for each of these elements is universal.[15] Anesthesiology residency programs should identify experiences within the six domains for their residents, define optimum behavior, and clearly identify behaviors that are unprofessional. Role modeling good behavior by staff and senior residents is essential to facilitate those elements of the professionalism competency that can be learned. Real-time assessment of behavioral performance, supplemented by case-based discussion and/or simulation, drives learning. Universally accepted key words for optimum medical professional behavior are known (Box 19.3), but teaching of this content is less relevant than experience-based learning combined with effective role modeling.

It is equally well known that there are key words for unprofessional behavior (Box 19.4) with the added caveat of learning from consequences of actions.

Other lists of domains of unprofessional behavior during graduate medical education (GME) have been published along with behavioral descriptors.[16] What is less clear is how these lists of defined behaviors become translated into resident learning.

Professionalism Curriculum

There are a variety of approaches to curricular design to achieve experience-based learning of medical professionalism for residents during GME. Aside from didactic lectures (which don't achieve the goal), several curriculum examples focus on review of real or

Box 19.3 Key words for optimum professionalism

- Altruism
- A commitment to excellence
- Sense of duty
- Integrity and character
- Tolerance
- Respect for all human beings
- Punctuality
- Honesty
- Sharing
- Waste avoidance
- Trustworthiness
- Lifelong learning
- Cost-effectiveness

Box 19.4 Key words for unprofessional behavior

- Abuse of authority
- Bias
- Sexual harassment
- Poor handling of confidential information
- Arrogance
- Greed
- Dishonesty
- Impairment
- Laziness
- Inappropriate use of valuable resources
- Complaining
- Avoidance
- "Attitude"
- Fraud
- Waste
- Conflict of interest
- Substance Abuse
- Intimidation

OR nurse in a manner similar to the senior attending, nicely demonstrating the hidden curriculum elements of role modeling bad behavior. Another curriculum example involved a review of clinical experiences that came from a collection of journal entries by medical students prompted to record clinical interactions that taught the student about professionalism.[17] Analysis of these journal entries revealed that it was the clinical care and case-based teaching as the most frequent themes for positive experiences (the great majority) and the negative experiences involved issues of conflict or disrespect, revealing these elements of the hidden curriculum. Most frequently, the students identified compassion and respect as the learning themes from these experience, and learned most from examples of effective teamwork.[18]

Although learning in the professionalism competency does not lend itself to the type of curriculum design that is appropriate for medical knowledge or subspecialized clinical care, this does not mean that curriculum design has no impact on the outcome. Linkage of appropriate assessment tools with unique elements of a curriculum can facilitate learning if real-time feedback is provided, especially reinforcing good behavior.[14]

Commitment of the faculty, the program, and even the specialty is an important element driving learning by example. The American Board of Internal Medicine created the Professionalism Charter, an ambitious example of a specialty that has defined *optimum professional behavior*.[19] The Professionalism Charter, a form of "Hippocratic Oath" for medical professionalism in internal medicine, is signed by almost every resident entering internal medicine training each summer, and creates learning by setting explicit expectations. Anesthesiology has also recognized the vital importance of professionalism. The ABA recognizes the role of behavior in evaluating residents. Gradually, the role of the "acquired characteristics" has increased in importance, and, in the present, any resident rated unsatisfactory for acquired characteristics must be rated unsatisfactory overall.

Creating learning by setting expectations (a culture change) is also found in the report by Suchman[20] at the Indiana University School of Medicine, where a commitment was made to change behavior systematically. They studied the issues and interviewed a broad sample of those involved including leadership, faculty members, residents, and medical students. Good and bad behavior was defined and a document was created

simulated clinical situations with examples of good and bad behavior in a setting to which the learners can relate. One example was a curriculum that started with more than 100 hours of taped interactions in the operating room (OR). These recordings captured conflict, most frequently created by the senior attending. When the senior attending was not present, there were instances where the resident was observed berating the with expectations focusing on respect, commitment, and collegial behavior. They completed this reflective cycle by observing the consequences of this intervention, documenting the broad range of cultural change. Most significantly, the expectations created eliminated the environment where the negative hidden curriculum had flourished.

This kind of change by setting expectations can occur at the residency program/department level if similar leverage is applied at all levels. Joyner[21] describes a transformative process in a urology residency program. The goal was improved professional behavior and the expectation was participation of all involved, including the faculty and departmental leadership. The behaviors were made explicit and performance was measured. The transformation was partly due to the measurement but also by virtue of the top-down commitment made by the sponsoring department. Appropriate assessment tools were used, and variability of the score (and hence, the behaviors?) decreased. This highlights the reality that professionalism is not a single entity but a complex array of interacting variables.[1] Teaching and assessing single elements of this array may miss the big picture.

The association of optimum professionalism with ideal patient care is also recognized and changes to optimize professional behavior are believed to improve patient care. The Center for Professionalism and Peer Support[22] at Brigham and Women's Medical Center in Boston is an example of a healthcare system that places value on building a culture in which mutual respect, teamwork, and trust are expected. This could also be regarded as effective curriculum support for positive elements of the hidden curriculum. Another source of transdisciplinary expectations is found in the American Medical Association Code of Medical Ethics, which defines optimum behavior for all physicians.[23] This code represents the ideal for role modeling within residency and good elements of the hidden curriculum. Lofty goals for professionalism are also identified by the American Society of Anesthesiologists[24] and can be the basis for role modeling as well as expectations for professional behavior.

Just as optimum behavior (professionalism) is associated with optimum performance during residency training, the converse is equally true. Lack of conscientiousness in medical students is associated with negative assessments during clinical rotations and even more ominously, disciplinary action during medical school is associated with a greatly increased probability of adverse action by state medical boards later in a physician's career.[25] A curriculum that highlights the concept of professionalism in the context of lifelong learning is important, as are structured consequences for unprofessional behavior. Teaching by the examples of negative outcomes, such as licensure actions, has a role in resident learning of professionalism.

Summary

In conclusion, there is a high level of interest in the teaching and assessment of professionalism within medicine, GME, and anesthesiology residency education. The association between optimum professionalism and model performance during residency has been made, leaving residency programs with a powerful incentive to create an ideal environment with case-based learning, and culturally supported optimum role-modeling of specialty-specific professional interactions with patients, surgeons, faculty, peers, and support personnel. Small, medium, and large entities have undergone cultural changes to eliminate negative elements of the hidden curriculum, and to reinforce positive behaviors. The result should be an appreciation for the lifelong learning of professionalism by anesthesiology residents, and optimum care for our primary mission – the patient.

References

1. D. A. Reed, C. P. West, P. S. Mueller et al. Behaviors of highly professional resident physicians. *JAMA* 2008; 300: 1326–33.

2. F. W. Hafferty, R. Franks. The hidden curriculum, ethics, teaching, and the structure of medical education. *Acad Med* 1994; 69: 861–71.

3. G. Boccaccio, G. Waldman, J. Usher. *The Decameron.* Oxford: Oxford University Press, 1993. Giovanni Boccaccio, The Decameron, Third Day, Seventh Story.

4. J. White, K. Brownell, J. F. Lemay, J. M. Lockyer. "What do they want me to say?" The hidden curriculum at work in the medical school selection process: A qualitative study. *BMC Med Educ* 2012; 12: 17.

5. J. Coulehan, P. C. Williams. Vanquishing virtue: The impact of medical education. *Acad Med* 2001; 76: 598–605.

6. F. W. Hafferty, E. H. Gaufberg, J. F. O'Donnell. The role of the hidden curriculum in "on doctoring" courses. *AMA J Ethics* 2015; 17: 130–9.

7. L. Loo, N. Puri, D. I. Kim et al. "Page me if you need me": The hidden curriculum of attending-resident communication. *J Grad Med Educ* 2012; 4: 340–5. (Additional content at www.jgme.org/doi/pdf/10.4300/JGME-D-11-00175.1; accessed November 17, 2017).

8. S. C. Mahood. Medical education: Beware the hidden curriculum. *Can Fam Physician* 2011; 57: 983–5.

9. S. P. Phillips, M. Clarke. More than an education: The hidden curriculum, professional attitudes and career choice. *Med Educ* 2012; 46: 887–93.

10. S. Hilton, H. B. Slotnick. Proto-professionalism: How professionalization occurs across the continuum of medical education. *Med Educ* 2005; 39: 58–65.

11. E. I. de Oliveira Vidal, S. Silva Vdos, M. F. Santos et al. Why medical schools are tolerant of unethical behavior. *Ann Fam Med* 2015; 13: 176–80.

12. M. Baker, J. Mayo. (2017, February 10). High volume, big dollars, rising tension. *The Seattle Times*. http://projects.seattletimes.com/2017/quantity-of-care/hospital/ (accessed November 17, 2017).

13. J. Abelson, J. Saltzman, L. Kowalczyk, S. Allen. (2017, February 10). https://apps.bostonglobe.com/spotlight/clash-in-the-name-of-care/story/ (accessed November 17, 2017).

14. I. Dorotta, J. Staszak, A. Takla, J. E. Tetzlaff. Teaching and evaluating professionalism for anesthesiology residents. *J Clin Anesth* 2006; 18: 148–60.

15. J. E. Tetzlaff. Professionalism in anesthesiology: "What is it?" or "I know it when I see it." *Anesthesiology* 2009; 110: 700–2.

16. A. G. Lee, H. A. Beaver, H. C. Boldt et al. Teaching and assessing professionalism in ophthalmology residency training programs. *Surv Ophthalmol* 2007; 52: 300–14.

17. O. Karnieli-Miller, R. Vu, M. C. Holtman et al. Medical students' professionalism narratives: A window on the informal and hidden curriculum. *Acad Med* 2010; 85: 124–33.

18. O. Karnieli-Miller, R. Vu, R. M. Frankel et al. Which experiences in the hidden curriculum teach students about professionalism? *Acad Med* 2011; 86: 369–77.

19. ABIM Foundation. American Board of Internal Medicine; ACP-ASIM Foundation. American College of Physicians-American Society of Internal Medicine; European Federation of Internal Medicine. Medical professionalism in the new millennium: A physician charter. *Ann Int Med* 2002; 136: 243–6.

20. A. L. Suchman, P. R. Williamson, D. K. Litzelman et al. Toward and informal curriculum that teaches professionalism: Transforming the social environment of a medical School. *J Gen Int Med* 2004; 19: 501–4.

21. B. D. Joyner, V. M. Vemulakonda. Making the implicit more explicit. *J Urol* 2007; 177: 2287–91.

22. Brigham Health. Center for Professionalism and Peer Support. 2015. www.brighamandwomens.org/medical_professionals/career/cpps/default.aspx (accessed November 17, 2016).

23. American Medical Association. AMA Code of Medical Ethics. www.ama-assn.org/delivering-care/ama-code-medical-ethics (accessed November 17, 2016).

24. American Society of Anesthesiologists. Ethics and professionalism. Ethical guidelines and statements. www.asahq.org/resources/ethics-and-professionalism (accessed November 17, 2016).

25. M. A. Papadakis, A. Teherani, M. A. Banach et al. Disciplinary action by medical boards and prior behavior in medical school. *N Engl J Med* 2005; 353: 2673–82.

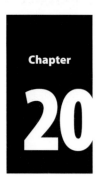

Providing Feedback

John D. Mitchell and Stephanie B. Jones

Scope of Feedback in Faculty Development

Much of the literature on feedback centers on best practices in providing feedback to learners; much less is known about effective faculty development strategies in this realm. While approaches to providing effective feedback will not be covered in this chapter, a summary table of key elements is provided here for concise review (Table 20.1).

Feedback provision, while important to the development of trainees, is notoriously difficult to teach or improve from baseline.[1] Instruction on feedback is often requested as an element of faculty development seminars.[2] Feedback skills do not improve simply with experience over time and workshop interventions alone also may not enhance feedback skills in faculty.[3]

In anesthesiology programs, two surveys have examined the issue of faculty development in feedback provision. The first, in 1999, demonstrated that only 20 percent of responding programs had any formal process to instruct faculty members in resident evaluation.[4] A follow-up survey in 2013 revealed that almost 90 percent of program directors indicated a need for faculty development in providing feedback, while only 48 percent had any resources to aid in this endeavor.[2] The addition of the Milestones[1] to the Accreditation Council for Graduate Medical Education (ACGME) evaluation system intensifies the need for available and consistent training on feedback. Professionalism Milestone 4 (Figure 20.1) specifically evaluates the resident's ability to both receive and deliver constructive feedback. Faculty modeling of feedback provision is an important mechanism for developing this skill in residents.

---

[1] www.acgme.org/Portals/0/PDFs/Milestones/Anesthesiology Milestones.pdf (accessed November 10, 2017).

Barriers to Effective Feedback

Barriers to effective feedback are numerous and must be addressed for faculty development to be effective. Responding to a survey about the need to teach communication skills, internal medicine faculty members cited their own lack of training, limited time, and the perception of a low priority at their institution as barriers to effective feedback provision.[5] A multispecialty survey that included anesthesiology residents suggested that time pressures, perceived inaccessibility of staff, and "discomfort with giving negative feedback" were the main obstacles.[6] Departmental culture may implicitly endorse avoiding confrontation or allow modeling of poor behaviors; this "hidden curriculum" can be particularly damaging in the context of teaching and providing feedback on professionalism or communication skills.[6,7] Anesthesiology educators in particular have limited opportunity to observe residents during key interactions with patients (see Chapter 6) and the perioperative team, have constrained time for feedback due to busy schedules, and often lack an appropriately private place to provide sensitive feedback.

Several obstacles created by learner limitations were proposed by Bing-You and Trowbridge. These include the learner's

- Ineffective self-assessment;
- Inability to process negative feedback because of intense affective responses; and
- Inadequate reflective skills.[1]

A recent model for feedback provision and reception encompasses many of these complex issues and suggests that the success of the interaction hinges on the environment and credibility of the parties involved. A coaching-type longitudinal relationship is emphasized along with timing of delivery and selection of feedback elements. The perceived credibility of the feedback providers is influenced not just by the quality

Table 20.1 Elements of effective feedback explained

Descriptors of the most common characteristics of effective feedback and their explanations are provided.

Characteristic	Explanation
Behavior oriented	Does not address traits that are not adjustable, focuses on observed behaviors that can be changed
Constructive	Containing useful information on how to improve
Detailed	Descriptive enough about an event to aid recall
Nonjudgmental	Does not assume negative motivation or traits underlie actions
Specific	Explains elements of an action that can be changed instead of generalities
Timely	Provided soon enough that the recipient can recall the event

Has not Achieved Level 1	Level 1	Level 2	Level 3	Level 4	Level 5
	Accepts constructive feedback, but occasionally demonstrates resistance to feedback while providing patient care	Provides constructive feedback in a tactful and supportive way to medical students to enhance patient care Accepts feedback from faculty members and incorporates suggestions into practice	Consistently seeks feedback, correlates it with self-reflection, and incorporates it into lifelong learning to enhance patient care Seeks out feedback from faculty members and other members of the care team	Provides constructive feedback in a tactful and supportive way to physician and non-physician members of the patient care team to enhance patient care	Effectively provides feedback in challenging situations (e.g. when there is resistance, there are adverse outcomes , or an experienced practitioner is involved)

Figure 20.1 The Anesthesiology Milestone Project. Professionalism 4: Receiving and giving feedback (from ACGME and the American Board of Anesthesiology. The Anesthesiology Milestone Project; www.acgme.org/Portals/0/PDFs/Milestones/AnesthesiologyMilestones.pdf [accessed November 10, 2017]).

of their feedback, but also by their perceived clinical competence. Environmental factors and patient interactions also play a role and form a complex ecosystem in which feedback must be managed dynamically (Figure 20.2).[8,9]

Characteristics of Experienced Feedback Providers

Sound faculty development programs should endeavor to teach or develop strategies used by successful feedback providers. A study by Wenrich and colleagues compared self-described approaches of novice and veteran teachers over time as they provided feedback for a group of medical students in the classroom setting.[10] The veteran teachers were more direct, transparent, and specific in their feedback, while novices tended to be general and positive. Veteran teachers could more easily immediately decide the subjects for feedback, and employed more than one approach to provide feedback. They were also more likely to cover

challenging topics in the realm of professionalism and communication. One important difference between the groups was the recognition that learners could be resilient in absorbing negative feedback, a reason why novices avoided criticism. Another study explored traits associated with faculty rated highly for their feedback skills.[11] This study of 300 physicians found that those faculty willing to address the emotional component of situations, deal with conflict, allow appropriate independence, and set "ground rules" and goals both for themselves and learners had the best ratings of their feedback skills.

Agencies of Feedback Training

Feedback training may be done at the level of the department, medical school, or through special groups like academies of educators or national organizations of educators. At the departmental level, Beth Israel Deaconess Medical Center (BIDMC) provides two one-hour sessions on feedback provision for all incoming anesthesia faculty, as well as reviews on the

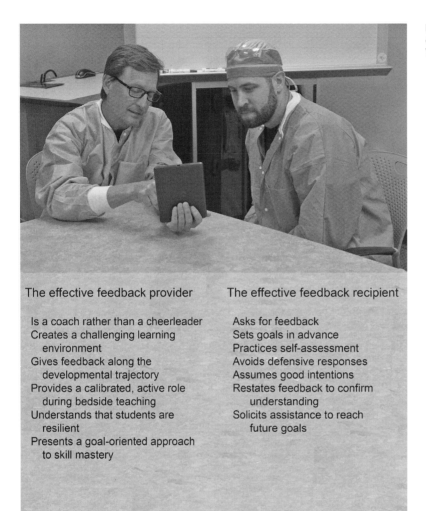

Figure 20.2 Providing and receiving effective feedback (adapted from Wenrich et al. *Acad Med* 2015; 90: S91–7).

The effective feedback provider

Is a coach rather than a cheerleader
Creates a challenging learning
  environment
Gives feedback along the
  developmental trajectory
Provides a calibrated, active role
  during bedside teaching
Understands that students are
  resilient
Presents a goal-oriented approach
  to skill mastery

The effective feedback recipient

Asks for feedback
Sets goals in advance
Practices self-assessment
Avoids defensive responses
Assumes good intentions
Restates feedback to confirm
  understanding
Solicits assistance to reach
  future goals

topic for the entire staff every two to three years.[12] Some schools provide structured, longitudinal faculty development courses for teachers of preclinical students that may include instruction on feedback provision. At the University of Washington, for example, the faculty development courses contain two, two-hour sessions on feedback provision. These courses, though in general not studied for efficacy, set the stage for faculty to learn about providing feedback.[10] Academies of educators are another source of faculty development on feedback provision for those interested in expanding their skills on an *ad hoc* basis. They often host workshops or other didactics on feedback delivery. National organizations like the American Association of Medical Colleges or the Society for Education in Anesthesia often offer workshops on

feedback provision as part of ongoing continuing medical education efforts for medical teachers. These organizations can help fill gaps for institutions lacking their own infrastructure or provide additional expert perspectives on this complex topic.

Modalities for Teaching Feedback

Across medical disciplines there are several training programs and curricula that aim to improve faculty feedback skills. These most commonly take the form of workshops, teaching consultations or evaluations, or participation in fellowships in medical education.[13] Across all specialties, a review of faculty development demonstrated that workshops are the most frequent method employed, followed by short courses, seminars, and longer-term didactics.[14] In internal medicine programs, the most common vehicles were small group discussions, lectures, and role play, with direct observation included in slightly more than 40 percent of programs. In anesthesiology, the most commonly utilized tools are lectures (27 percent), or seminars and courses (18 percent).[2] The reader is referred to the comprehensive literature review by Steinert and colleagues for a full selection of materials on this topic from 2006 and earlier.[14]

Duration of Training in Feedback

One significant question is how long training must be to ensure that feedback skills are appropriately developed. There is a wide range in the literature, from single-session interventions to programs lasting six months or longer.[5,13,15] While (in separate studies) undergraduate subjects demonstrated improvement in rating skills with multiple interventions over time, surgical faculty may be adequately trained on applying a rating scale with a single one-hour training session.[12,15] There are many possible explanations for this divergence including prior familiarity with similar rating tools, but this effect would be germane to experienced anesthesia faculty as well. While the evidence is far from conclusive, the literature tends to support the positive effects of multiple training sessions over time; this is consistent with established learning theory.[12,14]

Successful Programs for Teaching Feedback Skills

While resources do exist for faculty development of feedback skills, few are specific to anesthesiology or have been adequately studied or validated.[14] Most assessments consist of self-evaluation of participants obtained from immediate or near-term postintervention surveys.[16–18] Early studies suggested that the frequency of feedback encounters, and specific examples and detail incorporated into feedback could be improved.[14] As the rigor of assessment methodologies has improved over time, we will focus our discussion on more recent examples of these different types of faculty development tools.[17]

The most robust work to date in this area outside of anesthesia has been undertaken by Junnod Perron and colleagues. They first demonstrated that after a structured, six month series of interventions, staff perceived improvements in their feedback skills. Changes could also be detected in some dimensions of recorded performance in structured/simulated encounters as graded by trained raters. The course had elements that were adapted to address needs of participants from different specialties.[5] While it represents an important step to demonstrate impact of faculty development on feedback skills, the intervention is lengthy and complex. It also did not demonstrate transferability to a clinical environment. Therefore, the same group subsequently studied almost 30 faculty members who participated in a faculty development course of six months duration. This course focused on communication skills and teaching and was multimodal, incorporating elements such as structured teaching sessions, self-reflection of recorded performance, and role play with feedback. The outcome metric in this project was self-reported frequency of the teaching of communication skills. Measurements were made one month before and after the course; interviews were also completed to assess whether subjects had incorporated lessons from the course, including concepts like structured feedback. Overall, the subjects rated their experience positively and had subjectively increased comfort with providing feedback. They still noted issues with the work environment that limited their application of direct observation and immediate feedback. While these studies are innovative and valuable, they focused on teacher-centered outcomes and did not explore the learner's experience.

Multimodal teaching of feedback is also a theme in the work of Cole and colleagues.[16] This curriculum spanned nine months at three and a half hours per week and included multiple facets of teaching and learning, including feedback provision. They incorporated techniques such as review of recorded interactions, reflective work, and small group discussions. While self-assessment of teaching skills improved, there were no external measures provided. Another group incorporated portable resources, role-playing exercises, and discussion of recorded interactions over multiple sessions to accomplish their teaching of a group of staff and interns.[19] The result was improved comfort but not knowledge for staff, and slight improvements in both comfort and knowledge for the intern cohort.

Within anesthesiology, there are several approaches reported and some preliminary work ongoing. Utilizing a simulator-based intervention with structured debriefing, Minehart and colleagues were able to conduct a randomized, controlled trial involving a single-session faculty development workshop on feedback skills.[20] The session included a didactic lecture followed immediately by recorded interactions with a simulated resident (actor) and discussion/debriefing. A team of blinded raters was responsible for scoring using both a multi-item scale and an objective score sheet. Staff receiving the intervention scored higher in some areas including providing a safe environment for feedback, structuring the session, and examining performance issues. While not successful in enhancing all areas, this single-session model represents a potentially viable approach to feedback that deserves further evaluation in a clinical setting.

There is a growing interest in providing scoring and rating rubrics for evaluating complex behaviors such as professionalism. One such approach for professionalism evaluation and teaching was recently presented by Dorrotta and colleagues.[21] While this may enhance the consistency and reliability of ratings for this nebulous area, the authors do not provide suggestions on how to train faculty to apply their system. Furthermore, the system was global instead of more detailed and specific. The relationship of feedback to this evaluation tool is also unclear.

There are several ongoing efforts in faculty development for feedback provision for anesthesiologists at our institution, BIDMC. These efforts have been presented in abstract form, but have not yet been published in peer-reviewed journals and so should be interpreted with care. A full discussion of these projects is included elsewhere.[12] Efforts have focused on the establishment of a daily feedback system, engagement in issues of "difficult feedback," and auditing of feedback quality.

Prior to initiation of daily feedback, faculty were taught principles of feedback in a series of six lectures and workshops and then encouraged to provide feedback using cognitive aids on a single day of the week, "Feedback Wednesday."[22] The cognitive aid consisted of elements of the Mini-Clinical Evaluation Exercise (Mini-CEX), which was originally developed by the American Board of Internal Medicine (ABIM)[23] and adapted for anesthesiology use by Weller et al. The anesthesia version (Figure 20.3) consists of nine skill areas and overall clinical care rated on a nine-point scale).[24] Simulation-style facilitated debriefing techniques were incorporated and residents were encouraged to solicit feedback as well.

Elements of Mini-CEX and simulation-style facilitated debriefing (involving an open-ended conversation about what went wrong, what went well, and why it went that way) were incorporated.[25] Once this became an established part of departmental culture, we converted to a system of daily feedback. An e-mail link is sent to faculty each day reminding them to emphasize one thing the resident did well and one thing he or she needs to improve. There are no numbers, only narratives for formative feedback; clinical division designees complete monthly rotational evaluations separately. The value of face-to-face discussion is emphasized. This system has been in place for more than four years with stable quantities of faculty feedback; similar systems have been incorporated at University of Kentucky, University of Rochester, and University of California, San Diego.

Topics for which feedback is difficult, such as professionalism and communication, have received attention as well.[26] After an iterative process of testing for feasibility, a series of two faculty development workshops on providing feedback regarding professionalism and communication skills were tested at the four centers noted previously. These workshops incorporated video vignettes, role play, and interactive discussion.[27] A single session on receiving and soliciting feedback was provided concurrently for residents. Written feedback was assessed for quantity, quality, and utility using a structured scoring system and a global rating scale. While feasible, only one center showed improvements; this center had only enrolled new faculty, suggesting that perhaps this group is the most amenable to the intervention.[28]

We believe in the concept of continuous education and quality improvement; to that end we are starting to pilot random feedback auditing with the aim of helping faculty to improve the quality of their feedback to residents. The scoring system developed for use in the difficult feedback study is being applied to rate samples of faculty feedback. The ultimate goal is to retrain those with low-scoring feedback using interventions focused on their specific issues. Initial rater training and feasibility assessment is currently underway.

Multisource Feedback

It has been proposed that including groups such as patients or other healthcare professionals in the feedback process will help to triangulate, validate, or enhance assessments by faculty.

A group of internists from the University of Pennsylvania developed and piloted a patient survey

	Unsatisfactory			Satisfactory			Superior			*u/c
	1	2	3	4	5	6	7	8	9	
Patient assessment and preparation	0	0	0	0	0	0	0	0	0	0
Preparation for anesthesia	0	0	0	0	0	0	0	0	0	0
Management plan	0	0	0	0	0	0	0	0	0	0
Communication skills with patient	0	0	0	0	0	0	0	0	0	0
Communication skills with staff	0	0	0	0	0	0	0	0	0	0
Technical skills	0	0	0	0	0	0	0	0	0	0
Clinical judgment	0	0	0	0	0	0	0	0	0	0
Organization/efficiency	0	0	0	0	0	0	0	0	0	0
Professionalism	0	0	0	0	0	0	0	0	0	0
Overall clinical care	0	0	0	0	0	0	0	0	0	0
What did the trainee do well?										
Agree for improvement										
Agreed action										

Figure 20.3 Mini-CEX as modified for anesthesiology by Weller et al. (from J. M. Weller, A. Jones, A. F. Merry, B. Jolly, D. Saunders. Investigation of trainee and specialist reactions to the mini-Clinical Evaluation Exercise in anaesthesia: Implications for implementation. *Br J Anaesth* 2009 Oct; 103(4): 524–30).

tool that examined the professionalism and communication skills of Post Graduate Year 1 (PGY-1) residents.[29] After reviewing the literature, a 16-item instrument was developed. Most questions were adapted from existing sources, but two were new. They used a five-point scale with an "N/A" option to evaluate both individual and team communication. The survey, conducted at a single institution, had a reasonable (74 percent) completion rate by patients. While the patient evaluation failed to correlate with faculty evaluations, it did correlate weakly with standardized patient evaluations. It was estimated that 50 evaluations would be required to achieve an acceptable reproducibility coefficient of 0.57, but during the study period of 18 weeks, each subject was evaluated only 4.6 times on average. Thus, the instrument had significant limitations.

The ABIM created a tool called Teamwork Effectiveness Assessment Module (TEAM) to help assess interprofessional team performance.[30] TEAM builds on the Team Events Non-Technical Skills (TENTS) instrument, which is an observational checklist to be completed by a trained observer in an effort to assess health professional teamwork.[31] The TENTS checklist includes items on communication, leadership, situation monitoring, and mutual support/assertion, as well as overall teamwork and leadership.

TEAM is a more complex process that starts with identification of the interprofessional team members. The teamwork behavior survey is completed by the physician (self-assessment) and the team members. Finally, the physician reviews and reflects upon the results in a structured manner. The ABIM piloted this tool in 25 hospitals and received feedback that participants received "meaningful, actionable information that they could not have gotten otherwise."[30]

General practitioners in Belgium have been using video-recorded training since 1974, but recently began studying whether recorded patient sessions in real time with immediate peer and attending feedback would be feasible and acceptable to trainees.[32] Sixty-four percent of study subjects did not mind the peer evaluation, 68 percent of participants were positive about the recording experience, and 85 percent felt that the session improved their professionalism and nonverbal communication skills. Unfortunately, more than 60 percent said they believed patients were uncomfortable with the recording process and half felt that video-recorded interactions were not realistic. This area therefore requires refinement and study, but could be a beneficial approach for training residents in the future.

At BIDMC, we have incorporated patient assessment of resident communication skills into a curricular model that allows residents to target specific areas in need of improvement. We modified a survey instrument from the 4-Habits survey and initially conducted mailed surveys of patients for three months before and after an intervention. We were able to detect changes in overall program level scores after either simulation or web-based reflective interventions were employed to help residents improve on their specific communication deficiencies.[33] In a follow-up project, we adapted the survey to an iPad-based format and have demonstrated measurable changes in performance for residents who were not rated as perfect in the three-month preassessment phase. A manuscript has been submitted discussing these findings and is under review.

Summary

Unfortunately, there are few validated tools for helping faculty to improve their feedback skills. Those that do have evidence of effect involve lengthy courses that may not be feasible to apply in busy departments of anesthesiology. Minehart's work in simulated encounters holds promise for application as it required only a single-session intervention and involved practicing anesthesiologists, but transferability to the clinical setting remains to be demonstrated. Other interventions for anesthesiologists demonstrate potential in a single center, but could not yet be generalized to other institutions.

Standardized tools and cognitive aids may prove effective in enhancing feedback quality and consistency, but more work needs to be done. Based on our experience, we recommend incorporation of daily feedback, as it does seem to improve frequency of feedback encounters. Long-term follow-up and ongoing assessments of quality with continued education should be incorporated to avoid regression. We also value perspectives from other providers and patients, as it provides new, as well as corroborative, information that may not otherwise be available.

While the evidence remains scant, educators should heed the words of Dr. Eric Holmboe's group as they outline plans for faculty development for competency-based education systems: "We should not wait for research to find the perfect faculty development models ... we must build in ongoing research and learning as part of the process, using new methodological strategies to evaluate the effectiveness of faculty development as part of a continuous quality improvement project."[34]We must band together collaboratively to share and study best practices so that we may improve our abilities in this vital, but challenging, endeavor.

References

1. R. G. Bing-You, R. L. Trowbridge. Why medical educators may be failing at feedback. *JAMA* 2009; 302: 1330–1.

2. J. D. Mitchell, E. J. Holak, H. N. Tran, S. Muret-Wagstaff et al. Are we closing the gap in faculty development needs for feedback training? *J Clin Anesth* 2013; 25: 560–4.

3. A. Baroffio, B. Kayser, B. Vermeulen, J. Jacquet. Improvement of tutorial skills: An effect of workshops or experience? *Acad Med* 1999; 74(Suppl 10): S75–7.

4. M. A. Rosenblatt, S. A. Schartel. Evaluation, feedback, and remediation in anesthesiology residency training: A survey of 124 United States programs. *J Clin Anesth* 1999; 11: 519–27.

5. N. J. Perron, J. Sommer, P. Hudelson et al. Clinical supervisors' perceived needs for teaching communication skills in clinical practice. *Med Teach* 2009; 31: e316–22.

6. J. S. Brown, A. Collins, P. Duguid. Situated cognition and the culture of learning. *Educ Res* 1989; 18: 32–42.

7. R. R. Gaiser. The teaching of professionalism during residency: Why it is failing and a suggestion to improve its success. *Anesth Analg* 2009; 108: 948–54.

8. C. Watling, E. Driessen, C. P. M. Van Der Vleuten, L. Lingard. Learning culture and feedback: An international study of medical athletes and musicians. *Med Educ* 2014; 48: 713–23.

9. C. J. Watling. Unfulfilled promise, untapped potential: Feedback at the crossroads. *Med Teach* 2014; 36: 692–7.

10. M. D. Wenrich, M. B. Jackson, R. R. Maestas et al. From cheerleader to coach: The developmental progression of bedside teachers in giving feedback to early learners. *Acad Med* 2015; 90: S91–7.

11. E. P. Menachery, A. M. Knight, K. Kolodner, S. M. Wright. Physician characteristics associated with proficiency in feedback skills. *J Gen Intern Med* 2006; 21: 440–6.

12. L. M. Sulsky, D. V. Day. Frame-of-reference training and cognitive categorization: An empirical investigation of rater memory issues. *J Appl Psychol.* 1992; 77: 501–10.

13. L. Wilkerson, D. M. Irby. Strategies for improving teaching practices: A comprehensive approach to faculty development. *Acad Med* 1998; 73: 387.

14. Y. Steinert, K. Mann, A. Centeno et al. A systematic review of faculty development initiatives designed to improve teaching effectiveness in medical education: BEME Guide No. 8. *Med Teach* 2006; 28: 497–526.

15. B. C. George, E. N. Teitelbaum, D. A. Darosa et al. Duration of faculty training needed to ensure reliable or performance ratings. *J Surg Educ* 2013; 70: 703–8.

16. K. A. Cole, L. R. Barker, K. Kolodner et al. Faculty development in teaching skills: An intensive longitudinal model. *Acad Med* 2004; 79: 469.

17. H. Saedon, S. Salleh, A. Balakrishnan. The role of feedback in improving the effectiveness of workplace based assessments: A systematic review. *BMC Med Educ* 2012; 12: 25.

18. M. G. Hewson, M. L. Little. Giving feedback in medical education: Verification of recommended techniques. *J Gen Intern Med* 1998; 13: 111–16.

19. R. A. Brauch, C. Goliath, L. Patterson et al. A qualitative study of improving preceptor feedback delivery on professionalism to postgraduate year 1 residents through education, observation, and reflection. *Ochsner J* 2013; 13: 322–6.

20. R. D. Minehart, J. Rudolph, M. C. Pian-Smith, D. B. Raemer. Improving faculty feedback to resident trainees during a simulated case: A randomized, controlled trial of an educational intervention. *Anesthesiology* 2014; 120: 160–71.

21. I. Dorotta, J. Staszak, A. Takla, J. E. Tetzlaff. Teaching and evaluating professionalism for anesthesiology residents. *J Clin Anesth* 2006; 18: 148–60.

22. S. B. Jones, S. L. Muret-Wagstaff, L. J. Fisher, J. D. Mitchell. "Feedback Wednesday": A method to improve feedback to residents and ustain the gains. Association of University Anesthesiologists Annual Meeting. Cleveland, OH; 2012.

23. American Board of Internal Medicine. www.personalbesthealth.com/Literature%20for%20Web/Articles/Mini-CEX%20Guidelines.pdf (accessed October 10, 2017).

24. J. M. Weller, A. Jones, A. F. Merry et al. Investigation of trainee and specialist reactions to the mini-Clinical Evaluation Exercise in anaesthesia: Implications for implementation. *Br J Anaesth* 2009; 103: 524–30.

25. R. K. Dismukes, D. M. Gaba, S. K. Howard. So many roads: Facilitated debriefing in healthcare. *Simul Healthc* 2006; 1: 23–5.

26. J. D. Mitchell, M. Brzezinski, E. J. Holak et al. Teaching faculty to provide difficult feedback: A feasibility study. *Anesth Analg* 2012; 114(Suppl 5): 205.

27. J. D. Mitchell, C. Ku, L. J. Fisher et al. Assessing a multi-modal curriculum to develop resident professionalism and communication skills. HMS Medical Education *Day*. Boston; 2013.

28. J. D. Mitchell, A. DiLorenzo, S. Karan et al. Enhancing feedback on professionalism and interpersonal communication skills. *Anesth Analg [Internet]* 2015; 120: s–129. www.iars.org/education/annual_meeting/2015/ (accessed October 10, 2017).

29. C. J. Dine, S. Ruffolo, J. Lapin et al. Feasibility and validation of real-time patient evaluations of internal medicine interns' communication and professionalism skills. *J Grad Med Educ* 2014; 6: 71–7.

30. B. J. Chesluk, E. Bernabeo, B. Hess et al. A new tool to give hospitalists feedback to improve interprofessional teamwork and advance patient care. *Health Aff (Millwood)* 2012; 31: 2485–92.

31. S. M. Hohenhaus, S. Powell, R. Haskins. A practical approach to observation of the emergency care setting. *J Emerg Nurs* 2008; 34: 142–4.

32. T. Eeckhout, M. Gerits, D. Bouquillon, B. Schoenmakers. Video training with peer feedback in real-time consultation: Acceptability and feasibility in a general-practice setting. *Postgrad Med J* 2016; 92: 431–5.

33. J. D. Mitchell, C. Ku, V. Wong et al. The impact of a resident communication skills curriculum on patients' experiences of care. *A A Case Rep* 2016; 6: 65–75.

34. E. S. Holmboe, D. S. Ward, R. K. Reznick et al. Faculty development in assessment: The missing link in competency-based medical education. *Acad Med* 2011; 86: 460–7.

The Resident as a Teacher

Robert Gaiser

Introduction

According to the Accreditation Council for Graduate Medical Education (ACGME), "Residency is an essential dimension of the transformation of the medical student to the independent practitioner along the continuum of medical education. It is physically, emotionally, and intellectually demanding, and requires longitudinally concentrated effort on the part of the resident."[1] The transition from medical student to resident involves training in the six core competencies, one of which is Interpersonal and Communication Skills. Residency is also the period in which the individual transforms from a student to a teacher. Residents will teach other residents, medical students, nurses, and patients. The ACGME Common Program Requirements, applicable to residencies of all types, reads in part, "Residents are expected to: communicate effectively with patients, families, and the public; … communicate effectively with physicians, other health professionals; … work effectively as a member or leader of a health care team or other professional group; act in a consultative role to other physicians and healthcare professionals."[1] [1] The requirements for the core residency in anesthesiology simply reiterate those requirements.[2] While teaching may be intimated, it is not stated outright in either document. In contrast, the Anesthesiology Milestone Project[3] makes specific reference to teaching (Figure 21.1).

In addition, the requirements for pediatric anesthesiology clearly identify teaching as an outcome expected of all fellows. "Fellows must demonstrate the ability to effectively teach other resident physicians, medical students, and other health care professionals in the principles of pediatric anesthesiology, including management of patients requiring sedation outside the operating rooms, pain management, and life support."[4] Although the outcome of teaching is explicit only for fellows in pediatric anesthesiology, all residents must develop the skills of teaching as they will be teaching throughout their career regardless of whether they choose academic or private practice. For academics, teaching is an important component to the promotion process.

As the resident embarks on the path to becoming an effective teacher, several points must be considered. Residents have faculty on whom to model their teaching. Depending on the definition of a great teacher, the qualities for these teachers differ. If one were to assume a great teacher is one who teaches concepts and information that an individual may use beyond the acute teaching experience, the aspects of this type of teacher have been determined. In a study examining teachers' ratings by students and student performance, surprising results were obtained.[2] When examining students' performances at the end of a teaching session, those teachers with the higher ratings from the students produced students who performed better. This positive correlation between teacher ratings and student performance immediately following a teaching session has been confirmed in numerous studies. However, when performance of the student was determined later, there was a negative correlation. The students of the teachers who were

---

[1] www.acgme.org/Portals/0/PFAssets/Program Requirements/CPRs_2017-07-01.pdf (accessed November 18, 2017).

[2] www.acgme.org/Portals/0/PFAssets/Program Requirements/040_anesthesiology_2017-07-01.pdf?ver=2017-05-17-155314-547 (accessed November 18, 2017).

[3] www.acgme.org/Portals/0/PDFs/Milestones/AnesthesiologyMilestones.pdf?ver=2015-11-06-120534-217 (accessed November 18, 2017).

[4] www.acgme.org/Portals/0/PDFs/Milestones/PediatricAnesthesiology.pdf?ver=2015-11-06-120524-183 (accessed November 18, 2017)

Has not Achieved Level 1	Level 1	Level 2	Level 3	Level 4	Level 5
	Discusses medical plans and responds to questions from patients and their families Acknowledges limits and seeks assistance from supervisor	Explains anesthetic care to patients and their families Teaches basic anesthesia concepts to students and other healthcare professionals	Effectively explains subspecialty anesthetic care to patients and their families Teaches anesthesia concepts to students and other residents	Explains anesthesia care and risk to patients and their families with conditional independence Teaches anesthesia concepts, including subspecialty care, to students, other residents, and other health professionals	Serves as an expert on anesthesiology to patients, their families, and other healthcare professionals, (locally or nationally) Participates in community education about anesthesiology

Figure 21.1 Practice-based learning and improvement. Education of patients, families, students, residents, and other health professionals.

Table 21.1 Factors associated with increased difficulty of a teacher as assessed by students

Cover difficult concepts

Focus on concepts beyond the current course

Allow students to struggle while learning

Give frequent quizzes

Mix different kinds of problems together

Assign difficult problems in the homework

Give cumulative examinations

rated with low scores did not do as well on the initial assessment; however, these students outperformed the students taught by the highly rated teachers in assessments later. The challenge is how to explain the paradox. Ratings of an individual's teaching ability are based upon the perceived difficulty of the teacher by the student. The factors listed in Table 21.1 have been shown to increase the difficulty for the student and provide a greater challenge while resulting in a lower evaluation of the teacher by the students.

Yet, all these factors have also been proven to improve the learning by the student. These qualities also produce a more enduring understanding of the material. The major message from this study is that students do not enjoy being challenged but do learn more from those experiences. As such, the conundrum has been established – a resident who will be teaching must choose whether to increase the learning by the student at the cost of lower evaluations or to decrease the amount of learning but receive higher evaluations. The medical student may not like the questioning by the resident but will gain a greater appreciation of the material (Figure 21.2).

While the choice should be obvious, residents who select an academic career will be confronted by a promotion process in which evaluations by students are important; being an effective teacher (and receiving low evaluations from students) may be an impediment to promotion. Evaluations must be separated from the promotion process allowing teachers to challenge and correct students without the concern of jeopardizing promotion

Why Should a Resident Develop into a Teacher?

There are numerous reasons a resident must develop teaching skills. As residents care for patients, they will be required to obtain informed consent. Informed consent is the process by which the resident educates the patient on the procedure, the risks involved with the procedure, and alternatives to the procedure.[3] Residents also will be asked to teach medical students. All rotations in anesthesiology, including critical care and pain medicine, will have medical students working closely with residents. The resident will be asked to teach the medical student both concepts and procedures. As such, the resident will need to use different types of teaching. Effective teaching of medical students by the resident is important for recruitment of future residents to the specialty. Interactions between medical students and residents, including role modeling (by the resident), are the most significant factors in determining the choice of specialty by the medical student.[4]

An important point for the resident to know is that one of the best means for mastering the material is to teach it. In an experiment concerning a reading passage, learners who were informed they would be tested on the passage were compared to learners who were informed that they would be teaching

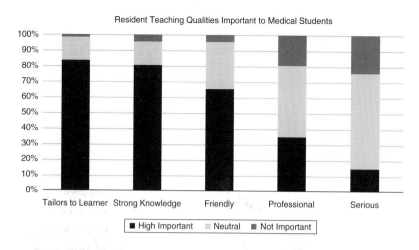

Figure 21.2 Resident teaching qualities important to medical students (from L. Melvin, Z. Kassam, A. Burke, P. Wasi, J. Neary. What makes a great resident teacher? A multicenter survey of medical students attending an internal medicine conference. J Grad Med Educ 2014; 6: 694–7).

the passage.[5] Regardless of the expectation, both groups of learners were tested. Those learners who thought that they would be just teaching produced better organized responses and had better recall of the passages, especially those concerning the major points. The importance of this study is that instilling an expectation to teach improves the learning of the individual. When mastering knowledge of anesthesia, the resident should have the expectation of teaching subsequent learners. This learning occurs because those who have the expectation of teaching know that they will be expected to effectively communicate the new material. While recall is improved in the participants expected to teach, more importantly, organization of the material and understanding of the major points was greater in this group. The explanation for this improvement is that the learners with the expectation of teaching place themselves in the mindset of a teacher, thus organizing the importance of the material and focusing on the major points. This study reinforces the importance of teaching in learning. Residents learn while they teach and while they prepare to teach. The importance to this study is that instilling an expectation to teach improves the learning of the individual. When mastering knowledge of anesthesia, the resident should have the expectation of teaching subsequent learners. This learning occurs because those who have the expectation of teaching know that they will be expected to effectively communicate the new material.

Many residents are reluctant to teach medical students as they feel that they do not have sufficient knowledge. As highlighted previously, teaching will improve the knowledge of the resident. The resident may be concerned about conveying inadequate knowledge to the medical student. In a survey administered to medical students following a rotation in family medicine, creation of a safe learning environment by the resident was more important than transfer of knowledge; in fact, the learning environment was deemed by the medical students to be the most important quality of the experience. Medical students want to have a safe, supportive environment created by the resident and are more forgiving if the resident does not have all the knowledge.[6]

Core Teaching Concepts for Residents

Residents have a plethora of information to assimilate during training. Given the emphasis (or lack thereof) on teaching by the ACGME, and the fact that information regarding teaching is unlikely to ever play a significant role in the high-stakes exams from the American Board of Anesthesiology (ABA), it is unreasonable to expect a resident to become an expert teacher. There are, however, a few simple guidelines that are likely to increase the efficiency of the resident as a teacher.

Relevance of Material

The most important task to improve learning by the medical student is for the resident to insure the relevance of the material. Too often, educators attempting to define relevance state that the material will be tested. This response is similar to a parent's response to a child's question with "just because." While this motivation may work for children, it will not be particularly effective for medical students. For adult learners, the material may be studied intensely for a short period to achieve a good grade on a test. However, the information will not be retrievable later when confronted with an unfamiliar problem that is based on the concept.[7] Effective acquisition of knowledge by the adult learner requires that the material be relevant to the individual. This is demonstrated by the fact that the most important quality of an individual resident teacher as determined by medical students was the clinical relevance of the material being taught.[7] (Figure 21.3).

As such, the resident must remember and adapt the teaching to the audience. This reasoning explains why a case conference provides much more effective learning than a lecture on the material. To enhance the learning of medical students, the relevance to the future needs of the student must be emphasized.

Information Retrieval Enhances Learning

The resident wants to improve understanding by the student or patient. Understanding may be enhanced by retrieval. Retrieval involves asking the student or the patient questions at various points. These questions will cause the individual to reflect upon the previous teaching. By internally examining the teaching, the patient or student is "retrieving" the knowledge and using it to answer the question. This point may be exemplified by studying. Following studying with a test or quiz to assess the learning produces greater recall and learning as compared to having one period of studying followed by another period of

studying.[8] The reason that a test enhances learning is that the quiz, questions, or test activates retrieval by the student. (See Chapter 18.) Retrieval involves a two-step process. The first step occurs when a question is posed to the student. At this point, the student reflects upon the question and previous knowledge to find the answer. The second step is when the knowledge from the question becomes further ingrained within the individual. While the second step is fairly clear, the first step has two possibilities. In one possibility, the learner must determine the correct answer without assistance, while another possibility occurs when an external source provides the answer following the individual thinking about the question. There was no difference in the subsequent learning whether the learner was able to recall it without assistance or required assistance. In other words, it was the question that instilled the learning as compared to achieving the correct answer without assistance. The results of this study are surprising as they suggest that the positive emotion associated with achieving the correct answer is not important in the learning process.

When educating a medical student, the resident must provide opportunities for the student to think about the information to determine an answer. It is not important if the answer is provided or if the student achieves the answer without assistance. The more important point in the learning process occurs during the time in which the learner is forced to think.

While these studies proved the importance of questioning in learning, it did not establish the

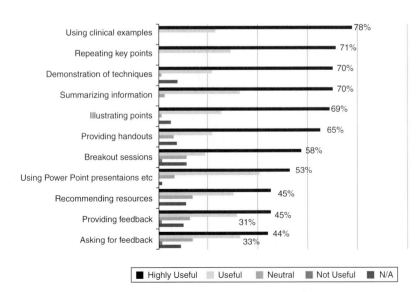

Figure 21.3 Resident teaching techniques (from L. Melvin, A. Kassam, A. Burke, P. Wasi, J. Neary. What makes a great resident teacher? A multicenter survey of medical students attending an internal medicine conference. J Grad Med Educ 2014; 6: 694–7).

optimal frequency of testing. Testing or questioning generates a stress response within the learner. In designing the learning environment, the stress accompanying questioning and testing must be considered, especially because the optimal frequency has not been determined. Being challenged by the resident will develop anxiety in the student. Anxiety is a normal response and allows the individual to adapt to the suspected danger. Anxiety may also become disabling, preventing learning from occurring. When confronted with something new, the individual must determine whether the suspected danger is real. This adaptation requires the individual to sample and to decide. If the individual refuses to explore, the anxiety will not be relieved and learning will not occur. If the individual explores the environment too much, this carelessness may lead to errors. The problem is that failure to explore is much more common than overexploration.[9] The resident must understand this concept when designing a learning environment and encountering a student who is experiencing anxiety. Understanding the underlying cause of the anxiety helps the learner. The educator must encourage the learner to explore the environment and to take chances. The learner must be reassured that it is all right to make mistakes. The learner won't understand that mistakes enhance learning but will be reassured to know lack of knowing the answer is permissible.

The resident should also use this type of learning when consenting patients for a procedure. After an explanation, the resident should ask about understanding. This question provides the patient the opportunity to think about the information. During this thinking and formulation of questions, the patient gains a better understanding of the information presented by the resident. As such, queries should be posed frequently during the process of obtaining informed consent. The questions may be as simple as "Does this make sense?" or "Do you need any additional information?"

Teaching Should Be Goal Driven

Residents encounter difficulty when designing a teaching opportunity for patients or for medical students. The typical approach is to decide upon a topic, design a learning opportunity, and then administer a means for assessment (Figure 21.4). While this

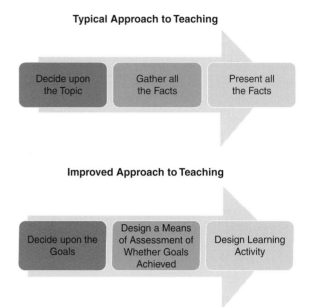

Figure 21.4 Approaches to teaching. The typical approach to a learning activity is to decide upon what should be taught and then design a learning activity. An optimal approach to teaching is to decide upon the goals of the teaching, decide upon a means of assessment as to whether the goals have been achieved, and then design a learning activity. The circle is completed when the results of the assessment are used to refine the goals, the assessment, and the learning activity.

approach may work, it is not optimal. The first step in teaching should be to decide upon the goals of the teaching. Goals provide the focus to the teaching exercise and allow the medical student to know what is expected. Goals also provide a means for the assessment of success of the teaching. It is for this reason that goals are generally presented first in any learning opportunity. With the goals, the learner knows the desired endpoint. Once the desired goals for the learner are set, a means for assessing whether the goals have been achieved is decided. This step, which is often neglected, provides the ability to assess and revise the teaching. By deciding upon the goals and assessments, the resident will prepare a teaching opportunity that is goal-centered as compared to an approach in which the teaching is created without any consideration given to the desired goals. This framework for education is known as "backward by design."[10] The inclusion of assessments provides the driving force for change as the resident is able to assess the success of the teaching and make appropriate adjustments (Figure 21.4).

The Hidden Curriculum Is Important

When a resident decides upon the information to teach, goals are established. However, medical students may learn unintended information during the interaction. This information is gained from the actions of and interactions with the teacher. These unintended teachings are known as the hidden curriculum – teachings never clearly stated but taught through the behavior of the residents (see also Chapter 19). These concepts, conveyed through one's actions as compared to one's words, reflect the culture in which the teaching and learning occurs. The hidden curriculum is the explanation for the impact of social interactions on the learner and the subsequent behavior of the learner. In the learning environment, much attention focuses on the intended teaching by the educator. The educator has designed learning goals, a means of assessment, and learning opportunities. The educator must also remember that additional learning occurs in the learning environment through the behaviors, attitudes, and beliefs of those who are teaching. The hidden curriculum explains the effect of both positive and negative role models. This hidden curriculum has a strong influence on certain aspects of learning, especially those concerning professionalism, behavioral modeling, and values. The hidden curriculum results from role models, rules and regulations, medical language, and hierarchy. In a qualitative study of 25 Harvard medical students, the hidden curriculum was described as an extremely powerful teaching experience as it was felt to impact survival of the learner. The most important finding was that the students internalized the hidden curriculum as they felt it contributed most to their identity as a physician.[11]

The hidden curriculum is influenced by the status of the teacher; the more senior the teacher is to the learner, the greater the influence. Residents always have a greater hierarchy compared to a medical student; as such, residents play an important role in the professional development of the medical student. In a review of the literature concerning the hidden curriculum, the studies mainly focused upon the negative effects, particularly the moral erosion of physicians.[12] A major theme among the articles was that the hidden curriculum was a significant contributor to the education of medical students and instructs them in what is valued in medical practice. It was also clear that this teaching was implicit, making the hidden curriculum difficult to identify and revise. One other prevalent theme was that humanism was secondary to scientific knowledge. A student who knows the "correct answer" is viewed more favorably on rounds as compared to a student who was respectful to the patient.

Given the importance of the hidden curriculum, change may only occur from those senior to the medical student, which includes residents. Currently, medical students are educated in professionalism and humanism. Given the importance of the hidden curriculum, it is the teachers who should receive the education in professionalism and humanism.

Spaced Teaching Is More Effective

When optimizing the learning experience, the resident must decide whether to consolidate the teaching into one or two long sessions or to provide the information over a longer period. Both approaches require the same time commitment. Other than minor considerations, the two approaches have minimal difference in the impact on the resident; the impact on the learner, however, is quite significant. The concept of massed learning versus spaced learning has been extensively studied.[13] If knowledge is measured by performance on a test, massed learning improves performance on an examination that is administered immediately after the session. This point is best exemplified by students who stay awake all night to cram for a test. On a test that is administered at a period delayed from the learning opportunity, spaced learning is optimal. There are several theories to explain the benefits of spaced learning. Critical to spaced learning is the process of forgetting. During spaced learning, there is the opportunity to forget some of the concepts before they are presented again. This forgetting allows the learner to generalize the concepts beyond the boundaries of the learning experience. The importance of forgetting is further highlighted by spaced learning of variable periods. Rather than presenting the material on a set schedule, expanding schedules allow for longer periods at certain times, thus increasing the probability of forgetting.[14]

As the resident instructs the medical student, the resident may teach at a fixed time each day. This approach is easier for the resident as it allows a set time for the teaching. If the resident wants the student to maximize the learning, the scheduled learning activities should occur on an expanded schedule, which means the time between learning activities changes. It is postulated that expanding schedules improve memory because of reactivation of material at optimal points on the forgetting curve (see Figure 18.1). In a study of children learning vocabulary, an expanded schedule produced greater retention of material on tests.[15] The spacing must occur at the period of consolidation, which may be one to three days. Thus, to effectively teach a concept it should be presented on day one, then day three, and then again on day seven as compared to presenting on days one, two, and three. In a separate study, expanded schedules for learning improved generalization of the information learned (ability to apply the information to new situations).[13]

Feedback Is Critical to Learning

Feedback is critical to learning; it formulates the positive associations allowing for the retrieval of knowledge. While feedback is important for learning, it does take time. In a situation of limited time, it decreases the time available for new teaching. This paradigm presents an interesting dilemma. The resident must decide upon whether to provide feedback or to continue with the lesson to ensure that all the information is presented. Medical students recognize this point. When learners are allowed to control feedback, they will skip certain aspects of feedback to allow for additional learning. Learners understand the constraints of a learning environment.[16] Residents should give feedback to those whose clinical experience is less than theirs; this feedback is generally well received and does not have the same connotations connected to when faculty provide feedback due to the concern of evaluations.

Feedback may occur immediately (right after a question is posed) or may be delayed. It stands to reason that immediate feedback should be superior. Immediate feedback does not allow the learner to remain with an incorrect idea. If feedback is provided immediately, the correct information may be learned. However, it also has been argued that spaced teaching enhances learning. Perhaps the persistence of processing the information may enhance the learning. In a study of a game designed to test learning, feedback was either provided immediately, one day later, or four days later.[17] In this study, delayed feedback was superior to immediate feedback. Furthermore, the delayed feedback of four days resulted in greater learning as compared to delaying the feedback by one day. There is a limit to the delay. There is a period in which the delayed feedback would match no feedback. This delay has not been determined for the game and certainly has not been determined for learning in anesthesiology. The importance of this study is that the resident may provide feedback later and not interfere with the learning process.

While the value of a failed test with immediate feedback has been demonstrated, the impact of the incorrect answer on subsequent learning requires further investigation. The previous study focused on the general concepts rather than the individual items. If a learner answers a question incorrectly, the learner may formulate an association that may impair future learning of the specific item. This notion is important when one considers errorless learning that postulates that learning is most effective when the learner does not make a mistake as compared to a false association being created by a mistake. In a study examining tests in which the learner would not be able to answer the question successfully, learning as documented by a test occurred to a greater extent than if the test had not been administered.[18] The tests were administered in which the learner was asked to attempt an answer and then with the test being administered with the answer being presented immediately without the learner generating an attempt. An unsuccessful attempt improved the learning of the material. Challenging students enhances learning. The time frame between the failed attempt and optimal learning is unclear. It is okay for students to fail as it stimulates further learning. After a failed attempt, feedback will improve the learning.

Teaching Procedures

The days of "see one, do one, and teach one" are over. Students still learn medical procedures but a majority of them are learned through simulation. To educate medical students in how to perform procedures, it is helpful to break the procedure into its individual steps. With this framework, the resident is able to teach the student and to provide feedback as to which step was not successful. This approach has been applied to epidural catheter placement.[19] (The procedure has been divided into groups of steps from obtaining consent, aseptic preparation, local infiltration, placing the epidural needle, locating the epidural space, placing a catheter, and securing the catheter. This framework is useful for teaching and for learning.) Any procedure that a resident would like to teach should be divided into its steps and provided to the student beforehand.

Residents as Teachers Curriculum

The education of residents as teachers is important for residency programs because residents serve as the major source of education for medical students. Several websites, some available only to individuals who become members of an organization or working group, provide information on a curriculum for this subject (Box 21.1).

Typically, a curriculum to instruct the resident regarding teaching will address issues surrounding running a small group, effective presentations, teaching procedures, and formative feedback. As with any effective teaching, the curriculum should be constructed using the previously discussed backward by design approach. A review of the literature determined there were 39 publications describing educating residents as teachers.[20] Of these 39, only one had goals and a curriculum that could be applied elsewhere. This study highlights that when designing a curriculum for teaching residents to teach, goals and assessments should come before the curriculum is designed.

Conclusion

Teaching is a valuable exercise for residents. It allows the resident to learn the material to a greater depth, while advancing knowledge of the specialty for the learner. To be successful, the resident must consider the concepts of teaching and learning that come from education theory. While teaching factual information or clinical decision-making is important, the greatest impact on the learner will come from the actions and interactions with the resident. Residents are the role models for medical students and other colleagues.

Box 21.1 Examples of websites related to resident as teacher

- www.im.org/page/residents-as-teachers-curriculum-modules (accessed November 18, 2017);
- www.ame.pitt.edu/Residents-as-Teachers.php (accessed November 18, 2017);
- www.uab.edu/medicine/home/residents-fellows/current/cert (accessed November 18, 2017);
- www.mededportal.org/publication/10152/ (accessed November 18, 2017).

References

1. Accreditation Council for Graduate Medical Education. Requirements in Anesthesiology. http://www.acgme.org/Portals/0/PFAssets/ProgramRequirements/CPRs_2017-07-01.pdf (accessed November 18, 2017).

2. N. Kornell, H. Hausman. Do the best teachers get the best ratings? *Front Psychol* 2016; 7: 570.

3. N. M. Bagnall, P. H. Pucher, M. J. Johnston et al. Informing the process of consent for surgery: Identification of key constructs and quality factors. *J Surg Res* 2016; 209: 86–92.

4. N. J. Borges, R. S. Manuel, R. D. Duffy et al. Influences on specialty choice for students entering person-oriented and technique-oriented specialties. *Med Teach* 2009; 31: 1086–8.

5. J. F. Nestojko, D. C. Bui, N. Kornell, E. L. Bjork. Expecting to teach enhances learning and organization of knowledge in free recall of text passages. *Mem Cogn* 2014; 42: 1038–48.

6. L. Melvin, Z. Kassam, A. Burke et al. What makes a great resident teacher? A multicenter survey of medical students attending an internal medicine conference. *J Grad Med Educ* 2014; 6: 694–7.

7. T. Montacute, T. V. Chan, Y. G. Chen et al. Qualities of resident teachers valued by medical students. *Fam Med* 2016; 48: 381–4.

8. N. Kornell, P. J. Klein, K. A. Rawson. Retrieval attempts enhance learning, but retrieval success (versus failure) does not matter. *J Exp Psychol Learn Mem Cogn* 2015; 41: 83–294.

9. F. Meacham, C. Bergstrom. Adaptive behavior can produce maladaptive anxiety due to individual differences in experience. *Evol Med Pub Health* 2016; 2016: 270–85.

10. J. McTighe, R. S. Thomas. Backward design for forward action: Using data to improve student achievement. *Educational Leadership* 2003; 60: 52–5.

11. J. Bandini, C. Mitchell, Z. D. Epstein-Peterson et al. Student and faculty reflections of the hidden curriculum: How does the hidden curriculum shape students' medical training and professionalization? *Am J Hosp Palliat Med* 2017; 34: 57–63.

12. M. A. Martimianakis, B. Michalec, J. Lam et al. Humanism, the hidden curriculum, and educational reform: A scoping review and thematic analysis. *Acad Med* 2015; 90: S5–13.

13. H. A. Vlach, A. A. Ankowski, C. M. Sandhofer. At the same time or apart in time? The role of presentation timing and retrieval dynamics in generalization. *J Exp Psychol Learn Mem Cogn* 2012; 38: 246–54.

14. H. A. Vlach, C. W. Kalish. Temporal dynamics of categorization: Forgetting as the basis of abstraction and generalization. *Front Psychol* 2014; 5: 1021.

15. H. A. Vlach, C. M. Sandhofer, R. A. Bjork. Equal spacing and expanding schedules in children's categorization and generalization. *J Exp Child Psychol* 2014; 123: 129–37.

16. M. J. Hays, N. Kornell, R. Bjork. The costs and benefits of providing feedback during learning. *Psychon Bull Rev* 2010; 17: 797–801.

17. J. Metcalf, N. Kornell, B. Finn. Delayed versus immediate feedback in children's and adult's vocabulary learning. *Mem Cognit* 2009; 37: 1077–87.

18. N. Kornell, M. J. Hays, R. A. Bjork. Unsuccessful retrieval attempts enhance subsequent learning. *J Exp Psychol Learn Mem Cogn* 2009; 35: 989–98.

19. D. J. Birnbach, A. C. Santos, R. A. Bourlier et al. The effectiveness of video technology as an adjunct to teach and evaluate epidural anesthesia performance skills. *Anesthesiology* 2002; 96: 5–9.

20. K. K. Bree, S. A. Whicker, H. B. Fromme et al. Residents-as-teachers publications: What can programs learn from the literature when starting a new or refining an established curriculum? *J Grad Med Educ* 2014; 6: 237–48.

Chapter 22

Teaching Quality and Safety

John H. Eichhorn

Introduction

Because patient safety and quality are fundamentally different from the fact-based "hard sciences" (e.g., pathophysiology, pharmacology) that anesthesia trainees need to learn, the approach to teaching safety and quality needs be somewhat nontraditional.

"Safety" in anesthesia practice traditionally referred to patient safety, as exemplified in the simple outcome-oriented vision statement of the Anesthesia Patient Safety Foundation (APSF) (Figure 22.1): "No patient shall be harmed by anesthesia."

"Quality" in anesthesia practice involves what is often referred to as "quality assurance" (QA; maintaining predefined standards for quality of care) or "quality improvement" (QI; a dynamic process of continually evaluating and implementing strategies to improve quality of care). The objective of both QA and QI is to stimulate attitudes and activities intended to promote high-quality care. The concept of quality incorporates all the classic three elements of any organized activity that performs a function and/or provides a service: structure, process, and outcome (Box 22.1).

Application of the World Health Organization (WHO) Surgical Safety Checklist[1] (Figure 22.2), including the preincision surgical time out is an excellent example of a process relevant to the quality of anesthesia care.

Importantly, both structure and process elements can be assessed more or less objectively. (Suction is or is not functional; the anesthesia machine is or is not plugged into an emergency power electric outlet; the time-out is or is not conducted completely and correctly.) Because of the objective answers to such questions, structure and process elements of care are relatively easy to observe and measure, leading to their use as representative "quality measures" to objectively assess the quality of care delivered.

"Outcome" is just that: the result of care. It is often argued that outcome is, by far, the most important element of quality. In most circumstances, however, outcome is more difficult to define and consequently more difficult to measure. Does the fact that a patient regains consciousness after general anesthesia or recovers peripheral nerve function after regional anesthesia mean, by definition, that patient received a high-quality anesthetic? Can a numerical score or a "grade" be generated for anesthetizing a given patient? Shifting focus to providers – does counting the number of patients experiencing adverse outcomes accurately reflect the actual quality of the anesthesia care provided? How is risk adjustment entered into the equation? These points can be debated endlessly. That debate yields some understanding of how the definition and measurement of quality will impact anesthesia practice.

In the United States, the patient safety movement was initially created in the mid-1980s through combined efforts of the APSF[2] and the American Society of Anesthesiologists (ASA). The focus was on attempting to eliminate preventable patient injuries from

---

Box 22.1 The three elements of quality

Structure: The constituent things needed to facilitate the practice of anesthesia: anesthesia professionals, anesthesia work stations, monitors, fully stocked carts (including medications, supplies, and equipment), electric power, medical gases, suction, and so forth.

Process: The mechanism of care delivery: protocols (some involving policies and procedures), rituals, habits, and related behaviors involved in the conduct of care.

Outcome: The result of care.

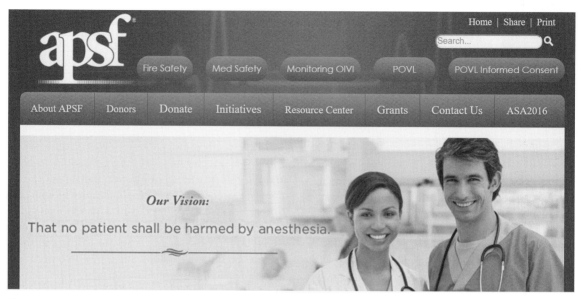

Figure 22.1 APSF no patient shall be harmed (www.apsf.org; accessed November 15, 2017).

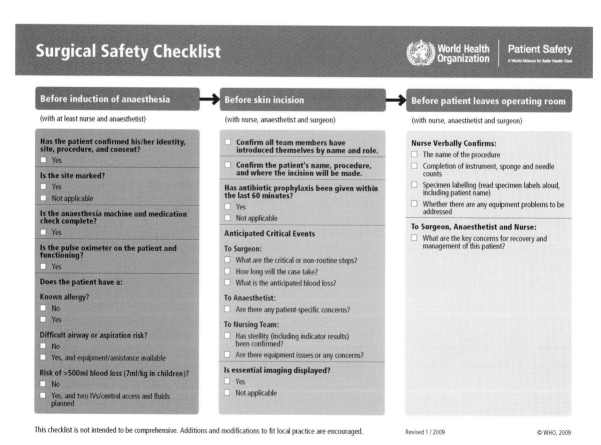

Figure 22.2 WHO surgical safety checklist (www.who.int/patientsafety/safesurgery/checklist/en/; accessed November 15, 2017).

anesthesia care as well as endeavoring to minimize the damage from adverse events that inevitably will occur. While there are differing opinions regarding whether anesthesia outcomes have improved, this is largely due to inconsistent definitions, nonparallel comparisons, the impossibility of any study employing a "no monitoring" patient control group, and small sample size. (Contrast the absence of a database for anesthesia-related adverse events with the Society of Thoracic Surgeons' [STS] database for outcomes after cardiac surgery. While the STS database addresses a relatively small number of surgical procedures on a relatively homogeneous population, a database for anesthesia outcomes would need to consider several operative procedures with an extremely diverse patient population undergoing multiple different anesthetic techniques.) There does appear to be agreement with the thesis[3,4] that catastrophic intraoperative anesthesia injuries to healthy patients have been reduced more than twenty-fold in the last 30 years.

Progress in anesthesia patient safety involves more than the seminal contribution of improved intraoperative monitoring using, particularly, the technical innovations of capnography and pulse oximetry that greatly extend the human senses by providing much earlier detection and warning of hypoxemia or hypoventilation. The concept of "safety monitoring"[3] also includes critical behavioral aspects, especially the requirement for *continuous* (rather than intermittent) attention to the patient's oxygenation, ventilation, and circulation as well as to critical functional aspects of the anesthesia delivery system. Contributions that have influenced the improvement in patient safety have included incremental improvements in:

- Quality of trainees entering the field;
- Literature and didactic sources;
- Information technology;
- Medications;
- All manner of equipment and supplies; and, importantly,

- Research (such as the ASA Closed Claims Study and the multitude of projects funded by the APSF).

Organizing a Curriculum

The challenge to developers of a safety/quality curriculum in an anesthesia training program is to incorporate the background and current concepts of patient safety in an impactful but manageable manner that equips the graduating trainee with the knowledge, habits, and tools to be a maximally safe practitioner.

As with any educational program, the first decision is what material should be taught. Suggestions for content can be obtained from multiple sources (Box 22.2).

Generic issues of patient safety and quality may be accessed through a multitude of sources. Even if the content is not specifically designed for anesthesia trainees, the topics covered by these organizations may be used to develop a framework for the curriculum.

- **National Organizations. Example**: The Institute for Healthcare Improvement (IHI; www.ihi.org; accessed November 15, 2017) offers multiple modules on quality and safety.
- **Accreditation Agencies.** Example: The Joint Commission (TJC; www.jointcommission.org/; accessed November 15, 2017). Provides content on patient safety. Furthermore, ABA written examinations often include TJC definitions (e.g., "sentinel event").
- **Large Healthcare Organizations. Example**: Duke University Health System (http://patientsafetyed. duhs.duke.edu/; accessed November 15, 2017). Motivated in part by the widely publicized, tragic situation in which a 17-year-old girl died following a heart and double-lung transplant of organs with the wrong blood type, Duke University Health System established a Patient Safety Center that has been extremely active.

Box 22.2 Some potential sources for content

- **Large healthcare organizations**: Large healthcare organizations frequently have free online resources available.
- **Accrediting agencies**: Agencies describe expectations for accreditation.
- **National organizations**: Multiple nongovernmental organizations provide quality and safety information.
- **American Board of Anesthesiology (ABA) "Content Outline"**: Serves as the basis for questions in ABA exams.
- **APSF**: Provides videos as well as the APSF newsletter; subjects of prior meetings may also prove useful.

Duke publishes a generic, online, six-module program on quality and safety program[5] that can be reviewed by anyone interested in any aspect of this subject area.

There is no model for a universal didactic curriculum for anesthesia quality and safety, but several sources can be potentially helpful for developing a syllabus.

- **ABA Content Outline.** The Content Outline has a section devoted to safety and quality (Box 22.3). The subject matter listed provides the basis for objective questions on the ABA exams.

- **APSF.** (http://apsf.org/; accessed November 15, 2017) The APSF provides a variety of online information on patient safety. In addition, APSF-sponsored meetings provide suggestions for appropriate content. One of the best other sources of potential course material on anesthesia patient safety is the *APSF Newsletter*, each issue of which contains relevant articles on a wide variety of patient safety topics, almost all of which would be appropriately sized for a videocast. Reports on the APSF-sponsored conferences, in 2016 on the threats of distractions in the operating room (OR) to patient safety and from "production pressure" in the OR schedule, would make excellent teaching topics. Likewise, the APSF has had multiple larger initiatives that would be suitable subjects within a patient safety curriculum. Recent programs have included:
  - Medication safety;
  - Technology training for anesthesia professionals;
  - Strategies for alarms on monitors;
  - Postoperative ventilatory depression from pain medication;
  - Anesthesia information management systems;
  - Vision loss from spine surgery;
  - Stroke associated with beach chair positioning; and
  - Fire safety in the OR.

  The instructional 17-minute video on preventing fires during monitored anesthesia care for superficial surgery on the chest, neck, and head[6] has been distributed, downloaded, or streamed many tens of thousands of times and is considered a definitive patient safety teaching tool, appropriate for every training program to present regularly to all trainees.

- **ASA** (www.asahq.org; accessed November 15, 2017). The ASA provides multiple resources relating to patient safety and quality, including an ever-expanding list of online Patient Safety Modules (Figure 22.3).

Box 22.3 Excerpt – American Board of Anesthesiology Content Outline *(Revised October 2016)*

E. Special Problems or Issues in Anesthesiology…

  4. g. Patient Safety

  1) Definitions: Medical Error, Adverse Event, Sentinel Event

  2) Medication Errors: Assessment and Prevention

  3) Reporting: Mandatory and Voluntary Systems, Legal Requirements

  4) Disclosure of Errors to Patients

  5) Safety Practices: Process-Based, Evidence-Based

  6) Root Cause Analysis

  4. h. Quality Improvement

  1) Quality Improvement Basics: Design, Analysis, Implementation of Quality Improvement Project

  a) Anesthesia Quality Institute; Data Entry; Information

  b) Lean Six Sigma; Assessing QI Methods; Approach

  c) Physician Quality Reporting System: Significance and Role in Practice

  d) Barriers to Quality Improvement

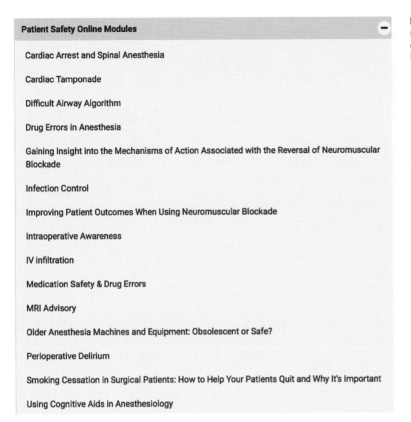

Patient Safety Online Modules

Cardiac Arrest and Spinal Anesthesia

Cardiac Tamponade

Difficult Airway Algorithm

Drug Errors in Anesthesia

Gaining Insight into the Mechanisms of Action Associated with the Reversal of Neuromuscular Blockade

Infection Control

Improving Patient Outcomes When Using Neuromuscular Blockade

Intraoperative Awareness

IV infiltration

Medication Safety & Drug Errors

MRI Advisory

Older Anesthesia Machines and Equipment: Obsolescent or Safe?

Perioperative Delirium

Smoking Cessation in Surgical Patients: How to Help Your Patients Quit and Why It's Important

Using Cognitive Aids in Anesthesiology

Figure 22.3 ASA online patient safety modules (http://asahq.org/education/online-learning/patient-safety; accessed November 15, 2017).

The ASA also offers a quality management and departmental administration "toolkit" with ten sections containing a panoply of topics suitable for inclusion in trainee teaching (Figure 22.4).

Further, the ASA is active in quality reporting activities, such as the Physician Quality Reporting System (PQRS) and the National Anesthesia Clinical Outcomes Registry (NACOR), and also with the NACOR subsidiary database/research organization, the Anesthesia Quality Institute (AQI). All this material could form the basis for elements of a curriculum for trainees.

Methods

Didactics

Whether the teaching vehicle involves traditional passive lectures, the flipped classroom model (see Chapter 15), videocasts (see Chapter 16), or any other means of communication, there will always be a need for trainees to be exposed to and absorb relevant didactic material. Standard anesthesia textbooks contain general material on the subjects of quality and safety. While making these assigned readings, even with scored objective testing on the material, is fine (and very traditional), they may be more effective as reference sources to answer questions that arise in a more streamlined and integrative approach. Likewise, there are brief treatments in anesthesia review books and exam-prep books. Because these books contain mostly broad highlights, they can be useful in serving as an outline for videocasts.

Dividing subject material during a didactic presentation into smaller packets (e.g., 10–20 minutes) has gained wide popularity. Not only is this based on sound educational principles, but it's much easier to find 10–20 minutes of time (e.g., while waiting for a patient to arrive in the holding area) than it is to find 45–60 minutes. Videocasts, usually based on a PowerPoint presentation with recorded audio elaboration (not unlike a lecture) can be recorded by a faculty member, posted on a server, and "consumed" anytime thereafter by a learner. Even when a traditional 50-minute-hour, face-to-face lecture period persists, presenters now often break the time into two or three

QMDA Regulatory Toolkit

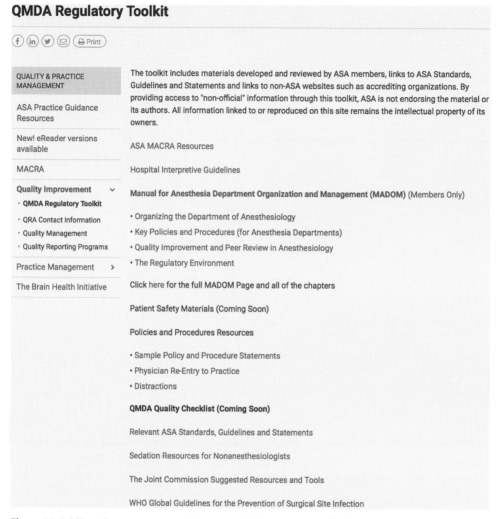

QUALITY & PRACTICE MANAGEMENT

ASA Practice Guidance Resources

New! eReader versions available

MACRA

Quality Improvement ⌄
 · QMDA Regulatory Toolkit
 · QRA Contact Information
 · Quality Management
 · Quality Reporting Programs

Practice Management ⟩

The Brain Health Initiative

The toolkit includes materials developed and reviewed by ASA members, links to ASA Standards, Guidelines and Statements and links to non-ASA websites such as accrediting organizations. By providing access to "non-official" information through this toolkit, ASA is not endorsing the material or its authors. All information linked to or reproduced on this site remains the intellectual property of its owners.

ASA MACRA Resources

Hospital Interpretive Guidelines

Manual for Anesthesia Department Organization and Management (MADOM) (Members Only)

 • Organizing the Department of Anesthesiology
 • Key Policies and Procedures (for Anesthesia Departments)
 • Quality Improvement and Peer Review in Anesthesiology
 • The Regulatory Environment

Click here for the full MADOM Page and all of the chapters

Patient Safety Materials (Coming Soon)

Policies and Procedures Resources

 • Sample Policy and Procedure Statements
 • Physician Re-Entry to Practice
 • Distractions

QMDA Quality Checklist (Coming Soon)

Relevant ASA Standards, Guidelines and Statements

Sedation Resources for Nonanesthesiologists

The Joint Commission Suggested Resources and Tools

WHO Global Guidelines for the Prevention of Surgical Site Infection

Figure 22.4 ASA quality management and departmental administration "toolkit" (http://www.asahq.org/quality-and-practice-management/quality-and-regulatory-affairs/qmda-regulatory-toolkit?_ga=2.174200546.1155189769.1510711733-1020287110.1445784851; accessed November 15, 2017).

distinct segments with distinguishably different subjects and a brief break between segments to facilitate rebooting learner's attention and receptivity.

A flipped classroom series of vignettes, each developed to illustrate an element of the preliminary reading (e.g., James Reason's "Swiss-cheese model" or any of the many cognitive bias issues that predispose to injury accidents) would be an excellent way to present human error theory, an element of patient safety that would be included in the curriculum of most safety and quality programs.

Especially acknowledging the current emphasis on quality in US healthcare, anesthesia trainees will need to learn about these and related functions.

Analogies

Use of analogies between new subject material and concepts the learner may already understand in a broader context can be an effective teaching tool. Specific analogies to anesthesia quality and safety principles offer creative educators interesting opportunities to illustrate key components of these topics in especially enlightening ways to anesthesia trainees.

• **Business:** All consumers of media and advertising are constantly bombarded with countless claims about the "best quality" this or that. Significant science and research have been devoted to the concept of quality. In commercial endeavors, QA is an organized plan or protocol to maximize efficiency while maintaining the expected quality standard of the involved product or service. The analogy to the throughput of patients in an OR is obvious, as are the central roles of the anesthesia professionals and their function. There is significant potential for a thought-provoking, flipped classroom discussion session after trainees absorb some basic information on industrial QA; such an interactive session would likely be a memorable class for trainees. Included in that or a companion class would be the issue of quality measures, specifically deciding what objective parameters can genuinely reflect the successful achievement of the desired quality result. This can be straightforward for a manufactured product meeting specifications and functioning correctly. Challenging the trainees to devise new and better ways to score or judge the quality of anesthesia care (far beyond the "times," e.g., "antibiotic administration time," we all know so well) not only emphasizes the relative roles of structure, process, and outcome in the quality paradigm, but also illustrates the conundrum that anesthesia care is uniquely difficult to evaluate objectively.

Although incorrectly frequently used interchangeably with QA, QI is different and somewhat more complex. The thesis of QI is that the focal point (whether structure, process, or outcome) can be improved. There may be a clear disruptive/obstructive "problem" in the endeavor that needs to be remedied to return to a baseline acceptable function. Or, the problem may be that the focal point or the entire endeavor is just not good enough and, thus, needs improvement. The classic QI paradigm consists of four steps:

○ Problem identification;
○ Problem investigation;
○ Problem resolution; and
○ Verification of resolution.

Usually, the goal is "zero defects," such as in the "lean process improvement model" (Toyota "kaizen") or the "Six Sigma" approach (originally from manufacturing and referring to the normal distribution curve – results six standard deviations above a theoretical mean: 99.99966 percent perfect, only 3.4 errors per one million occurrences). A key feature of classic QI efforts that specifically target changes intended to improve outcome has been the "plan-do-study-act" (PDSA) continuous activity cycle (or "Deming cycle"). The PDSA cycle concept has been widely adopted in healthcare (see Figure 22.5).

Voluminous literature on QI exists in commercial settings and a basic primer article or chapter on the general overview would be sufficient background to facilitate another lively discussion about applying those techniques to the overall function of an OR suite. As anesthesia practice and healthcare in general become increasingly complex and with progressively more emphasis being placed on quality, it is incumbent upon programs to ensure that their trainees have a reasonable understanding of these concepts.

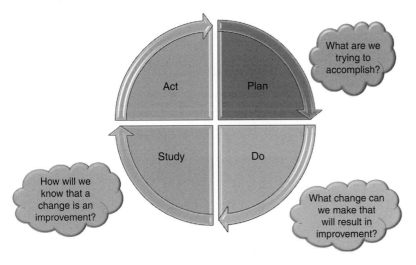

Figure 22.5 PDSA cycle (https://innovations.ahrq.gov/qualitytools/plan-do-study-act-pdsa-cycle; see also: www.ihi.org/resources/Pages/HowtoImprove/default.aspx; accessed November 15, 2017).

- **Aviation.** Patient safety in anesthesia has been blessed (or, some say, cursed) with an especially relevant analogy to safety efforts and programs in commercial aviation. Analogies between piloting a jumbo jet and conducting a general anesthetic abound; the most obvious of these are:
  - Preflight = preoperative evaluation of patient and preparation of equipment;
  - Takeoff = induction;
  - Cruising = maintenance phase; and
  - Landing = emergence.

The original connection came from a landmark recognition[7] that anesthesia professionals (pilots) can make errors that might injure patients ("critical incidents" or actual crashes) that then can be investigated with a "root cause analysis" (RCA). In the aviation industry, the National Transportation Safety Board (NTSB) dissects the antecedents to any accident in meticulous detail. Generally speaking, as the accident is analyzed in progressively greater detail it will be determined that more than one factor contributed to the outcome. After determination of the contributing causes, the NTSB makes recommendations for changes that might have averted the accident or even other factors that may not have contributed to the accident but pose a risk. The Joint Commission follows a pattern similar to that used by the NTSB (Figure 22.6).

All this is specifically relevant to overt intraoperative anesthesia accidents, not only for the prototypical case of unrecognized esophageal intubation causing a patient's catastrophic injury or death, but also to a host of other less severe, but still important, complications.

Problem-Based Learning

Problem-based learning (PBL) has assumed a large role in many anesthesia residency training programs. Using PBL in a quality/safety curriculum for anesthesia trainees requires knowledge of the subject area, insight, reasoning, clinical judgment, communication skills, and, in some cases, self-assessment abilities. Trainees soon learn that beyond the few absolute truths in anesthesia care (e.g., "put the tube in the hole in front," "verify an abnormal vital sign before responding"), there are many roads to the same destination. Different approaches can often all lead to successful resolution of the clinical problem, although the

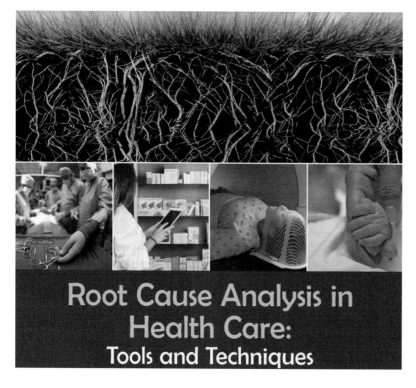

Figure 22.6 Joint Commission root cause analysis (www.jointcommissioninternational.org/assets/1/14/EBRCA15Sample.pdf; accessed November 15, 2017).

heuristic, normative tendency of a group to converge opinions and exclude more complex or less familiar solutions can limit this realization. Trainees need to learn this dynamic balance in problem solving, both in general and particularly in the areas of quality and safety. These problems are more perceptual, demanding insight and judgment, not just remembering the dose of amiodarone in the treatment of ventricular tachycardia with hypotension. Accordingly, it is incumbent on instructors addressing anesthesia quality and safety to take the extra time and effort to maximize the benefit of PBL sessions by devising scenarios that sometimes can elicit multiple "right" answers and then encouraging wide-ranging discussion. To date, there is not a published compendium of such case scenarios regarding anesthesia quality and safety, creating the opportunity for a dedicated teacher to devise one and thus make a significant contribution to anesthesia education.

Simulation

High-fidelity human mannequin simulation originated with anesthesiologists as a teaching tool.[2] Simulation, the topic of Chapter 17, has now been adopted throughout all healthcare fields. The analogy to commercial aviation persists because pilots for commercial airlines "fly" simulators for a great many hours before they ever enter the cockpit of a real airplane. Consideration of whether anesthesia trainees should have the same type of experience and spend, for example, the entire CA-1 year exclusively anesthetizing simulator mannequins before they ever touch a live patient, is beyond the scope of this chapter. The reasonably significant experience most anesthesia trainees have in simulation not only is very valuable, but also has noteworthy positive implications for their education in patient safety. Continuing the analogy to airline pilots' training to deal with in-flight emergencies, simulation can be used to expose anesthesia trainees to a whole host of rare and/or dangerous developments that test their knowledge, clinical perception and judgment, and susceptibility to human-error pitfalls.

Airline pilots train in crew resource management while anesthesia trainees working in simulation scenarios train in "crisis resource management"[8] (organizing and deploying people and effort during an acute event). Specific interactive scenarios are an excellent vehicle to engage anesthesia trainees in understanding and incorporating patient safety principles. Trainees can practice critical skills, including "speaking up to power" when circumstances of the scenario force them, for example, to challenge the surgeon, such as with impending hemorrhagic shock. Some simulation centers may be willing to share their simulation scenarios with training programs starting up a new simulation component. Further, as of this writing, the ASA is developing a virtual online simulation program[1] that will provide an immersive environment to enhance anesthesia education in a new format.

Some trainees initially state they are intimidated by the high-fidelity mannequin simulation milieu of having their actions recorded and reviewed as the basis for evaluation. Others report being apprehensive working in front of their peers (who become the actors playing the role of other personnel involved in the scenario, with each resident getting an opportunity to be in the "hot seat"). Overcoming these anxieties is a very valuable development in the patient safety education of a trainee, helping to form habits and attitudes that cannot be readily learned in a classroom and that, one day, may well help a graduate successfully resolve a life-threatening, intraoperative emergency. Most trainees eventually acknowledge the great value of their simulation sessions and many even seek out more opportunities to be challenged in developing their clinical prowess.

Investigations, Observations, Surveys

Because, as noted, the subject areas of anesthesia quality and safety do not involve as much hard science as traditional topics, exercises are possible to illustrate, emphasize, and imbed many core principles in quality and safety.

Outcomes of anesthesia care (beyond the obvious parameter of a patient emerging from general anesthesia) can be difficult to define and even more difficult to measure. A challenge can be issued to a program's trainees to attempt to define and then test new quality measures that more accurately reflect the actual quality of anesthesia care. Because of the inherent difficulty in that assignment, however, limited challenges are probably more realistic. (Nonetheless, even engaging in the thought process will be educational.) Many anesthesia organizations attempt to keep a central

---

[1] www.asahq.org/education/simulation-education (accessed November 15, 2017).

record or listing of patient events/complications. An excellent quality project with additional patient safety implications for an anesthesia trainee, or group of trainees, would be to pick one of the events on the standard list, such as reintubations in the postanesthesia care unit, and then conduct a "focused review" of the medical records of each patient who required reintubation. Then the trainee investigator(s) would create a spreadsheet or comparison chart including patient demographics and characteristics, surgical procedure, anesthetic technique, medications used and their timing, vital signs, intraoperative events, and so forth. Examination of these data for commonalities, differences, trends, outliers, and any red flags would then facilitate conclusions about contributory factors of the specific event studied. From there, the "problem resolution" phase would involve recommendation of some type of change (e.g., policy or practice) to reduce or eliminate that event. Follow-up over a subsequent time interval would reveal whether the change resulted in improved outcomes. Potential examples for projects abound, and they do not need to address only major, reportable complications. One example would be corneal abrasions occurring during lengthy robotic abdominal surgery with the patient in steep head-down position. Not only are these "real-life" demonstrations of the QI process, but any project of this type will be an important learning tool for all the trainees involved.

While retrospective investigations are common in the QI armamentarium, prospective observational studies can be even more dramatic in the "teaching by doing" approach to quality and safety in anesthesia. Engaging trainees in recognizing clinical quality and safety issues ("problem identification" in the QI paradigm) creates opportunities for observational evaluations that will be instructional for the trainees and valuable to the department. Without carrying clipboards or publicizing their mission, trainees can simply appear in various ORs and observe exactly what really occurs. Is the time-out conducted correctly and sincerely, with genuine involvement of the anesthesia professional(s) present? If the WHO Surgery Safety Checklist is employed in the institution, is it completed fully? Using the results of this analysis to implement a change that produces an increase in compliance with the designated processes would have resulted in the first three steps in the QI process. A repeat survey the following year would verify results of the QI project. Many other examples are possible. (An example of a simple QI project involved ensuring that the nurse in the holding area placed the pulse oximeter probe on the same side as the IV. While the subject seems mundane, it resulted in some savings of pulse oximeter probes but, more importantly, provided instruction to the residents in terms of the QI process.) One ancillary feature of such a program is demonstration of the Hawthorne Effect, wherein subjects of a study alter or improve their performance due to awareness that they are being observed and evaluated. This phenomenon is especially important in studies involving quality and safety. Knowledge of its implications will make the trainees better investigators and more discriminating consumers of reported research.

Documenting widespread compliance with proven safety protocols is a positive quality-of-care reassurance to the department. Alternatively, discovering partial or little compliance with policies and procedures designed to enhance quality and safety clearly is an identified problem that is suitable for application of the subsequent steps of the QI process. Again, the trainees will see and experience this as quality management in action, and will likely learn more from this participation than from attending a lecture or reading a chapter.

Similarly, structured projects for trainees can involve classic "failure modes and effects analysis" (FMEA) in which a structure or process is analyzed prospectively to identify where and how components might fail and the effects of such failures. The ultimate intent is to prevent the failures and resulting problems. Originally developed for use in military planning, this technique has been adapted to medical care as evidenced by the fact that IHI publishes a model FMEA protocol.[9] Potential examples for its application in anesthesia practice abound, from something as simple as the function of a lightbulb in a traditional laryngoscope blade to more complex challenges, such as the transfer of a critically ill, postoperative patient with a left ventricular assist device to a distant intensive care unit.

Another type of related exercise for a trainee project is to construct a Fishbone (aka Ishikawa and "cause and effect") Diagram in which an identified problem is inscribed on the right edge of a very large piece of paper at the end of a horizontal arrow (Figure 22.7).

At least six contributing factors (people, methods, equipment, materials, measurements, and environment) are side branches of the main arrow. Participants enter all possible component elements of each factor in

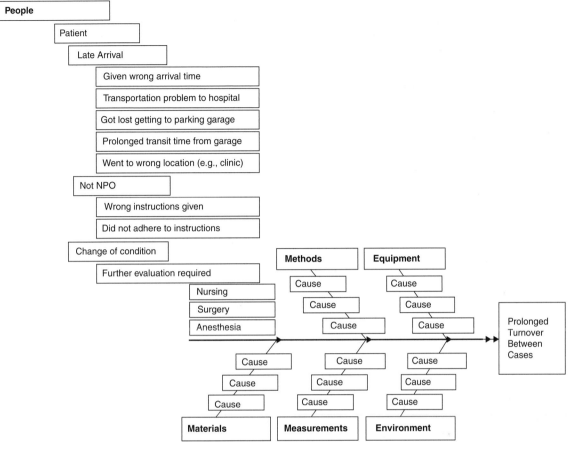

Figure 22.7 Fishbone (aka Ishikawa and "cause and effect") diagram.

a search for the true original etiology of the ultimate problem. Details on FMEA and the others included in the "seven basic quality tools" (Box 22.4), as well as an exhaustive list of wide-ranging topics related to quality, are available on the website of the American Society for Quality (www.asq.org; accessed November 15, 2017).[10]

A different type of engagement activity for trainees is designing, executing, analyzing, and reporting surveys of their fellow trainees and/or other members of the department. Making contact and receiving results anonymously online could facilitate classic questions such as circumstances surrounding "close calls" (Box 22.5).

Asking anesthesia professionals, or trainees in particular, what specifically annoys them (e.g., inadequate supply of drugs or supplies, slow response to urgent requests, unrealistic performance expectations) in their anesthesia practice could lead to a list of topics that would be potential subjects of QI activities.

Assembling a list of these issues in detail would likely provide significant subject matter for many QI projects initiated by trainees for the benefit of the entire department.

Box 22.4 Seven basic quality tools

- Cause-and-effect (Ishikawa) diagram;
- Check sheet;
- Control charts;
- Histogram;
- Pareto chart;
- Scatter diagram; and
- Stratification.

Source: From http://asq.org/learn-about-quality/seven-basic-quality-tools/overview/overview.html (accessed November 15, 2017).

Box 22.5 Examples of survey questions related to "close calls"

- Have you had any "close calls" in the OR?
- What was the circumstance?
- Were you distracted before noticing a problem?
- What did you do to remedy the situation?
- After it was over and "no harm done," did you report it to anyone?
- Why or why not?
- What did you say?

Requirements for Residents

The quality and safety topics in the ABA Content Outline on which residents will be tested in the written ABA exams (thus making them required curricular elements) have already been presented (see Box 22.3). With the possible exception of root cause analysis (which can effectively be taught by example), the topics are relatively broad. Beyond that, curriculum planners will need to extrapolate the relevant subheadings in the outline to maximize resident exposure to required material.

Anesthesiology residents are usually required to complete at least one QA/QI project (individually, or as a member of a small group) during their three years of clinical anesthesia training. Essentially any of the topics, and, particularly, the methodologies outlined throughout this chapter would provide an excellent format for completion of this requirement.

One section of the Anesthesiology Milestone Project, sponsored by the American Council on Graduate Medical Education (ACGME) and the ABA describes five levels of expectations related to patient safety and QI for evaluating and grading the progress of an anesthesiology resident through the training program (Figure 22.8).[11]

In addition to the milestones that apply to each resident as an individual, all residency training programs and their sponsoring institutions are evaluated and accredited by the ACGME, based in part on the Clinical Learning Environment Review (CLER) Program.[12,13] Quality and safety are prominently featured in this program and comprise three of the six CLER focus areas (Box 22.6).[13]

These expectations for all residents in all programs include the fundamental quality and safety concepts contained within the milestones for individual anesthesiology residents, but extend the engagement of the residents specifically to the interaction between residents and the institution and healthcare system as well as the community in which it functions. While program directors and curriculum planners can be creative in finding and assigning quality and safety topics that meet these expectations, the likely more valuable heuristic would be to challenge the residents to identify and pursue quality and safety activities and projects with institutional, system, and community implications. Residents who do so would have the optimal opportunity to gain genuine insight and appreciation of the huge role the concepts of quality and safety will play throughout their entire anesthesiology practice lives.

Conclusion

Contents of this brief treatment represent the mere tip of an iceberg of a fascinating and important field of study that easily could merit its own complete textbook.

Safety is best exemplified by the APSF vision statement, "No patient shall be harmed by anesthesia." Quality includes structure, process, and outcome. Although defining quality may be easy, because quantitating quality is much more difficult, organizations tend to focus on surrogate markers (e.g., timely administration of antibiotics) purporting to reflect

Box 22.6 Excerpt – ACGME: Areas of focus for the CLER program

- **Patient safety:** Including opportunities for residents to report errors, unsafe conditions, and near misses, and to participate in interprofessional teams to promote and enhance safe care.
- **Quality improvement:** Including how sponsoring institutions engage residents in the use of data to improve systems of care, reduce healthcare disparities, and improve patient outcomes.
- **Transitions in care:** Including how sponsoring institutions demonstrate effective standardization and oversight of transitions of care.

Systems-based Practice 2: Patient Safety and Quality Improvement					
Has not Achieved Level 1	Level 1	Level 2	Level 3	Level 4	Level 5
	Describes common causes of errors Describes team-based actions and techniques designed to enhance patient safety Participates in established institutional safety initiatives Follows institutional safety policies, including reporting of problematic behaviors or processes, errors, near misses, and complications Incorporates national standards and guidelines into patient care	Uses the safety features of medical devices Participates in team-based actions designed to enhance patient safety, (e.g., briefings, closed-loop communication) Identifies problems in the quality of healthcare delivery within one's institution and brings this to the attention of supervisors Incorporates anesthesiology-specific national standards and guidelines into patient care	Describes and participates in systems and procedures that promote patient safety Identifies departmental and or institutional opportunities to improve quality of care Participates in quality improvement activities as a member of an inter-professional team to improve patient outcomes Takes patient preferences into consideration while promoting cost-effective patient care that improves outcomes	Applies advanced team techniques designed to enhance patient safety (e.g., 'assertiveness') Participates in formal analysis (e.g., root cause analysis, failure mode effects analysis) of medical error and sentinel events with direct supervision Indentifies opportunities in the continuum of care to improve patient outcome and reduce costs	Leads multidisciplinary teams (e.g., human factors engineers, social scientists) to address patient safety issues Provides consultation to organizations to improve personal and patient safety Proactively participates in educational sessions prior to using new advanced medical devices for patient care Defines and constructs process and outcome measures, and leads quality improvement projects Effectively addresses areas in anesthesiology practice that pose potential dangers to patients

Figure 22.8 ACGME Anesthesiology Milestone Project.

anesthesia quality. Instructing residents in safety and quality initially involves determining the objectives of the program. Multiple resources are available that can be used to help select appropriate topics. Paramount in the decision-making process is awareness of the ABA Content Outline. Once the content of the curriculum has been determined, conventional didactic presentations, including PBL sessions, should be supplemented with investigations in the form of prospective analysis of processes, retrospective review of complications, or surveys.

References

1. World Health Organization. Surgical Safety Checklist. 2009. http://apps.who.int/iris/bitstream/10665/44186/2/9789241598590_eng_Checklist.pdf (accessed November 15, 2017).

2. J. H. Eichhorn. The Anesthesia Patient Safety Foundation at 25: A pioneering success in safety; 25th anniversary provokes reflection, anticipation. *Anesth Analg* 2012; 114: 791–800.

3. J. H. Eichhorn. Prevention of intraoperative anesthesia accidents and related severe injury through safety monitoring. *Anesthesiology* 1989; 70: 572–7.

4. J. H. Eichhorn. Effect of monitoring standards on anesthesia outcome. In D. Roystan, T. W. Feeley, eds. *Monitoring in Anesthesiology – Current Standards and Newer Techniques.* International Anesthesiology Clinics. Boston: Little Brown, 1993; 31(3): 181–96.

5. Duke University Health System. Patient Safety – Quality Improvement. http://patientsafetyed.duhs.duke.edu/ (accessed November 14, 2017).

6. Anesthesia Patient Safety Foundation. Prevention and Management of Operating Room Fires. 2010. www.apsf.org/resources/fire-safety/ (accessed November 15, 2017).

7. J. B. Cooper, R. S. Newbower, C. D. Long, B. McPeek. Preventable anesthesia mishaps: A study of human factors. *Anesthesiology* 1978; 49: 399–406.

8. D. Gaba, K. Fish, S. Howard, A. Burden. *Crisis Management in Anesthesiology*, 2nd edn. Philadelphia: Elsevier Saunders, 2014.

9. Institute for Healthcare Improvement. Failure Modes and Effects Analysis (FMEA) Tool. www.ihi.org/resources/pages/tools/failuremodesandeffectsanalysistool.aspx (accessed November 15, 2017).

10. American Society for Quality. Learn About Quality: Quality Topics A to Z. http://asq.org/learn-about-quality/ (accessed November 15, 2017).

11. Anesthesiology Milestone Group. The Anesthesiology Milestone Project. 2015. www.acgme.org/Portals/0/PDFs/Milestones/AnesthesiologyMilestones.pdf (accessed November 15, 2017).

12. K. B. Weiss, R. Wagner, T. J. Nasca. Development, testing, and implementation of the ACGME Clinical Learning Environment Review (CLER) Program. *J Grad Med Educ* 2012; 4: 396–8.

13. ACGME. CLER Pathways to Excellence: Expectations for an optimal clinical learning environment to achieve safe and high quality patient care. www.acgme.org/Portals/0/PDFs/CLER/CLER_Brochure.pdf (accessed November 15, 2017).

Chapter

23

Teaching Residents How to Critically Read and Apply Medical Literature*

Brian S. Donahue, Brian J. Gelfand, and Matthew D. McEvoy

It is almost taken for granted that resident physicians should become skilled readers of the medical literature. Young physicians are those who will move our practices farthest into the future, so knowing how to critically evaluate and apply the literature should be an essential part of resident training. On philosophical grounds, Hautz et al. recently listed characteristics that make a doctor a scholar, including lifelong learning, critical appraisal of evidence, and application of evidence to patient care.[1] The mention of lifelong learning is significant and timely, as it represents a recent paradigm shift in medical education, a move away from traditional categorization of time-based education periods and toward identification of all physicians, not just academicians, as perpetual students.[2]

Despite clear understanding among educators and authors that knowing how to critically review the literature is important,[1,2] formal exposure to this subject during residency is frequently limited. Reading primary source literature during residency often provides very good *exposure to content*, without necessarily having any training in the *appraisal of content*, or how research findings should be understood and then incorporated into practice. The issue is further complicated by lack of objective outcome measures. Unlike board scores or case logs, which have measurable training goals, universal standards by which resident skills in critical reading of the literature can be objectively quantified are not available. Programs that use multiple-choice questions are able to demonstrate improvement over the course of residency when the topic is didactically and intentionally addressed.[3,4] Without universally accepted metrics, however, it may sometimes be difficult to define just what return is being generated from the investment of precious time and resources in this domain. This chapter will discuss

what we believe all residents should learn about research while in training, including an understanding of different types of research studies and statistical methods, how to critically appraise the research findings presented in current medical literature, and how to apply those findings in their practice.

Current Resources

Resident training programs interested in following a more formal treatment of critical literature review have multiple resources available to assist them.[5–9] The *British Medical Journal* published a series of ten articles beginning in 1997 entitled *How to Read a Paper*,[10] which covered a wide range of common study designs. With an emphasis toward teaching, the *Canadian Medical Association Journal* offered a series of six articles from 2004 to 2005 entitled *Evidence-Based Medicine Teaching Tips*.[9] Likewise, the *Journal of General Internal Medicine* published a more concise series entitled *Tips for Teachers of Evidence-Based Medicine*, which began in 2008.

Most prominently featured in this genre is the very comprehensive literature reading course devised by authors of the *Journal of the American Medical Association* (*JAMA*). In 1993 a working group was formed to compose a series of articles entitled *User's Guide to the Medical Literature*.[11] Each article was to feature a specific type of research study with a detailed discussion of the limitations and applicability of the conclusions. The result was series of 32 papers appearing in JAMA from 1993 to 2000. Guyatt and colleagues compiled and edited the series into a textbook entitled *Users' Guide to the Medical Literature: A Manual for Evidence-Based Clinical Practice*, which was first published in 2002. The third edition of this popular work was printed in 2015.[7] Many other excellent textbooks on the subject are available, with a partial list included in the online content associated with this chapter.

---

* An appendix to this chapter showing session outlines is available at www.cambridge.org/9781316630389.

The Use of Journal Clubs

As with many academic subjects, critical reading skills can be taught through various mechanisms including a series of formal lectures or directed readings. While the optimal pedagogical approach for teaching this subject during residency is unknown, the journal club setting represents an Accreditation Council for Graduate Medical Education (ACGME) program expectation for organized clinical instruction and an excellent mechanism for the formal teaching of critical reading of the literature.[12] "Journal club" is a popular term used to identify a series of formal, focused meetings, where a small number of published papers are presented and discussed. Journal club has been identified as a venue for practice-based learning,[12] based on a 2005 review of the literature. Although journal clubs vary in their structure and formality, it is logical to assume that the most educationally profitable journal clubs are those with the more organized approaches including the presence of written objectives, a structured review process, teaching faculty participation, and a formalized meeting structure and process. To further enhance the learning process, some programs report the inclusion of novel adjuncts to journal club curricula, including use of social media for making announcements, distributing content, and creating hashtag communities.[13] The focus of a journal club series can be defined along various axes such as recent findings, historical landmark studies, and specific content relevant to subspecialties.

Recognizing the importance of becoming a skilled reader of the medical literature, we developed a journal club program within the anesthesiology residency program at Vanderbilt University to formally teach critical reading of the medical literature to our residents. The curriculum was based roughly on the concept outlined in the published series mentioned in the preceding text.[9–11] Namely, each monthly journal club session would focus on a specific genre of research study (e.g., case-control study, randomized trial, propensity analysis, meta-analysis). A general description of the study genre would be presented along with a list of specific criteria for evaluating the credibility, applicability, and limitations of a typical paper within the specific study genre. Example articles (two to three per session) would then be presented from the current literature, and each example would be measured against the established criteria.

Development of the Curriculum

The first decision in creation of such a program involves the length of the course and the selection of topics for each session. A program such as Guyatt's,[7,11] though very comprehensive, would last longer than the 36-month residency and contain topics of greater relevance to internal medicine than to anesthesiology. We decided on the 16-month list of topics listed in Table 23.1. The sessions were originally scheduled monthly, but because of interfering events such as holidays and required administrative sessions, this 16-session course fit well into a two-year cycle. Although there is some overlap within the curriculum (e.g., some randomized trials involve survival analysis, and propensity analysis is a type of regression), we felt this outline provided the residents with a critical process by which to approach nearly every study they might encounter in the anesthesiology literature.

After deciding on the overall scope and length of the program, the next step involved the construction of learning objectives and the content for each session. These were developed by summarizing the published series on each type of research study,[9–11] and by suggestions from available textbooks, accompanied by teaching examples with particular applicability to anesthesiology. Often, it was helpful to begin with a historical example of how specific studies evolved. Although some topics focused on statistical methods, we chose not to concentrate on details of statistics because we directed this course toward all residents,

Table 23.1 Course outline for journal club: How to critically read the literature

1. Introduction and Classification of Evidence
2. Retrospective Cohort Studies
3. Case-Control Studies
4. Randomized Trials I: Drug Trials
5. Randomized Trials II: Treatment Trials
6. Studies Using Linear Regression
7. Studies Using Logistic Regression
8. Survival Analyses
9. Genetic Association Studies
10. Studies Using Propensity Analysis
11. Quality Improvement Studies
12. Economic Analyses
13. Use of Consensus Guidelines
14. Computer-Based Decision Support Studies
15. Meta-Analyses and Systemic Reviews
16. Summary and Exercises in Study Review

not specifically those targeted toward academic careers. We did, however, feel it was necessary for residents to understand the applicability and limitations of commonly used statistical methods to facilitate the development of trainees as lifelong learners who could rightly apply the literature for years to come.

Finally, we selected example papers from the current literature to evaluate. This provided a tangible, focused exercise on literature review. Resident participation in the evaluation augmented the learning experience. We found that assigning residents to prepare presentations of the sample papers was excessively burdensome, considering the general task load of residency, with little educational return for the time invested. After the first few sessions, the faculty course director made the presentations of the sample papers, with resident participation in the review process. This decision removed any barrier to participation for the residents and engaged them more thoroughly in the learning process rather than in just completing another assignment.

At each session, the residents were provided with printed, laminated cards summarizing the approach to any article within the selected study genre. (See appendix to this chapter.) By the end of the 16-month course, each resident then had a box of cards for quick reference applicable to review an article when the need arose in the future. We believe that practice using these cognitive aids during discussion sessions will increase the likelihood of their use after graduation.

Example of a Session: Quality Improvement Studies

One of the sessions in the journal club series dealt with quality improvement (QI) studies. The topic was chosen because such studies are appearing more frequently in the anesthesiology literature. With increasing focus on outcome metrics and resource utilization, this trend is likely to continue (see Chapter 22). Of note, the goal of this session was not to train residents on how to do QI projects, but rather on how to evaluate articles reporting the results of such projects.

The historic example of Ignaz Semmelweis was used to introduce the subject. Semmelweis is widely credited with recognizing the importance of hand washing (between the morgue and the delivery ward!) for preventing puerperal sepsis, notably before Pasteur's discovery of microbes. His data showing the efficacy of implementing this practice constitute an early form of a QI study. The discussion next focused on the multiple possible sources of bias in a QI study, and what can be done to limit or overcome such bias. The applicability of results arising from a QI study was then discussed, which are outlined in Table 23.2. The recent papers selected as examples provided a focus for practical application of these points. The residents then were able to identify which potential sources of bias were relevant to these papers. The outline in Table 23.2 was printed on laminated cards (see appendix to this chapter) that were given to the residents for this session.

Program Refinement – Feedback and Future Developments

Verbal feedback from residents and fellows has been positive. Several residents have mentioned that the cards were useful in subsequent sessions where they were tasked with evaluating a journal article for other journal club series. Faculty from our department and residents from departments other than anesthesiology have requested to attend the sessions. The administration of Vanderbilt University School of Medicine has expressed interest in making this series available to all departments in the medical center, as part of our institution's commitment to continuing medical education.

As is characteristic of nearly all educational programs, we expect that this series will become edited and refined in the future, synchronously evolving with the overall forward-looking educational mission of our department. We plan to consider the suggestions for improvement arising from the residents and faculty, adding or dropping specific sessions as necessary. Likewise, we envision incorporating critical literature reading skills into the performance metrics of the milestones assessment of individual resident progression across the educational continuum. As well, a defined, objective measure of resident competency in the ability to critically review the literature is likely to be forthcoming.

We advocate for the development of common anesthesiology residency program criteria for evaluating resident competency in these subject areas. Knowing how to critically appraise and apply the literature is a core component of delivery of excellent patient care and one that will hopefully reduce the current publication to application gap of more than 15 years.[14] Accordingly, we feel it would benefit the specialty to

Table 23.2 Example of a journal club session discussion outline: Quality improvement studies

QI initiatives:
- Target provider behaviors and practices
- Endpoint is often improved adherence to a standard
- If standard does not exist, or outcome evidence lacking, studies must show improved outcome

QI studies:
- Often are local, dependent on practices and environment
- Often are not randomized or blinded
- Often are observational

Limitations of QI studies:
- Degree of bias
- Applicability of results

Sources of bias in QI studies:
- Local bias
  - Results specific to a unique practice location
  - Characteristics of locale make generalization difficult
  - Overcoming local bias:
    - Selection of appropriate study practice
    - Make interventions generalizable
    - Demonstrate reproducibility in other populations
- Hawthorne effect
  - Persons will alter their behavior simply from participating in a study
  - Overcoming Hawthorne effect:
    - Demonstrate that quality care was provided before intervention
    - Document consistency of care
    - Demonstrate sustainability of benefit
    - Reproducibility of results in other groups over time
- Nonrandomization and unidentified confounders: Overcome by:
  - Demonstrating groups are similar in meaningful ways
  - Demonstrating outcomes independent of study did not change across the interval
  - Demonstrating that included covariates account for a significant amount of variability
  - Demonstrating sustainability across time
  - Demonstrating reproducibility in other populations
- Unblinded investigators: May be overcome by:
  - Arguing that the study could not be accomplished without some unblinding
  - Demonstrating that remaining blinding efforts were effective
  - Demonstrating that unblinding did not result in differential treatment between groups
    - Pilot data
    - Additional control groups
    - Comparison with historical controls
- Data quality issues
- Conflicts of interest

Applicability of results:
- Best when aligned with randomized controlled trials (RCTs)
  - Outcome data possibly not needed when RCT data extensive
  - Compliance is probably sufficient
- Context of site
- Duration of follow-up
- All important outcomes considered?

Cost/benefit analysis

eventually have components of the American Board of Anesthesiology Staged Examination and Maintenance of Certification in Anesthesiology process dedicated to testing specific knowledge, not just of clinical content and basic statistics, but of the principles of critical literature review. Such changes would emphasize this essential skill set for effective lifelong learning, and concepts requisite to the scientific rationale underlying safe, clinical management and decision-making throughout one's professional career.

Conclusion

Knowing how to critically evaluate and apply the literature should be an essential part of resident training. While primary source material provides information about content, the residents need to know how to evaluate the article and then determine if or how to incorporate the results into their practice. Series of articles from the *British Medical Journal, Canadian Medical Journal, Journal of General Internal Medicine,* and *JAMA* provide useful information on interpreting the medical literature. In addition, the *JAMA* articles were combined into *Users' Guide to the Medical Literature: A Manual for Evidence-Based Clinical Practice.* These resources can be used as the foundation for establishing a curriculum on interpreting the medical literature. In practice, the journal club is the most commonly used venue for teaching critical analysis of the medical literature. When using that format, it is important to provide the residents information about the expectations as well as a framework to be used for evaluating the articles being reviewed.

References

1. S. C. Hautz et al. What makes a doctor a scholar: A systematic review and content analysis of outcome frameworks. *BMC Med Educ* 2016; 16: 119.

2. V. N. Naik, A. K. Wong, S. J. Hamstra. Review article: Leading the future: Guiding two predominant paradigm shifts in medical education through scholarship. *Can J Anaesth* 2012; 59(2): 213–23.

3. J. A. Kellum et al. Teaching critical appraisal during critical care fellowship training: A foundation for evidence-based critical care medicine. *Crit Care Med* 2000; 28(8): 3067–70.

4. R. S. Moharari et al. Teaching critical appraisal and statistics in anesthesia journal club. *QJM* 2009; 102(2): 139–41.

5. S. Gehlbach. *Interpreting the Medical Literature,* 5th edn. New York: McGraw-Hill, 2006; 293.

6. T. Greenhalgh. *How to Read a Paper: The Basics of Evidence-Based Medicine,* 5th edn. West Sussex, UK: Wiley Blackwell, 2014; 284.

7. G. Guyatt et al. *Users' Guide to the Medical Literature: A Manual for Evidence-Based Clinical Practice,* 3rd edn. New York: McGraw-Hill, 2015; 697.

8. R. Riegelman, M. Rinke. *Studying a Study and Testing a Test,* 6th edn. Philadelphia: Lippincott Williams and Wilkins, 2012; 340.

9. P. C. Wyer et al. Tips for learning and teaching evidence-based medicine: Introduction to the series. *CMAJ* 2004; 171(4): 347–8.

10. T. Greenhalgh. How to read a paper: The Medline database. *BMJ* 1997; 315(7101): 180–3.

11. G. H. Guyatt, D. Rennie. Users' guides to the medical literature. *JAMA* 1993; 270(17): 2096–7.

12. A. G. Lee et al. Using the Journal Club to teach and assess competence in practice-based learning and improvement: A literature review and recommendation for implementation. *Surv Ophthalmol* 2005; 50(6): 542–8.

13. A. D. Udani, D. Moyse, C. A. Peery, J. M. Taekman. Twitter-augmented journal club: Educational engagement and experience so far. *A A Case Rep* 2016 Apr 15; 6(8): 253–6.

14. Z. S. Morris, S. Wooding, J. Grant. The answer is 17 years, what is the question: Understanding time lags in translational research. *J R Soc Med* 2011; 104(12): 510–20.

Further Reading

1. D. Buck, R. Subramanyam, A. Varughese. A quality improvement project to reduce the intraoperative use of single-dose fentanyl vials across multiple patients in a pediatric institution. *Paediatr Anaesth* 2016; 26: 92–101.

2. J. Forister, J. Blessing. *Introduction to Research and Medical Literature.* Burlington, MA: Jones and Bartlett Learning, 2015.

3. S. Gehlbach. *Interpreting the Medical Literature,* 5th edn. New York: McGraw-Hill, 2006.

4. T. Greenhalgh. *How to Read a Paper: The Basics of Evidence-Based Medicine,* 5th edn. West Sussex, UK: Wiley Blackwell, 2014.

5. P. F. Kotur. Introduction of evidence-based medicine in undergraduate medical curriculum for development of professional competencies in medical students. *Curr Opin Anaesthesiol* 2012; 25: 719–23.

6. G. S. Letterie, L. S. Morgenstern. The journal club: Teaching critical evaluation of clinical literature in an evidence-based environment. *J Reprod Med* 2000; 45: 299–304.

7. B. Lytsy, R. P. Lindblom, U. Ransjö, C. Leo-Swenne. Hygienic interventions to decrease deep sternal wound infections following coronary artery bypass grafting. *J Hosp Infect* 2015; 91: 326–31.

8. C. M. Miranda, T. L. Navarrete. Semmelweis and his outstanding contribution to medicine: Washing hands saves lives. *Rev Chilena Infectol* 2008; 25: 54–7.

9. W. S. Richardson, M. C. Wilson, S. A. Keitz. Tips for teachers of evidence-based medicine: Making sense of diagnostic test results using likelihood ratios. *J Gen Intern Med* 2008; 23: 87–92.

10. R. Riegelman, M. Rinke. *Studying a Study and Testing a Test*, 6th edn. Philadelphia: Lippincott Williams and Wilkins, 2012.

11. S. E. Straus, W. S. Richardson, P. Glasziu, R. B. Haynes. *Evidence-Based Medicine: How to Practice and Teach It*, 4th edn. Edinburgh: Churchill Livingstone, 2010.

12. A. D. Udani, D. Moyse, C. A. Peery, J. M. Taekman. Twitter-augmented journal club: Educational engagement and experience so far. *A A Case Rep* 2016; 6: 253–6.

Index